A practising dietitian and nutritional consultant in Chelsea, Jane Clarke treats prominent clients for a wide range of food-related problems, from eating disorders to fatigue. She writes regularly on nutrition for *You Magazine*, and has presented her own six-part television series. She is also a consultant to the World Cancer Research Fund.

Body Foods for Women

EAT YOUR WAY TO GOOD HEALTH

Jane Clarke

ORION

An Orion paperback

First published in Great Britain by
Weidenfeld & Nicolson Ltd in 1996
This paperback edition published in 1997
by Orion Books Ltd, Orion House,
5 Upper St Martin's Lane, London WC2H 9EA

A CIP catalogue record for this book is available
from the British Library.

ISBN: 0 75280 922 9

Printed and bound in Great Britain by
Guernsey Press Co. Ltd, C.I.

Editor Maggie Ramsay
Illustrations Daniel Pudles

for Mum, Dad, Annie and Paul

Contents

Introduction

Our lifestyles and eating habits have changed drastically over the last ten to twenty years, so drastically that they would shock our ancestors, yet the technological and economic developments that have brought an increase in disposable income, food processing machinery and the equipment to produce meals effortlessly has not brought about positive nutritional changes. More and more women are overweight, suffering from cancer, depression or constipation, or living in an eating disorder 'jail'.

At the same time women are spending hundreds of hours on diets and hundreds of pounds on food supplements. Real food is out there, in the fields, markets and shops, but we don't seem to know how to get the best from it to help, rather than hinder, our bodies. Food can make you feel fantastic: 'A good chef is half a physician,' wrote Andrew Boorde, an English doctor, in the 16th century, but the emphasis in Western society is not positive. We are forever hearing about what we shouldn't have, rather than all the things we can enjoy. This book aims to redress the balance. I will explain what your body needs to feel and perform well and how to organize your life so that food regains its rightful place as a pleasurable pastime.

Although there were flaws in the diets of our mothers and their mothers before them, their way of life and of cooking – eating simple, unadulterated foods in season – made them a much healthier and happier population. They appreciated the fruits of the earth and looked forward to the first strawberries of summer and apples of autumn. Eating disorders were rare and obesity was nowhere near as prevalent as it is today.

Shops now sell the same foods virtually all year round, which on one hand means that we have the resources to pick and choose what we eat, but on the other hand seems to have led to unbalanced over-indulgence, and the meal table commonly featuring a ready-made 'convenience' dish. The criticism is not meant to be levied at you the consumer, but rather at the food manufacturers, the supermarkets and the press. Between them they have managed to make us think that cooking is time-consuming and that it's much easier for woman the worker or woman the mother to grab a ready-made meal and pop it in the oven.

Convenience foods have their place, but they don't contain all the nutrients we need and unfortunately contain many substances we would do better to avoid. Sugar, salt, fat, preservatives and other additives don't help our bodies to feel well and in some cases, if taken in excess, lead to health problems such as high blood cholesterol levels, heart disease, breast cancer and irritable bowel syndrome.

We should look afresh at the foods Mother Nature puts before us, learn how they react with our bodies and enjoy eating them. There are so many delicious foods out there that will enhance your quality of life. All you need to do is consider your goal and begin to plan your food accordingly. Do you want to become and stay healthy or do you have a specific problem which needs your eating habits to be finely tuned? Either way, this book will help.

Once you've defined your goal, you need to set aside the time. Time is all we have and yet we seem to rush through life. Sadly, the women who really seem to value time are those who either don't have unlimited time because of a health problem or those who have lost someone they care about and wish they'd spent more time with them. We should take steps before we're in this situation.

Lack of time is one of the main reasons women give for not cooking or looking after their bodies. We expect our bodies to go on functioning, even when we don't fuel them properly or give them time to recover from illness. Women turn to antibiotics and other medication because they haven't got time to be ill. The problem with this is that if our bodies are exposed to drugs and supplements on a long-term basis, they can become inefficient at healing themselves, and may even begin to 'complain' and malfunction.

It would be much better if we looked at the supplements and artificial substances in our foods and asked ourselves if we could do without them if we gave ourselves some time. In a lot of cases the answer is yes, especially if we make sure that everything we put into our bodies is as natural as possible.

Many women run into digestive problems when they have a diet high in refined and force-grown produce. When they change to a healthy eating pattern incorporating unrefined, organic produce whenever possible, the bowel behaves much more efficiently and they feel a lot better. I am not saying that all non-organic produce is bad, but I am turning against it more and more as I see, for example, perfect-looking tomatoes that have no taste whatsoever.

We are on this earth to taste and enjoy everything we put in our mouths. Ignore the articles telling you what you shouldn't eat and learn to love food. I hope that this book turns you on to eating so much that you want to cook more. As James Beard, the great American chef and writer said, 'Good food has a magic appeal. You may grow old, even ugly, but if you are a good cook, people will always find the path to your door.'

While it is healthy to make a positive choice over the food and drink you're consuming, food should not become the sole focus in your life. Overly focusing on food and controlling your eating habits can become an obsession, which can far too easily escalate into an eating disorder such as anorexia or bulimia, if there are underlying insecurities. The pressures on women to be thin and in control of their eating habits are phenomenal in our society. All women have the right to live healthily, happily and without guilt attached to food.

I hope that this book will help you feel positive about food and the delightful effect it can have on your body.

Jane Clarke

You and your food

Developing a healthy relationship with food can help you maximize fitness while enjoying everything you eat. In this section I shall look at the physical and psychological aspects of eating.

• BODY RHYTHMS

Not everyone feels hungry at the same time. Hunger pangs can be caused by many things, including association with a certain time, place or smell. Some women need to eat first thing in the morning to stop themselves from feeling lousy, while others cannot face breakfast. You may also find that your hormonal and stress levels affect whether or not you feel hungry. While it is good to get into the habit of having three meals a day, these don't have to be three large meals at set times, they could be five smaller meals. Don't stress yourself about eating or not eating. See how your body responds by eating three or five meals a day, then try to build a healthy regular eating pattern around your conclusions. You may find that you feel like having something light such as yoghurt and fresh fruit mid-morning, when you have got up and given your system longer to wake itself up. Others may feel better if they have a large breakfast and then have a couple of lighter meals during the day.

The one thing I would encourage you to do is to take a little time to think what you would like to eat, rather than eating the same as everyone else, just because the food is there. I am not suggesting you become selfish, but at breakfast time for instance, many women eat what everyone else is eating rather than taking a few moments to think what they would like and what would feel good in their body.

Food is not digested any differently at nine o'clock in the evening than at nine o'clock in the morning. The only thing you should realize about late eating is that you should leave time for the food to partially digest, usually an hour or so before you lie down, as you may

*'Spread the table and
contention will cease.'
English proverb*

find it settles heavily in the stomach and could cause indigestion. There is no truth in the saying 'breakfast like a king, lunch like a queen and dine like a pauper'. You should eat as you feel comfortable.

• DIGESTION AND THE FREQUENCY OF MEALS
The time food takes to be broken down, absorbed and passed through your digestive system differs in everyone, taking anything from 12 to 36 hours. This is partly why some people find that they have to have a little something every two to three hours, while others are content with three meals a day. Whatever you feel, you shouldn't go for long periods without eating. Not only can this harm the digestive system by leaving it exposed to acids produced by the stomach, it also makes you feel desperate and more inclined to eat inappropriately or overeat. Overeating after a period of starvation can take your digestive system by surprise: the production of digestive juices slows down when you don't eat; if you then eat a lot there aren't enough juices to digest the food properly. The food may then sit undigested in your stomach, making you feel uncomfortable and bloated, or it can pass through the system partly digested, which can cause other gut problems such as diarrhoea or constipation.

• RELAX AND GIVE YOUR DIGESTIVE SYSTEM
TIME TO WORK PROPERLY
The digestive system is a collection of glands and muscles. As with other muscles, it needs to be treated with respect. It needs a plentiful supply of oxygen and the appropriate hormones to enable it to work properly. If you get up and rush around immediately after eating, or eat on the move, oxygen is diverted away from the stomach to other muscles, which means that the stomach and the rest of the gut become slightly lacking in oxygen. This hinders digestion. Mother Nature tries to stop us from doing this by releasing hormones that make us feel sleepy immediately after a meal. Don't fight this – the Mediterranean habit of taking a little

siesta after a meal is a good one. You don't have to sleep, just rest for 10 to 15 minutes before rushing off. You may say that you haven't got time to sit down and eat and relax, three times a day. My answer would be to look at how efficient you are when you're feeling satisfied and well, and how much time you lose through feeling sluggish and unwell. A little relaxation is vital for the health and happiness of your body.

• POSITION OF EATING
Sitting upright places your stomach in a position where gravity helps rather than hinders. If you have a tendency towards indigestion or discomfort, first look at your posture.

• PLACE YOURSELF IN AN ENVIRONMENT THAT ENCOURAGES YOU TO ENJOY YOUR FOOD
Instead of just seeing eating as a quick nutrient fix, think of it as an enjoyable pastime. Value meals not only for their content, but also their setting. Take winter picnics, for example, with flasks of steaming soup and warm rolls which have been kept in an insulated box. (A coolbox will also keep things warm, as long as there is little room for air to circulate.) Don't try to take warm meats such as sausages or chicken dishes, however, as they carry a risk of food poisoning. Food can taste delicious when you are sitting on a rug overlooking the cliffs, or on top of the Yorkshire Dales. Just take your jumpers and plan a route home via a little coffee shop!

Also think about where you eat in the house. Set the table with candles for a romantic or relaxing touch. Have a meal on a tray, but don't just eat in front of the television; if you're with a friend, talk. Have breakfast in bed. Don't see these as things you only do on special occasions – make every day a special day.

• SEE FOOD AS ART
Think about its presentation, beginning with the colour of the plate. A good colour combination can start the saliva flowing even before a morsel has passed your lips.

Generally the simpler the pattern, the more attention is paid to the food's colours and textures. Think about whether the food would look better in a deeper dish or glass bowl. The size of the plate is important too: food should be neither lost nor crowded on a plate. Place small portions of food on the plate; you can always go back for more.

Create something that looks good and attracts you to devour it. Think about the colours of foods and include variety and compatibility. For example, a salmon trout's pink colour is enhanced by bunches of watercress, or you could use edible flowers such as nasturtiums to scatter on salads and cold platters.

• SERVE FOOD AND WINE IN A WAY THAT WILL ENABLE YOU TO FULLY APPRECIATE THE GOODNESS

We tend to lose out on a lot of the flavours of food because we serve them at such extreme temperatures. Cold foods develop their flavours when they are left to come a little closer to room temperature after they have been take out of the refrigerator or freezer and hot foods taste better when they are left to cool slightly. In either case you need to be careful about food poisoning, but you will be surprised how much tastier cheese is if it is left for an hour or so after it has come out of the refrigerator before you eat it. Equally wines should be served at the correct temperature if you are to enjoy them at their best.

You should chill white wines in the refrigerator for an hour or so before serving. Leave reds at room temperature, apart from young, light, fruity reds such as Beaujolais, which can also be enjoyable lightly chilled.

As a rule, the sweeter the wine, the more chilling it can take. If an hour in the refrigerator demands more foresight than you normally apply, you might invest in a cooling sleeve that you store in the freezer and simply slip on to the bottle five minutes before you intend to drink it, which is about the time it takes to get the glasses out and find a corkscrew. The better white wines should not be chilled too much, or we miss their subtleties. The converse applies too: if somebody has brought a dread-ful bottle by way of a gift, get it as close to freezing as possible and you'll hardly notice what it tastes like!

Just as 'refrigerator temperature' is an approxima-tion, so is 'room temperature' for reds. In both cases, what we should aim for is a temperature that simply feels right, but in general reds give of their best around 15°C/60°F, slightly lower for light wines, slightly higher for Cabernet Sauvignons and other 'big' wines. If in doubt about the temperature, keep it on the low side, and warm the glass gently in your hand as you drink.

• CHOOSE FOOD YOU LOVE AND FEEL EMPOWERED

The production of saliva increases when you think about, choose and eat food and drink you like. It is futile to munch your way through something you don't fancy, leaving yourself dissatisfied and looking for something else. All the 'diet, slim-line, low-fat, diabetic, reduced this, that and the other' foods are a wasted eating experience, unless you love them of course. Whatever health problem you have, if any, there is always something delicious you can eat.

• DON'T USE FOOD AS A CURRENCY

Food is there to be enjoyed, but it should always be kept in perspective in your life. Food should not become an obsession, or something that is used as the only tool of affection. Parents who withdraw food when they are displeased or make children eat quantities of food to show that they care for them, are heading for problems. Women who take it very personally if their partner or child doesn't eat the food they have prepared should try to communicate in other ways. Because food is one of the few things we can control in life, it can become a destructive weapon to be used against us, sowing the seeds of an eating disorder such as obesity, anorexia nervosa or bulimia.

Above all, don't let food become a negative issue: think of all the wonderful things you can eat which provide positive pleasure and comfort.

The appetite mechanism

It's not until you understand how your appetite mechanism works that you will be able to glean maximum benefit from food. By understanding hunger and satiety (the feeling you get when you're happily full) you will be able to feel well after eating, both in body and in mind. Bad eating habits don't just mean bad food, they also mean being out of harmony with the way you eat: excess weight, indigestion and many other problems occur when women don't listen to their bodies and eat properly.

The first thing is to learn to be tuned in to the satiety value of eating. Satiety, or sensory satisfaction, encompasses physical properties such as smell, taste, texture and temperature, and the emotional and/or psychological perceptions of eating. The greater the degree of satiety, the more we enjoy what we eat and drink.

Appetite is co-ordinated in an area of the brain called the hypothalamus; this same area controls a lot of our emotions, which is why emotions and feeding are so closely linked. The 'feeding' centre within the hypothalamus is sub-divided into 'hunger' and 'satiety' or 'fullness' centres. The number of signals reaching these centres dictates whether you feel hungry or full. If you feel pleasantly full and contented after your meals you'll be less likely to binge or pick on inappropriate foods.

THERE ARE BASICALLY FOUR STAGES DURING EATING WHEN YOU SEND SIGNALS BACK TO THE 'SATIETY' CENTRE

• CHEWING

Within the jaw are stretch receptors, which respond when you chew. The more you chew and the more time you take over eating, the greater the perception of satiety.

• STIMULATING THE TASTE BUDS

Both taste and tactile stimulation within the mouth lead to greater satiety. If you have exciting flavours, varying temperatures and textures within a meal, your mouth has a greater opportunity to register satisfaction. The foods with the highest satisfaction value are those with several organoleptic properties, in other words they stimulate more than one sense: they look good, smell good, feel good in the mouth, taste good and even sound good – think of sizzling bacon, the crackle of roasting chestnuts or the snap of the sugar crust on a crème brûlée.

Think about this when planning meals. If you eat similar foods all the time, your mouth gets used to the taste and texture, and to some extent 'switches off'. The production of saliva and other digestive juices increases when you choose food you love and therefore both your body and your mind recognize the experience of eating.

See eating as a sensual and enjoyable occasion. It is hopeless to choose food or place yourself in a situation you're not going to enjoy, as your mouth and sensory recognition mechanism will switch off and you won't feel as if you've eaten. Notice your food, concentrate on eating and avoid needless consumption when your mind is distracted.

• LIFTING THE ARM TO EAT

The more often you lift your hand to your mouth, delivering food, the greater the satiety. Take smaller mouthfuls and take little breaks while you're eating a meal. Eat slowly and cut food into small pieces using a knife and fork. For example, rather than holding a whole apple permanently up to your mouth, slice it and fan it on a plate with a few orange segments. The orange will enhance the apple's colour, texture and taste, and picking up the slices individually will ensure that your brain recognizes an enjoyable eating experience.

• ACKNOWLEDGING YOUR STOMACH

Within the stomach wall are stretch receptors, which send signals of fullness to your brain when there is food in your stomach. If you take in foods that are low in bulk they pass through the stomach quickly, so you don't have many signals sent back to the satiety centre, therefore you don't feel full for very long and you are likely to take in more food before feeling full. Nutritionally this occurs when you eat fatty, sugary or refined foods and alcohol, as there is not a lot of bulk to them. The converse occurs when you eat high-fibre foods, such as fresh fruit and vegetables, pulses and wholegrain bread, pasta and rice. These have thick cell walls and are more difficult for the body to break down; they stay in the stomach for a lot longer, swell and send lots of signals back to the satiety centre in the brain, making you feel full and contented.

It is also very important to relax when you're eating. Sitting calmly allows your body to concentrate its blood supply and fully acknowledge the stomach. Eating when there are stress hormones such as adrenaline in your bloodstream causes the majority of blood to go to your limbs: stress hormones are some-times called 'fight or flight' hormones because they prepare the body to run. This situation does not help you gain satiety from the eating experience.

What your body needs

In order to become and remain healthy, our bodies need good food and the time and energy to process it and use it to help us feel well. A healthy eating lifestyle provides all the necessary nutrients to create and repair tissues, to sustain a healthy immune system and to enable the body to execute daily tasks with ease. To understand how you should structure a healthy eating lifestyle, it is important to know which types of food you need to eat and why.

CARBOHYDRATES

Carbohydrates in the diet, along with fats (see page 15), provide our bodies with vital energy. Some carbohydrates also contain fibre, which adds healthy bulk to our diet, along with many other benefits (see page 11).

There are two types of carbohydrate; sugar and starch. The latter, when made up in a particularly complex way that the body is unable to break down, forms fibre. Sugars and starches may be refined or found in a more natural form, which is generally healthier.

• Natural sugars are found in fruits and vegetables, and in fruit and vegetable juices.

• Refined sugars (which include honey and both white and brown sugar) are found in soft drinks (squashes, cordials and canned drinks), cakes, biscuits, jams and other preserves.

• Natural starches are found in wholegrain and wholemeal breakfast cereals, wholemeal flour and breads (from the dark pumpernickel types to the seeded, lighter wholemeal loaves), wholewheat pasta, brown rice, potatoes, lentils, chickpeas and beans (all varieties, including kidney, borlotti, haricot and cannellini), bananas, parsnips and many other fruits and vegetables, especially root vegetables.

• Refined starches are found in sugary, processed breakfast cereals, white flour and white bread (all varieties, such as the Italian ciabatta and focaccia, French baguette, English milk loaves), pasta, white rice, sugary biscuits and cakes.

• **WHY UNREFINED, NATURAL CARBOHYDRATES ARE BEST**
While refined carbohydrates are not in themselves bad for us, they don't enable the body to work as efficiently as the unrefined or natural types. All carbohydrates taken in by the body first have to be digested and converted into a type of sugar that the body can use. The refining of carbohydrates (for example when brown rice has its outer husk removed to become white rice) involves breaking them down into simpler parts, doing work that in natural carbohydrates is done at a steady pace within the body. Simpler carbohydrates in foods are digested and absorbed into the blood very quickly. At this point an organ called the pancreas secretes insulin, a hormone that helps take the sugar into the cells for them to use. If the cells receive more sugar than they need, the body stores some of the sugar as glycogen, either within the liver or in fat around the body. Then when you do need energy, a hormone called glucagon breaks down the glycogen in the liver to be used by the cells. So sugar metabolism is a cycle of sugar, insulin and glucagon reactions.

The gentler these reactions are, in other words the slower the release of the sugar and hormones, the more stable you will feel. Rapid changes adversely affect your energy and mood levels.

When making up your daily eating plan you should base each of your meals on a starch food such as potato, rice, beans, pasta or bread. These provide energy at a slower, steadier rate than sugary foods. If you can include some wholegrain versions, so much the better for your body – you should feel a lot healthier. Starch foods are not fattening until you load them up with butter or deep-fry them.

The natural sugars found in fruits and vegetables come as a complete package with fibre, vitamins and

*'When one has
tasted water melons,
one knows what
angels eat.'
Mark Twain*

minerals, but refined sugary foods are of very little nutritional benefit, and of course they contribute to tooth decay, so you should keep your intake of them low. I don't mean that you should cut them out completely as they can be delicious, but save them for special treats. If you fancy something sweet, think of a juicy orange, a ripe peach or a handful of grapes.

FIBRE

The benefits of fibre are explained in more detail in the chapters on constipation, cholesterol and cancer, but in simple terms fibre is needed to:
• Stimulate the bowel to excrete waste products on a regular basis
• Ensure that the absorption of nutrients from our foods occurs in a controlled and gradual fashion, thereby avoiding energy and mood crashes
• Stimulate the body to produce substances that limit free-radical damage. Free radicals are a group of highly reactive substances that increase the risk of developing cancers, heart disease and other health problems. They are discussed in more detail in the chapter on Skin.

If fibre is going to work efficiently in your body you need to drink at least two litres (four pints) of water every day. This helps the fibre to swell and carry out its functions. Without water the fibre will just lie in your stomach, doing very little apart from possibly causing constipation.

The main providers of fibre in our diet are, firstly, cereals (edible grains) such as wheat, corn (maize), oats and rice and foods made from them, preferably whole-grain or wholemeal types, including bread, pasta and breakfast cereals. The other great fibre providers are vegetables (including fresh or dried beans and lentils, known as pulses) and fruits.

In addition to fibre, fresh fruits, vegetables and wholegrain products provide us with vitamins and minerals which not only help keep our body healthy, but

FLAVOURED OILS
There are many
flavoured oils on
the market, such as
Chinese chilli oil,
garlic oil and truffle
oil, which is fabulous
sprinkled over pasta
and potato salads.
Apart from truffle oil,
you can easily make
your own flavoured
oils. They add
delicious flavours
to salads and other
dishes and also make
lovely gifts.

Take a clean glass
jar and fill it with a
good (but not very
fine or expensive)
oil such as olive or
sunflower. Add fresh
herbs, chillies, cloves
of garlic, peppercorns
or whatever takes
your fancy. Leave the
oils to infuse for
about a week, giving
the jar the occasional
shake, before using.

also help to prevent the above and other diseases. Women who have diets rich in these foods are much less likely to suffer from a variety of problems, including constipation, diabetes, mood swings and infertility.

• VEGETABLES AND FRUITS

In order to gain the maximum benefit from the fibre, vitamins and minerals so abundant in fruit and vegetables, it is strongly recommended that you eat five good-sized portions of fresh fruits or vegetables every day. Including vegetables with your main meals, either as a salad or chargrilled, roasted, steamed or quickly boiled, and fresh fruit after every meal, easily makes up five portions throughout the day.

The type of fruit or vegetable is entirely your choice, but you should aim to get plenty of variety. It doesn't really matter whether they are raw or cooked (a combination of the two is best).

Women should not worry that vegetable hot pots and similar dishes that have been left to cook slowly in the oven may not provide much in terms of beneficial nutrients. While some vitamins and minerals are lost with long cooking times, the benefits of the nutrients and fibre that remain outweigh the losses.

When choosing your vegetables and fruits, think whether you would like them to be organic (see below). Even if you do not choose organic, you need to make sure that, as far as possible, you remove the pesticides, waxes and other substances from the skins of fruits and vegetables. If not removed, these substances can lead to free-radical damage within your body's cells, causing cancer, heart disease and premature ageing. Exhaust fumes contain similarly damaging substances, so you should wash produce brought from road-side stalls.

• ORGANIC PRODUCE

Organic fruits and vegetables can be both tastier and healthier, but this is hotly debated. I think that organic produce is preferable because no pesticides and chemicals are used in its production. Surely, the fewer chemicals we put in our bodies the healthier we will be: our guts are not used to the levels of pesticides used in some non-organic produce. I see many women with problems such as the skin condition urticaria, or irritable bowels, whose symptoms disappear once their gut is fed organic produce rather than non-organic.

Organic vegetables and fruit are not as widely available as non-organic produce, although thankfully as demand increases more suppliers are popping up around the country. There are some wholesale co-operative companies who deliver nationwide. At the moment organic produce is a little more expensive, but the price will come down if there is greater demand. I recommend that you read Henrietta Green's book, *Around Britain*, which lists various outlets. You could also contact the Soil Association for names of suppliers.

PROTEIN

Protein is needed to help the body build strong muscles, repair tissues and maintain an effective immune and hormonal system. Proteins in the diet are broken down by digestive enzymes and absorbed into the blood as amino acids, often called the 'building blocks' of protein. These are then either taken to repair muscles and other body tissues, or used to build a strong immune system. Any extra may be used for energy or stored as fat.

There are two types of amino acids: essential and non-essential. The body can produce non-essential amino acids from other sources, but essential amino acids must be obtained directly from food. You therefore need to make sure that your daily diet contains an adequate supply of essential amino acids.

• SOURCES OF ESSENTIAL AMINO ACIDS
Meat, poultry, game, fish and shellfish, eggs and dairy products, as well as soya products (soya milk, tofu),

contain all the essential amino acids. Beans and other pulses, grains, nuts, seeds and manufactured vegetable protein foods contain protein, but don't contain all the essential amino acids. However, in combination – for example pulses with grains or pulses with nuts – they can be used by the body to meet its daily protein requirements. They do need to be carefully balanced in the diet, so make sure that you eat a good quantity and variety of these foods every day.

Since the proteins found in cereal products such as wholegrain bread help the body to use the protein from pulses, some good examples of meals that contain no animal foods are: baked beans on wholegrain toast, lentil curry with rice, or the Caribbean dish of rice and peas.

As far as quantity is concerned, we need approximately 1 gram of protein per kilo of body weight. Too little protein can compromise your health but, as with carbohydrates and fats, if you eat too much protein your body stores it as fat.

If you have a very physically active job or are involved in rigorous sports training, you may need more protein in your daily diet. Seek the advice of a dietitian.

• For the average woman, all you need is a piece of lean protein about the size of a breast of chicken for your main meal, plus an additional portion, half this size, in a smaller meal or snack. To name just a few delicious examples of lean protein foods: chicken, poussin, turkey, quail, pheasant, rabbit, venison, ham, beef, smoked or fresh salmon and trout, sole, halibut, monkfish, tuna, swordfish, oysters, mussels, prawns, lobster, eggs (chicken, duck or quails' eggs).

• Vegetarians should aim to include a protein food together with a cereal food (pasta, bread, rice) in their main meals, and consider combinations of these foods for other meals and snacks: beans and pulses (baked beans, haricot, black-eyed, broad, butter, mung, aduki, soya and kidney beans; chickpeas; red and Puy lentils); nuts (Brazil, cashew, hazel and walnuts), tofu, Quorn, eggs, cheese. See page 39 for specific advice for vegetarians and vegans.

For a number of health reasons, which are discussed throughout this book, it's best to choose a lean protein, i.e. one without noticeable fat, rather than fatty or processed protein products such as sausages and pies. For variety of flavour, use herbs, spices and wines for marinating and in cooking.

• OILY FISH

Oily fish such as salmon, mackerel, mullet and sardines contain beneficial fish oils called omega-3 fatty acid and omega-6 fatty acid, which help to prevent heart disease and some types of cancer. They have also been shown to improve skin conditions such as psoriasis. To gain maximum benefit, try to include oily fish once or twice in your weekly eating pattern; there are a number of recipe ideas in this book.

FAT

Fat provides a very concentrated source of energy. The body also needs to store some fat in order to prevent excessive loss of body heat. Women with very low body fat levels, such as anorexics or serious athletes, can have problems keeping warm. Fat is also needed to produce and carry the sex hormones oestrogen and progesterone around the body. Too little body fat can cause you to stop menstruating and can also make you more prone to developing osteoporosis, a disease that causes brittle bones (discussed in more detail in the chapter on the menopause).

Today, when the fashion is to be thin, I see many women who suffer from too little body fat, without realizing the long-term implications. Magazines and model agencies don't tell you about the down sides of being too thin. Most women know that too much body fat can cause you to develop high blood pressure and heart disease, and aggravate joint problems such as osteoarthritis, but are less aware of the problems associated with too little body fat. You should try not to let your body fat level go too high or too low. See page 44 for details on how to measure your body fat level.

Some fat is essential in every woman's diet. Foods that contain fats not only provide energy but also contain the fat-soluble vitamins A, D, E and K, which are vital in the development and maintenance of a healthy body and mind. The problem in Western society is that many people eat too much and very often the wrong type of fat. This is all too easily done, partly because fat carries a lot of the flavour in food.

There are two main types of fat, saturated and unsaturated. Unsaturated fats can be further divided into mono- and poly-unsaturated fats. The fats are digested by enzymes secreted by the pancreas and gall bladder, absorbed through the intestine and then carried to various parts of the body to fulfil specific functions such as energy production, hormone metabolism or tissue repair. The fact that the various fats are metabolized in slightly different ways means that we can bring about positive health changes – for example, reducing blood cholesterol and triglyceride levels – by choosing a certain type of fat in preference to another. This is discussed in more detail in the chapter on high blood cholesterol.

• SATURATED FATS

These come mainly from animal products such as butter, lard, suet and dripping, meat, eggs, full-fat milk, cheese and full-fat yoghurt. They are also found in hard margarines, which contain trans-fatty acids (see below). Therefore most cakes and biscuits, made with butter or hard margarine (hydrogenated vegetable oil), are likely to be high in saturated fats. Be aware that coconut oil and palm oil are also high in saturated fats.

• UNSATURATED FATS

These come from vegetable sources, namely oils such as olive, sunflower, safflower, rapeseed, soya, peanut and sesame. Soft margarines labelled 'high in polyunsaturates' and oily fish (sardines, herrings, tuna, mackerel) also contain unsaturated fats.

• TRANS-FATTY ACIDS

I would not recommend that you use the hard margarines containing hydrogenated vegetable oil, as they contain trans-fatty acids, which have been linked with heart disease and cancer. Hydrogenation of fats entails changing the vegetable oil into a solid fat, by changing its chemical structure. It was once thought that all vegetable fats, solid or liquid, had fewer detrimental health effects than animal fats, but we now know that trans-fatty acids can cause free-radical damage within the body's cells. If you really need a hard fat for cooking, stick to butter.

• DAILY FAT INTAKE

Even if we don't eat any noticeably fatty foods, we generally consume enough fat to meet most healthy women's requirements. This is because there are hidden fats in a number of foods, including meat and fish. A balanced diet, with meals rich in lean protein, wholegrain starches, fresh fruits and vegetables, will provide an acceptable fat intake. The only women who expose themselves to lack of fat in their diets are those with strange eating habits such as those on permanent restrictive diets or who suffer from anorexia.

In the majority of cases it is far too easy to over-consume on fats. Excess fat in our diet usually leads to an increase in the amount of body fat deposited under the skin, causing weight gain. An excess of saturated fats can deposit in the blood vessel lining; this can cause serious problems such as heart disease.

We should all watch our total fat intake, whether it be from animal or vegetable sources. Keep the quantity of fat you consume as low as possible. If you don't have a medically diagnosed cholesterol problem, choose the fat you like, whether it's butter or olive oil, and use just a small amount of it.

Choose lean sources of protein rather than fattier meats such as lamb, sausages, pies, pâtés and salamis. Instead try to eat plenty of chicken, turkey, lean ham, fish, shellfish, pulses and other non-meat protein sources.

• FATS IN COOKING

If you get into the habit of using fats sparingly and investigate ways of flavouring and cooking foods other than with fat, you will reap the benefits in a healthier body. Recipes and menus often refer to butter. I use this as a 'catch-all' word to represent fats of all sorts. If you don't want to use butter, then substitute your preferred fat. Low-fat spreads, whatever they say, cannot be used for cooking: the water content is too high and it simply disappears, burning the bottom of the pan. I wouldn't advocate that you use them in any case, as they are inferior to the more natural butter or oil. A small amount of fat in cooking is fine, just don't use lashings of it.

WATER, THE ESSENCE OF LIFE

Humans can survive for quite a time without food, but only a few days without water. Water is needed to keep the body flushed of waste products, the skin, hair and body organs healthy, to produce digestive enzymes and to enable the body to glean all the beneficial nutrients from the food and drinks we consume. In a healthy diet, water works in conjunction with fibre (see page 11) to prevent constipation. Lack of water can also cause dry, wrinkly skin, dull hair and fatigue. We lose water mainly through our skin and kidneys. We also lose a lot of water when we suffer from sickness, diarrhoea or any infection that causes fever.

Since a lot of women live in centrally heated houses and work in offices with heating and air conditioning, we lose a lot more water through our skin than women in the past. It is very important that you do not allow your body to dehydrate, by making sure that you drink plenty of fluids.

Most women should try to drink two to three litres (about four or five pints) of water every day.

• BOTTLED OR TAP?

Many women wonder whether bottled or tap water is best. Each has its pros and cons.

• Tap water in many areas has fluoride added, which helps reduce tooth decay.

• You should be aware that the bacterial content of bottled water is not regulated by any official 'body', but tap water is regulated and undergoes stringent checks. I think the choice of water depends primarily on taste. Some tap water tastes of chemicals such as chlorine and is not very pleasant to drink. You can buy filters to improve the taste of tap water, but make sure that you follow the manufacturer's instructions on using the filter, and change the filter regularly. Old filters can contaminate the water.

Away from the home it can be more convenient to carry bottled water around with you. What you should not do is to open a bottle of mineral water and then leave it in the refrigerator with the seal broken for a few days. This enables unwanted bacteria to grow, so use opened bottles within a day of opening.

If you prefer sparkling water you may choose bottled water or you can buy water 'sparklers' to fit to your tap.

• PLAIN OR FLAVOURED?

Pure water is the best drink: it quenches thirst more effectively than other drinks. Plain water can be jazzed up with a variety of flavourings. On a hot day, still or sparkling water is delicious chilled and flavoured with fresh mint leaves, a few drops of orange blossom water or a little elderflower cordial. The same flavourings can be added to hot water. There is a huge choice of herb and fruit teas and tisanes on the market. These can either be drunk hot or can be prepared and then chilled in the refrigerator.

Although carbonated fizzy drinks are all right in themselves, watch out for caffeine in cola-based drinks and sugar in most sweet drinks. The label might say dextrose or fructose, but don't be fooled: these are just other types of sugar, in addition to sucrose and glucose. Try not to drink too many fruit squashes, canned drinks, syrups and sweetened herbal-type drinks, as the sugar content of all these is quite high. Too many sugary drinks cause energy balance problems, headaches, mood swings, weight problems and tooth decay. Excessive amounts of caffeine cause a number of health problems; see page 60 for more information. 'Diet' drinks contain artificial sweeteners and additives that, while not harmful in small amounts, are not as good, healthy or refreshing as simple water.

VITAMINS

The possibility of vitamin and mineral deficiencies should not be ignored, but they are not as common as health supplement manufacturers would like you to believe. I frequently see women who suffer from iron-deficiency anaemia, but other deficiency conditions such as scurvy (caused by a lack of vitamin C) are normally found only in women with extreme eating habits or very unbalanced diets, who are very heavy smokers or who have a complicating health condition such as gut malabsorption problems. For most healthy women there is really no need for vitamin or mineral supplements, as long as you are eating a good balance of fresh foods in sufficient quantity and not drinking excessive amounts of tea or coffee. The caffeine in tea, coffee and other drinks inhibits the absorption and increases the excretion of vitamins and minerals. I sometimes see women who become deficient in vitamins and minerals because they drink so much coffee, but this is quite rare.

There are two types of vitamins: water-soluble (C and B complex) and fat-soluble (A, D, E and K). Water-soluble vitamins cannot be stored by the body, so foods containing these should be eaten daily. They can easily be destroyed by overcooking, especially by boiling vegetables or fruit in lots of water. To preserve these vitamins you should try to eat the foods lightly cooked, for instance steamed, or raw, in salads.

VITAMIN A

This vitamin is essential for growth, healthy skin, good vision and healthy tooth enamel. If you eat a well-balanced diet you should easily receive sufficient vitamin A from your food. You need about 750–800 micrograms a day, increasing to 1200 micrograms if you are breastfeeding.

Vitamin A (also known as retinol), is found in animal products: oily fish such as salmon, tuna, mackerel; offal such liver and kidneys; milk, eggs, cheese, butter and margarine.

Beta-carotene, a substance found in orange, yellow and green vegetables and fruit, is converted into vitamin A within the body. Foods rich in beta-carotene include: carrots; dark green vegetables such as spinach, broccoli, Savoy cabbage, watercress, asparagus, lettuce (especially Cos lettuce); apricots and peaches (fresh and dried); oranges; tomatoes, red and yellow peppers; sweet potatoes; squash, pumpkins; yellow-fleshed melons (e.g. cantaloupe).

Vitamin A preparations are sometimes used externally to treat skin conditions, but under no circumstances should you take a vitamin A preparation or supplement without medical supervision. An excess of vitamin A (vitamin A toxicity) causes liver problems and is extremely serious.

VITAMIN B COMPLEX

The term 'B vitamins' covers a group of substances: B1 (thiamin), B2 (riboflavin), B3 (nicotinic acid), folic acid, B5 (pantothenic acid), B6 (pyridoxine) and B12 (cobalamin). These vitamins are essential for growth and the development and maintenance of a healthy nervous system. They also help digest food and convert it into energy.

Luckily there are several foods that are rich sources of the majority of them, so you do not need to become obsessed with them individually. Just for your information, recommended daily allowances are:

B1 (thiamin)	0.7–1.1 milligrams (depending on age, active or sedentary lifestyle, pregnancy and lactation)
B2 (riboflavin)	1.3–1.8 milligrams
B3 (nicotinic acid)	15–21 milligrams
Folate (folic acid)	300–500 micrograms

B5 (pantothenic acid), B6 (pyridoxine) and B12 (cobalamin) have no recommended dietary allowance: in a regular well balanced diet you should get enough of them in combination with the other B vitamins, but since B12 is found mainly in foods of animal origin, vegetarians and vegans may need to take a supplement (see page 32): lack of this vitamin may cause a form of anaemia.

There has been a lot of interest in the role that the B vitamins, especially vitamin B6, play in the alleviation of pre-menstrual tension and mood swings. Unfortunately the studies are inconclusive and can encourage women to take unnecessary vitamins, potentially causing toxicity. Vitamin B6 toxicity gives symptoms of extreme lethargy, numbness in the fingers and toes and lack of appetite, as well as serious liver problems. Toxicity has been found in women taking 200 milligrams a day, which is easily done taking over-the-counter preparations.

Instead of taking vitamin supplements, I recommend that you eat foods rich in the B vitamins. No foods except for liver and yeast extract contain them all. Since the majority of us don't eat these in large quantities, I suggest you boost your overall intake of the following foods, which contain a significant amount of them: meat, especially meat juices (so use them in a sauce or gravy) and liver; dairy produce – milk, yoghurt, cheese, butter, eggs; fish; wholegrain cereals and wheatgerm; dark green vegetables such as broccoli and spinach; potatoes; yeast extract (e.g. Marmite); nuts such as brazils, pistachios, walnuts; beans; bananas.

• FOLIC ACID

So much has been written about women's need for folic acid, that I thought it worth looking at this vitamin in greater detail. Folic acid is needed to create healthy blood cells, therefore if lacking in the diet it can cause anaemia. In addition it is needed to enable the body to absorb iron, itself a vital nutrient for strong blood; lack of iron results in the most common form of anaemia, iron-deficiency anaemia. Women frequently have a low folic acid intake because the folic acid intake of foods decreases greatly both with cooking and storage times, as well as in processing. Various medications such as aspirin and birth control pills hinder the absorption of folic acid, so it might be worth considering changing to another form of contraception if you have a poor level of folic acid in your body; ask your doctor for advice. In pregnancy, when your body is rapidly producing new cells, your requirement for folic acid increases, and it is important to bear in mind that folic acid deficiency has been linked with birth defects; this is covered in more detail in the chapter on pregnancy.

Since many of us rely heavily on foods that have travelled from further afield than the back garden, by the time we get the food on the table the folic acid content may be low. The major sources of folic acid in the diet are the dark green leafy vegetables such as Savoy cabbage and spring greens, asparagus, curly kale, spinach, fresh orange juice and wheatgerm (found in wholemeal bread and cereals). In order to keep the amount of folic acid high you should keep cooking time to a minimum and eat the foods freshly cooked; if you store and then reheat them the folic acid content drops significantly.

VITAMIN C

As with the other vitamins, vitamin C is needed for growth and healthy body tissue; it is also important in the healing of wounds. In addition, it helps the body to absorb iron, a very important mineral (see page 28).

Vitamin C (also known as ascorbic acid) is one of the most common supplements taken by women. It is one of the antioxidant vitamins (see page 32), and may prevent or reduce the severity of the common cold. The recommended daily intake is 60 milligrams but, contrary to popular belief, consuming more than 1000 milligrams per day does not have clearly proven benefits. This is mainly because vitamin C is a water-soluble vitamin, therefore the body cannot store excess amounts. If you consume more than 1000 milligrams a day your body will simply excrete it. I sometimes find that women who take excess vitamin C suffer from sensitive and irritable stomachs and mouth ulcers. Vitamin C is, after all, ascorbic acid.

The main sources in the diet are fresh fruit and vegetables. I try to encourage women to have five portions of fruit or vegetables every day, as this will easily meet their body's requirements. An average bowl of strawberries contains about 180 milligrams of vitamin C; half a plate of steamed broccoli contains 150 milligrams; 1 kiwi fruit contains 75 milligrams; and a large orange contains 70 milligrams. You can therefore realistically reach the 60 milligrams recommended intake.

Other rich vegetable sources of vitamin C are: spinach, curly kale, Brussels sprouts, cabbage, leafy greens and cauliflower, red, green and yellow peppers, tomato juice, potatoes, green peas, asparagus. Fruits high in vitamin C, besides oranges, strawberries and kiwis, include: grapefruit, lemons and other citrus fruits, blackcurrants, rosehips, melon, papaya.

• THE EFFECT OF COOKING ON VITAMIN C CONTENT

The debate continues as to whether our vegetables have any vitamins and minerals left in them by the time we eat them. There is very little difference in the vitamin C content of raw and cooked foods, as long as they are not overcooked. Problems occur if you boil vegetables for hours, as by the time you eat them all the vitamin C will have dissolved in the water.

If you try to choose fruit and vegetables that are as fresh as possible and eat them raw or lightly cooked you should get sufficient vitamin C from your diet. Keep the cooking time down to a minimum; experiment with vegetables stir-fried, steamed, baked or boiled just until 'al dente' (to the tooth), in other words they retain plenty of texture when you bite into them.

There can be quite a lot of vitamin C in frozen and tinned fruits and vegetables. The time that elapses between the food being picked and frozen or tinned is often a lot shorter than the time it takes for so-called 'fresh' foods to get from field to shop shelf or market stall.

VITAMIN D

Vitamin D works in conjunction with the mineral calcium (see below); both are essential for proper bone formation. Vitamin D is found in a few foods, listed below, but it is chiefly made by the skin in the presence of sunlight. This is one of the reasons why it is important to get out in the fresh air every day, if possible.

Sources of vitamin D in the diet include: oily fish such as tuna, salmon, mackerel, sardines; liver; oils and margarine; eggs; dairy produce – milk, butter, yoghurt, cheese.

VITAMIN E

Vitamin E is needed to help develop and maintain strong cells, especially in the blood. It is one of the group of antioxidant vitamins (see page 32), which have been shown to decrease the incidence of heart disease and some cancers. Many women feel that they need to take an antioxidant tablet containing vitamin E, but this is unnecessary; it is much better to enjoy a well-balanced diet that includes some of the following foods: avocado, blackberries and mangoes, nuts and seeds; wheatgerm, wholewheat bread and wholegrain cereal; soft margarine and vegetable oils such as olive oil.

VITAMIN K

The role of this vitamin is mainly that of helping the blood to clot to the naturally healthy degree, and maintaining strong bones. It is found in small quantities in most vegetables and wholegrain cereals but it is mainly produced by healthy bacteria in the gut. If you don't have a healthy bacterial population in your gut, your production of vitamin K and other anti-disease substances will be affected. Women who have problems such as irritable bowel syndrome or chronic constipation, or who take antibiotics on a long-term basis, should make a particular effort to encourage healthy gut bacteria by eating a well-balanced diet. If you are able to tolerate acidophilus and bifidus, it can be of great benefit to eat a small pot of 'live' (bio) yoghurt every day, but if you have gut problems you should talk to your doctor first.

CALCIUM

Calcium is needed for strong bones and teeth. Lack of calcium has been linked with the development of osteoporosis, a disease that causes brittle bones. For more information on preventing osteoporosis, see the chapter on the menopause. All women benefit from a diet that meets their calcium requirement throughout childhood and well into adulthood. Young children need approximately 525 milligrams per day and this increases to 800 milli-grams for adult women, or 1,200 if you are pregnant or breastfeeding.

• **DAIRY PRODUCE**

The primary source of calcium in the diet is dairy produce. The recommended daily requirement is found in 660 ml (just over 1 pint) of semi-skimmed milk or 100 g (3½ oz) of Cheddar cheese or 400 g (14 oz) of natural yoghurt. You can easily obtain sufficient calcium if you incorporate some milk in drinks and cooking and some other dairy products in your cooking every day.

All milk, from skimmed to rich Jersey milk, is high in calcium; so are most types of cheese and cream, but some of these are also high in fat, so watch the quantities. Yoghurt is another good source, whether it be a full-fat or low fat-version. The yoghurt should ideally be live, but other yoghurts, especially the delicious thick Greek sort, are also rich in calcium.

• **OTHER SOURCES OF CALCIUM**

If you don't like dairy products, other food sources include spinach, okra, curly kale, watercress, broccoli and pulses, dried apricots, figs and peaches, oysters, canned fish with soft, edible bones (sardines, salmon, pilchards and mackerel) and sesame seeds. A regular source could be breads and flour, especially white flour, as this may be enriched with calcium. This is a legacy of World War II, when dairy products were scarce; the Government decided to fortify white bread to help prevent calcium deficiency.

However, you need to eat a lot more of these foods because they contain 'salts', chemical substances that bind the calcium and reduce the amount that can be absorbed into your blood. It is doubtful that the majority of women would be able to meet their daily requirement of 800 milligrams from non-dairy sources of calcium alone: they would need to eat the equivalent of at least 400–500 g (about 1 lb) of raw spinach or 1 kg (over 2 lb) of dried apricots to derive enough calcium for one day! In this situation, therefore, you should seek professional advice about meeting the shortfall with a supplement.

There are many different calcium supplements on the market and you should check with your doctor or dietitian before you choose one. This is important because several medical conditions, including kidney problems, can be aggravated by supplements.

If you are taking a supplement, you should try to ensure that your calcium intake is around 1000 milligrams a day, rather than the 800 milligrams recommended above. The reason for the difference is that the body does not absorb as much from a supplement. You should still eat as many calcium-rich foods as possible.

It is also important to look beyond the calcium level in your supplement or diet, as it can be affected by complementary and aggravating factors such as vitamin D and vitamin C intake, smoking and caffeine.

IRON

Iron is needed for healthy blood and muscles. Some women can become deficient in iron, especially if they lose a lot of blood in heavy periods, which leaves them feeling tired and generally 'run down'. If this goes on for any length of time, it can develop into iron-deficiency anaemia. If you suspect that you are anaemic, I suggest you read the separate chapter on anaemia.

There are two main sorts of iron in food: haem iron, found in animal foods such as lean red meat and offal, and non-haem iron, derived from some plants, grains and nuts (see page 25). Unfortunately the vegetable sources of iron also contain 'salts' (oxalates and phytates) – substances that obstruct the absorption of iron, meaning that your body cannot absorb the iron from these sources as effectively. You therefore need to eat a lot more of them to obtain sufficient iron. Egg yolks and oily fish are quite rich in iron, but they too contain substances that prevent the body from absorbing it as efficiently as the iron from red meat sources.

The body absorbs approximately 5–20% of the iron from vegetable sources whereas it absorbs 20–40% of the iron available in red meat and offal. If we eat a mixed diet including fruits, vegetables, meat and fish we are thought to absorb approximately 15–20% of the iron in our food.

As with all nutrients in the diet, iron relies on a healthy gut to absorb it. Some women with digestive problems such as irritable bowel syndrome or chronic constipation can have slightly disrupted iron absorption. If you have a specific bowel problem see your dietitian or doctor for advice.

Iron needs vitamin C and folic acid(associated with the B vitamins) to help the body absorb it. It is therefore important that you look at the overall balance of your diet when trying to maximize the absorption and utilization of iron and other nutrients.

• SOURCES OF IRON

Most women need 12–15 milligrams of iron in their diet every day. The primary source is lean red meat, game and offal: beef, lamb, venison, hare, pheasant, pigeon, grouse, liver and kidney.

Other iron-providers include: eggs, spinach, curly kale, watercress, broccoli, Savoy cabbage and other dark green leafy vegetables; lentils, beans (including baked beans) and peas; oily fish such as tuna, mackerel and sardines; oysters; dried fruits (especially figs, apricots and raisins); canned blackcurrants; wholegrain cereals; black treacle; nuts; liquorice and chocolate (yes!).

MAGNESIUM

This mineral has a variety of functions in the body, including building strong bones, releasing energy from your muscles and regulating your body temperature. It also helps the body absorb and metabolize various other vitamins and minerals such as calcium and vitamin C. Magnesium deficiency can cause high blood pressure and, in extreme cases, heart attacks.

Good sources include wholewheat cereal products such as wholemeal and granary bread, leafy green vegetables, milk, yoghurt, meat, apricots, bananas.

POTASSIUM

This mineral works with sodium to regulate the body's water balance, heart rhythm, nerve impulses and muscle function. Potassium and sodium levels within the body work rather like a pair of scales. When the potassium level increases the sodium level decreases and vice versa. An increase in sodium can cause the body to retain fluid, which may cause puffy eyes, swollen ankles and the general bloated feeling many women experience at some time (see the chapter on periods). It is generally a very good idea to make sure that your potassium intake is substantial, because most of us consume too much sodium in the form of salt. A low potassium intake can ultimately cause high blood pressure or your heart to beat erratically, a medical condition known as arrhythmia.

Good sources include potatoes, bananas, orange juice, winter squash, dried apricots and prunes, natural yoghurt.

ZINC

Zinc has many functions in the body, and deficiency may result in sexual problems such as low libido, sterility and birth defects, a poor immune system, skin problems or lack of appetite. Zinc deficiency is quite common in women who have been taking the contraceptive pill for any length of time. Everyone should try to include some zinc in their daily healthy eating plan, and it is particularly important if you have just come off the pill or you are unwell in any way.

I offer a warning against supplementing your zinc intake. As with other minerals and vitamins, many people think that if you boost your diet with a supplement this will improve your health. Over and above the recommended daily allowance of 15 milligrams, zinc supplements can actually make your body more susceptible to bacterial infections. This is important to bear in mind if you have a blood test to screen for vitamin and mineral deficiencies. Many clinics tell you you're zinc deficient, but this is not a bad thing in certain circumstances, because the body purposely lowers your blood zinc level so that you don't get a secondary infection. There are cases for zinc supplements, but they need individual advice.

The majority of women simply need to include the following zinc sources in a well-balanced diet: shellfish such as oysters, mussels, crab and lobster; canned sardines; turkey; lean red meats such as beef and lamb; parmesan and other hard or crumbly cheeses such as Cheshire; wholegrain cereals.

• VITAMIN AND MINERAL SUPPLEMENTS

In general, I advise people to be wary of taking proprietary nutritional supplements. Ideally they should be taken only on the professional advice of someone who is not motivated by selling the product: your doctor or dietitian. Many supplements are a waste of money and, worse, are a potential cause of toxicity and related problems. I have seen several women with toxicity symptoms ranging from mouth ulcers to liver failure, as a direct result of taking inappropriate supplements. Unfortunately, many of us tend not to think twice before taking yet another pill, which we feel is going to make a 'new woman' of us. Throughout this book I hope to show you that there is more to life than swallowing pills; our bodies were designed to chew real food.

Over the last few years there has been a lot of exciting research into antioxidants, a group of substances that includes vitamins C and E and beta-carotene, which the body converts into vitamin A. Antioxidants are believed to reduce your likelihood of developing cancer, either through the production of anti-cancer substances or more generally by boosting the immune system, and also the risk of heart disease, by preventing blood fats from oxidizing and depositing in the blood vessels (see the chapter on high blood cholesterol).

So the question arises as to whether you should take a supplement. Recent studies have shown that if you take one supplement, for instance beta-carotene, a well-known antioxidant, your prognosis in the case of cancer can be worse than if you don't take any supplements. The reason lies in what I refer to as the 'domino effect'. If you have too much of one vitamin or mineral, some natural advantageous hormonal and cell reactions can be disturbed, which can then lead to other problems. It is far better to concentrate on deriving all the good-ness you can from fresh food, rather than delving into the supplementary pill market, tempting though the array of bottles might be, with all their promises of good health and well-being.

• ANTIOXIDANTS

Good sources of antioxidant-rich foods can be found below vitamins A, C and E. In addition, the mineral selenium is an antioxidant needed in tiny, but regular, amounts. It is found in skimmed milk, skinless chicken, lean meat and offal, seafood, most vegetables, whole-grain cereal and wholewheat bread. Bioflavonoids also act as antioxidants. These compounds are pigments in fruits and vegetables and are concentrated in the peel, skin or outer layers of plants. Orange and other citrus fruits contain approximately 50–100 milligrams of bioflavonoids per 100 grams (3½ oz) of fruit.

• GARLIC

Perhaps the perfect health supplement, garlic (*Allium sativa*) is a complex of substances displaying anti-cancer, immunity-boosting, anti-viral, anti-bacterial, anti-blood-clotting, decongestive, digestive and cholesterol-reducing properties. Much research on animals in the laboratory has shown that garlic contains chemicals that block cancers of every type, including breast, liver and colon. John Pinto, of Memorial Cancer Center in New York, reports that a specific garlic compound suppressed prostate cancer cells in test tubes by about 25%. Obviously this is not of direct relevance to women, but other tests have proved interesting. A recent study of 42,000 older women in Iowa, USA, found that those who ate garlic more than once a week were half as likely to develop cancer of the colon as non-garlic eaters. Garlic can be effectively included in your diet, not just as a flavour enhancer but as a vegetable in its own right (see my recipes for Garlic bean soup and Baked garlic bruschetta).

• For anti-cancer effects, garlic can be eaten raw or cooked. Cooked garlic is gentler on the stomach, as more than three raw cloves a day can cause wind, bloating, diarrhoea and even fever in some people.

• Garlic also reduces the incidence of cardiovascular disease and has decongestive properties, which can be useful when you're full of cold.

• The garlic bulb should be stored in a cool, dark, airy place. A special earthenware garlic jar with holes around the sides is best.

• Cloves of garlic will last well if peeled, put in a glass jar, covered with white wine and kept in the refrigerator.

• BACTERIA

Exciting recent research suggests that we should reconsider the bacteria within our guts. The gut normally contains a collection of flora (bacteria), which help to produce vitamins and energy, as well as substances believed to be beneficial in preventing many diseases, including heart disease. New nutritional research surrounds the theory that if we boost the level of two particular bacteria with-in the gut – acidophilus and bifidus – by including more in our diets, we can positively reduce the incidence of some cancers and heart disease, and generally improve our immune system.

These bacteria should feature regularly in the diet, particularly if you have been taking antibiotics or eating a diet heavily based on over-refined foods. Antibiotics kill the good bacteria that live in the gut and thereby expose the gut to an overgrowth of 'bad' bacteria, which can cause irritable bowels, thrush and fatigue. Diets rich in fatty and sugary foods can also adversely change the balance of gut bacteria. Taking in regular quantities of good bacteria helps to redress this balance. Bowel symptoms frequently disappear as soon as you do this.

You can take acidophilus and bifidus in various forms, but I think they are most easily and effectively absorbed from natural yoghurt. Look out for the 'live' or 'bio' yoghurts containing these substances. A good daily dosage would be 20 milligrams, which provides around 20 million live organisms. This quantity can usually be found in a small pot of yoghurt. Alternatively you could ask your dietitian to suggest another source.

A word of warning: people who have a sensitive immune system or gut, including those with irritable bowel syndrome, Crohn's disease or arthritis, should seek advice from their doctor before taking these flora, as they are potentially irritating to the gut and immune system in certain cases.

Healthy eating for life

Having established that your body needs a well-balanced diet, with a good supply of carbohydrates, especially high-fibre foods, water, vitamins and minerals, and a certain amount of protein, fat and bacteria, you need to know how to put it into practice. First you need to know the ingredients and principles around which you should base your food intake. With this knowledge you can enjoy choosing foods and shopping.

Much media attention is focused on foods thou shalt not have, yet there has been very little to tell women how they can use food to enhance their life rather than make it more difficult. Shopping has become a nightmare for many women, as they feel that they have to read the label on every packet, without knowing exactly what they should be looking for. Forget the labels: every figure is relative and food manufacturers are frequently very selective about what they tell you, making your task of deciding what is right for you an impossible one. Instead build on the following guidelines.

• **RESPECT YOUR MOUTH AND BODY; GET INTO THE HABIT OF ONLY EATING THINGS YOU LIKE AND NEED**
Before you put anything in your mouth, ask yourself three questions: Do I want it? Do I like it? Do I need it?

If you want it and like it then go ahead and enjoy it; if you don't, why bother wasting the eating experience? Throw all the boring, unnecessary eating out of your life.

The worst thing you can do with food is to feel guilty about eating it. If you have eaten something that you know is not the healthiest but you really fancied it or were in a situation where you didn't have any choice, enjoy it and forget about it. Don't beat yourself up with guilt. Guilt is a negative emotion, which is likely to lead you to bingeing on comfort foods. This can then get you into a negative sugar or salt cycle in which you eat more of these foods, which in turn makes you feel even more guilty. You might then decide it's not worth continuing with your healthy eating lifestyle. It is always worth persevering. Remember that life is for living and food is there to help us, not hinder us.

Deciding whether you need the food is a little more difficult. Usually when women start thinking about need, the issue of weight comes up. This is discussed in detail on page 43. Are you the correct weight for your height? The table on pages 46–47 will help you decide.

• AIM TO EAT FIVE PORTIONS OF FRESH FRUITS AND VEGETABLES EVERY DAY

This provides your body with a good source of vitamins, minerals and fibre, to maintain your body in peak condition to fight diseases. Fibre helps your food to move effectively through the body, keeps you feeling pleasantly full and satisfied and in control of your eating habits, and your energy levels steady.

• EAT THREE MEALS A DAY

This is usually made up of one main meal, a smaller snack or lunch-type meal and breakfast. You may, however, feel that you need two smaller snacks, such as a piece of fruit, a small sandwich or a piece of cake, in between two smaller meals. It all depends on your body rhythms. Meals should be based on carbohydrates, such as pasta, wholemeal bread, wholegrain cereals, rice or potatoes, along with fruits and/or vegetables. The 'main' meal should include a source of lean protein, along with carbohydrate and plenty of vegetables and fruits.

• CHOOSE LEAN SOURCES OF PROTEIN

Fish, shellfish, lean red meat, game, poultry, eggs or pulses meet your body's protein requirements without overloading on fats.

• TRY TO GET INTO THE HABIT OF USING JUST A SMALL AMOUNT OF FAT

You can use butter, olive oil, sesame oil or walnut oil to enhance the flavour of your food or for cooking, but do try to keep the quantity low.

• KEEP YOUR INTAKE OF REFINED SUGARY FOODS LOW

Too much sugar disrupts your natural energy balance, and can cause headaches, mood swings and – if eaten in large quantities – sugar sensitivity problems such as hypoglycaemia and diabetes mellitus. It is much better to get into the habit of using the natural sugars in fruits to provide sweetness. This doesn't just mean eating a piece of fresh fruit. You can make fruit shakes (see page 72) or purée fruits such as strawberries, raspberries, blackcurrants, peaches and apricots to spread on bread or use as a sauce.

• INCLUDE SOME DAIRY PRODUCTS OR ANOTHER SIGNIFICANT SOURCE OF CALCIUM IN YOUR DAILY DIET

This has far-reaching benefits for all women.

• DRINK TWO TO THREE LITRES (FOUR TO FIVE PINTS) OF WATER EVERY DAY

Water helps the fibre in your food to swell and perform its duties. It also helps to metabolize other nutrients from your food, keep your skin and hair healthy and prevent your body from becoming dehydrated.

• TRY NOT TO DRINK MORE THAN THREE CUPS OF COFFEE, TEA OR COLA-BASED DRINKS A DAY

All such drinks contain caffeine, which inhibits the absorption of vitamins and minerals from the gut, causes your body to excrete vital nutrients and interferes with the fluid and energy balance mechanisms in your body. Caffeine also causes your body to be stimulated in an artificial way, which in the long run has the opposite effect of suppressing your performance and general feeling of well-being. Enjoy the caffeine-free drinks on page 62.

• INCLUDE SOME 'GOOD' BACTERIA IN YOUR DAILY DIET, IN THE FORM OF 'LIVE' YOGHURT CONTAINING BIFIDUS AND ACIDOPHILUS

A small pot of 'bio' yoghurt a day should help to keep a healthy balance of good and bad bacteria in your gut. If you don't like or are unable to eat live yoghurt, seek the advice of your dietitian.

• TRY TO EAT REGULARLY AND IDEALLY NOT LEAVE YOUR STOMACH EMPTY FOR MORE THAN FOUR TO FIVE HOURS

This helps to keep your gut functioning effectively. Regular eating helps your gut maintain a steady supply of digestive enzymes, protects it from excess acid secretion and enables it to metabolize food in the most efficient way, to keep your energy level and moods on an even keel.

• KEEP YOUR ALCOHOL INTAKE MODERATE

Some drinks, especially young red wines such as Beaujolais, contain anti-oxidant vitamins and minerals, which can help to reduce the risk of heart disease and some cancers. Beers and Champagnes can also provide beneficial nutrients. Drinking can be a very pleasurable part of a healthy lifestyle, but drinking to excess can cause liver damage, mood and energy-balance problems. Try not to drink on an empty stomach as this can cause your blood sugar levels to crash.

• FOOD COMBINING/SEPARATING

The issue of whether you should eat proteins and carbohydrates at the same meal is one that regularly crops up in the media. Some diet consultants feel strongly that proteins and carbohydrates should be separated, and advocate that proteins should be eaten only with vegetables and fruit, not mixed with carbohydrates. Many people feel that their body functions better if they put this into practice; it is commonly known as food combining.

From the physiological and nutritional viewpoint, proteins (meat, chicken, fish, eggs, cheese, nuts, pulses) provide the body with amino acids, used as building blocks within muscles and other tissues. Carbohydrates provide energy and fibre. If you eat proteins on their own, without carbohydrate present, the protein can be broken down into energy, rather than used for building body tissue. Proteins also have other important functions to perform in maintaining body health and carbohydrates protect proteins, enabling them to fulfil these functions.

The choice is yours, but there is no physiological reasoning behind food combining, and I have never recommended it. I believe that food is there to be enjoyed. Women should not have to agonize over whether they are 'allowed' to eat certain things at certain times.

VEGETARIANS AND VEGANS

Before considering the nutritional issues of being vegetarian or vegan, let's clarify a few terms.

A vegetarian diet is one that excludes all animal flesh (meat, poultry, fish and shellfish) and other products derived from the animal carcass, such as gelatine and lard. Some vegetarians also avoid animal-derived rennet, which is used to make many hard and soft cheeses. Some refuse to eat foods that have cochineal (derived from insects) added as a red or pink food colouring.

There are many types of vegetarian diet: the most common variation is lacto-ovo-vegetarian, where animal flesh is excluded but the diet includes milk, milk products and eggs. Lacto-vegetarians exclude eggs. Many women, whether for moral or health reasons, decide that they don't want to eat red meat, but are happy to eat poultry, fish and shellfish.

A vegan diet completely excludes all forms of animal foods, including milk, milk products, eggs and honey. Some vegans also avoid food additives that may be of animal origin, such as vitamin D, whey and lecithin.

The Vegetarian Society (see page 256) keeps a comprehensive list of products that are completely free from animal products.

The majority of vegetarian women I see are lacto-ovo-vegetarians, so I shall concentrate on helping you to eat healthily as this sort of vegetarian.

• ENERGY
One of the key issues is whether vegetarian women derive enough energy from their food. If you are under-weight or of normal body weight and don't want to go

any lower, you may find that if you fill yourself up with mainly vegetables and fruits you might begin to lack energy and lose a little too much weight. To keep your energy level up and avoid any undesirable decrease in body weight, making sure that you include a wide range of the following foods, in addition to basics such as bread, pasta, rice and other cereals: pulses such as chickpeas, lentils and beans (borlotti, haricot, kidney and baked beans), cheese, avocados, bananas, nuts (and peanut butter) and olive oil. If a blood test has revealed high blood lipids, you should read the chapter on high blood cholesterol.

• PROTEIN

When you decide not to eat fish, poultry or meat, it becomes slightly more difficult to make sure that your body receives enough protein every day. Some vegetarians have eggs, milk and cheese as protein sources, but if you exclude all animal products you need to give a bit more thought to your protein intake. The protein in non-animal foods does not contain all the essential amino acids (see page 15) the body needs, unless foods of various types are eaten together. For example, the proteins you find in pulses help the body to absorb the proteins from cereal products such as wholegrain bread and wholewheat pasta. A small meal of baked beans on toast is a good example of how vegetarians and vegans can take in protein.

Eating a good quantity and variety of the following foods every day should make sure that your protein needs are met:
• Beans and other pulses – lentils (red, green or brown), chickpeas, split peas, borlotti, haricot, cannellini, flageolet and kidney beans
• Soya products – soya beans, milk and cheese, tofu (bean curd)
• Cereal and grain foods – wheat and rye breads, muffins and scones, wheat and buckwheat pancakes, pasta and noodles, rice and bulgar wheat

- Seeds – sunflower, sesame and pumpkin seeds
- Nuts – cashew, peanuts, walnuts, almonds
- Other vegetable protein foods such as Quorn.

• VITAMINS AND MINERALS

Vegetarian women are likely to lack iron, zinc, calcium and vitamins B12 and B2. There are various steps you can take to avoid deficiencies.

Among the best sources of iron and zinc for vegetarians are eggs, whole-grain cereals, pulses (peas, beans and lentils) and green leafy vegetables such as spinach, kale and dark Savoy cabbage (see page 28 for other sources). However, the gut does not absorb the minerals from these foods as easily as it would from animal foods, therefore you need to eat a lot more of them to gain the right amount of iron and zinc. You can help the body to absorb iron and zinc by including some vitamin C in the same meal. Vitamin C is found in fresh fruits and vegetables, especially citrus fruits, tomatoes, kiwis, mangoes, peaches and cranberries, so it's a good idea to get into the habit every meal-time of having a glass of freshly squeezed fruit or tomato juice or a piece of fresh fruit after the meal.

You can also help increase the amount of iron and other nutrients that are available to your body by limiting the amount of tannin and caffeine you consume. These substances inhibit the absorption of a number of nutrients. I would certainly suggest that you don't round a meal off with a cup of coffee and that you try to keep your intake of tea and coffee down to a couple of cups a day.

For most women, the main source of calcium in the diet is milk, cheese and other dairy products. Dairy foods also provide vitamins B12 and B2. If you feel you need to make up a shortfall in B vitamins, yeast extract (Marmite) is usually fortified with all the important B vitamins, so use it in savoury dishes or just spread it on bread and add some sliced tomato or grated cheese for a nutritious snack.

• HOW TO PLAN A HEALTHY VEGETARIAN DAILY DIET

As with non-vegetarians, you should have one portion of protein-rich food at your main meal and half a portion in your smaller meal every day. A portion could be 1 egg, about 150 g (5 oz) cooked weight of pulses, 90 g (about 3 oz) of nuts or 225 g (8 oz) of tofu.

A good intake of milk and other dairy products provides calcium, protein, vitamins B12 and B2 among other nutrients. In a typical day you should try to include 600 ml (1 pint) of milk or its equivalent. As a guideline, a small glass of milk of about 125 ml (4 fl oz) would be the equivalent of 25 g (1 oz) of a hard cheese such as Cheddar, Stilton or double Gloucester, or 250 ml (8 fl oz) of yoghurt.

For two people, you could make a stilton and spinach soufflé, using two eggs, 300 ml (½ pint) of milk, a large bunch of fresh spinach and 50 g (2 oz) of cheese (and a pinch of mustard and nutmeg to enhance the cheese and spinach flavours). Serve this with a warmed wholegrain walnut roll and you have a perfect meal.

WHAT TO DO IF YOU'RE VEGAN

There are many excellent books on how to be a healthy vegan, and you might also like to seek the advice of a dietitian. Although a vegan diet can be a healthy diet, if not carefully executed it may lead to malnutrition. I see quite a few young women who have decided, usually for moral reasons, to become vegan. They start to eat vegetables and fruits with a few cereal foods, but they fail to balance their diet and end up with problems such as extreme fatigue or iron-deficiency anaemia. It is important to understand where a vegan diet needs particular attention.

• PROTEIN
The advice is the same as for other vegetarians.

• CALCIUM

As a vegan eating no dairy produce, you may not be taking in sufficient calcium. Some soya milks and cheeses have added calcium, so look out for these. Sesame seeds and tahini (sesame seed paste, used to make hummus) are a good source of calcium, as are almonds and green leafy vegetables such as spinach. However, the calcium in green vegetables is not as easily absorbed by the body as the calcium in milk products, so you may require a calcium supplement. See page 26 for further information.

• VITAMINS B12 AND B2

Since these are found primarily in animal foods, vegans may have a problem getting enough of these vitamins. Some soya milks are fortified with vitamins B12 and B2; this is one of the few instances where I support the action of food manufacturers.

Yeast extract, dried fruits such as apricots and figs, pulses, green leafy vegetables and nuts also contain B vitamins, but again this is one of the rare situations when I think you might need a vitamin B complex supplement. The reason for taking a general B complex supplement is that the B vitamins help each other to be absorbed. See your dietitian or doctor before you proceed.

WEIGHT

How much should you weigh? This is a complex subject and before reaching any decision it is important to consider firstly how happy you are with your body and secondly the ratio of fat to muscle.

Many women won't pay any attention to ideal weight charts if they are not happy with their bodies. Changes in weight can help you to feel more positive about yourself, but you need to work at the underlying reasons why you ended up being over- or underweight.

If you know that it was caused by overeating or eating the wrong types of food, then this can be relatively easily corrected once you understand which foods are best and ways to change your eating habits to include them. If, however, you know that unhappiness and emotional issues caused you to lose or gain weight, these need to be addressed if you are to be able to enjoy the body you aim to achieve.

The feeling that you need to just lose a few more pounds before you can feel really happy is a very common thought in many women's minds. Fortunately the majority of women don't have the deep-rooted insecurities that lead to the serious eating disorders anorexia and bulimia.

Weight charts fail to take into consideration that the weight on the scale does not tell you whether you are carrying too much or too little body fat. Healthwise there are more risks for people who carry too much fat; for example there is an increased risk of heart disease. There are fewer worries associated with having too little body fat, other than if your body fat level becomes so low that it interferes with your hormone metabolism and general health. Most women are not particularly worried about having too much muscle; far more are upset by carrying excess fat. Measuring the level of fat in your body is a specialized skill, which requires your dietitian or fitness instructor, doctor or physiotherapist to take skin fold measurements. I suggest you seek their advice as they will be able to tell you whether or not your fat levels are appropriate. However, if you take your skin in your hand and can pull a lot of fat away from your body, it is highly likely that you need to lose some fat.

• IDEAL WEIGHT CHARTS

Tables are useful as a rough guide to what you should weigh in relation to your height, but remember that you are an individual and no table can really tell you something you don't already know. Tables of ideal weights are drawn up by insurance companies concerned with whether you are putting your health at risk by being outside of the ideal range. Not everyone will fit precisely into their ranges.

The ideal weight is calculated most effectively by working out your body mass index. To do this you need to convert your weight into kilograms and your height into metres. Body mass index = weight (kg) divided by height (m) squared. Don't bother getting out your calculator: the table on the following page does this for you.

The ideal body mass index is between 20 and 25. Below 20 is the under-weight category, 25–30 is the slightly overweight category and a body mass index of more than 30 is in the significantly overweight range. A lot of the young women I see like to have a body mass index below 20. While 19 or 18 is not necessarily too low, if your body mass index is this low or lower you run the risk of suffering from conditions such hormonal imbalance, lack of periods, osteoporosis and malnutrition.

Whether you decide you want to stay the weight you are and use this book to build a better relationship with food or want to lose weight, you need to bear in mind your weight history. Don't expect your body to become something it's never been. A woman who has always been light for her height, with a body mass index of 18, with parents of similar stature, will not easily reach a body mass index of 23. Equally, a woman who has always struggled with her weight being over the ideal range shouldn't really expect herself to get down to a body mass index of 18 or 20, unless she has been eating very inappropriately for a long time. Remember also that the shape of your body generally stays the same whether you gain or lose weight. Women are generally either an 'apple' or a 'pear' shape. The only difference lies in the size of the apple or how toned the pear is.

If you decide that you need to lose weight, I suggest you read the chapter on weight loss. If you simply want to eat healthily then I suggest you follow the guidelines beginning on page 35.

IDEAL BODY WEIGHT

Obesity Grade	Body Mass Index	Weight (kg) to the nearest 1kg									
	45	101	104	107	110	112	115	118	121	124	127
	44	99	102	104	107	110	113	115	118	121	124
3	43	97	99	102	105	107	110	113	116	118	121
	42	95	97	100	102	105	108	110	113	116	119
	41	92	95	97	100	102	105	108	110	113	116
	40	90	92	95	97	100	102	105	108	110	113
	39	88	90	93	95	97	100	102	105	108	110
	38	86	88	90	93	95	97	100	102	105	107
	37	83	86	88	90	92	95	97	100	102	104
2	36	81	83	85	88	90	92	95	97	99	102
	35	79	81	83	85	87	90	92	94	96	99
	34	77	79	81	83	85	87	89	91	94	96
	33	74	76	78	80	82	85	87	89	91	93
	32	72	74	76	78	80	82	84	86	88	90
	31	70	72	74	75	77	79	81	83	85	88
	30	68	69	71	73	75	77	79	81	83	85
	29	65	67	69	71	72	74	76	78	80	82
1	28	63	65	66	68	70	72	74	75	77	79
	27	61	62	64	66	67	69	71	73	74	76
	26	59	60	62	63	65	67	68	70	72	73
	25	56	58	59	61	62	64	66	67	69	71
	24	54	55	57	58	60	61	63	65	66	68
0	23	52	53	55	56	57	59	60	62	63	65
	22	50	51	52	54	55	56	58	59	61	61
	21	47	49	50	51	52	54	55	57	58	59
	20	45	46	47	49	50	51	53	54	55	56
Under weight	19	43	44	45	46	47	49	50	51	52	54
	18	41	42	43	44	45	46	47	48	50	51
	17	38	39	40	41	42	44	45	46	47	48
Height	m	1.50	1.52	1.54	1.56	1.58	1.60	1.62	1.64	1.66	1.68
Height	ft in	4.11	5.0	5.0¾	5.1½	5.2¼	5.3	5.3¾	5.4½	5.5½	5.6

Body Mass Index (BMI) = $\dfrac{\text{Weight in Kilograms}}{(\text{Height in Metres})^2}$

This is an ideal body weight chart which gives you a rough idea of the weight you should be. Remember the most important thing is how you feel in yourself.

Weight ((kg) to
the nearest 1kg)

130	133	136	139	143	146	149	152	156	159	162	166	169	173
127	130	133	136	139	143	146	149	152	156	159	162	166	169
124	127	130	133	133	139	142	146	149	149	155	159	162	165
121	124	127	130	130	136	139	142	145	145	152	155	158	161
119	121	124	127	127	133	136	139	142	142	148	151	154	158
116	118	121	124	127	130	133	135	138	141	144	148	151	154
113	115	118	121	124	126	129	132	135	138	41	144	147	150
110	112	115	118	120	123	126	129	132	134	137	140	143	146
107	110	112	115	117	120	123	125	128	131	134	136	139	142
104	107	109	112	114	117	119	122	125	127	130	133	136	138
101	104	106	108	111	113	116	119	121	124	126	129	132	134
98	101	103	105	108	110	113	115	118	120	123	125	128	131
95	98	100	102	105	107	109	112	114	117	119	122	124	127
93	95	97	99	101	104	106	108	111	113	116	118	120	123
90	92	94	96	98	100	103	105	107	110	112	114	117	119
87	89	91	93	95	97	99	102	104	106	108	111	113	115
84	86	88	90	92	94	96	98	100	103	105	107	109	111
81	83	85	87	89	91	93	95	97	99	101	103	105	108
78	80	82	84	86	88	89	91	93	95	98	100	102	104
75	77	79	81	82	84	86	88	90	92	94	96	98	100
72	74	76	77	79	81	83	85	87	88	90	92	94	96
69	71	73	74	76	78	80	81	83	83	87	89	90	92
67	68	70	71	73	75	76	78	80	80	83	85	87	88
64	65	67	68	70	71	73	75	76	76	79	81	83	85
61	62	64	65	67	68	70	71	73	73	76	77	79	81
58	59	61	62	63	65	66	68	69	69	72	74	75	77
55	56	58	59	60	62	63	64	66	67	69	70	72	73
52	53	55	56	57	58	60	61	62	64	65	66	68	69
49	50	52	53	54	55	56	58	59	60	61	63	64	65
1.70	1.72	1.74	1.76	1.78	1.80	1.82	1.84	1.86	1.88	1.90	1.92	1.94	1.96
5.6¾	5.7¾	5.8½	5.9¼	5.10	5.10¾	5.11¾	6.0½	6.1¼	6.2	6.2¾	6.3¾	6.4½	6.5¼

FRAME

Light frame	Heavy frame	
<15	-	Seriously under nourished
15	19	Underweight
20	25	Acceptable/Desirable
26	30	Slightly overweight
31	40	Seriously overweight
-	40+	Dangerously overweight

Woman the shopper

Food shopping doesn't have to be a nightmare. Many women think that the only way to shop healthily is to stand for hours reading the sides of every packet, analysing the nutritional information. Of course labels can be helpful on occasions, for example if you need to avoid a particular ingredient such as lactose, but the normal woman shouldn't need to go to this extreme. Besides which, food manufacturers tend to tell you only the information they want you to see. Every figure is relative and with only a little knowledge the information can mislead and confuse you.

Instead you should stick to the basic list of foods you need to have in your diet and enjoy shopping for simple fresh ingredients. Don't get hassled by labels and rest assured that simple food is the secret to success.

• STOCKING UP

In trying to become and remain healthy, it is important to be prepared. Stock up your cupboards, refrigerator and freezer, so that you have a store of things you can throw together to make good food fast. Don't feel guilty about sometimes using frozen vegetables or tinned foods; they can play a supporting role in your healthy lifestyle. This book is full of ideas for quick things you can cook. All it takes is a little knowledge and an organized pantry. Think about how good you feel after you've eaten something freshly prepared, in comparison to a ready-cooked meal.

• SHOP AROUND

If you have the time, try to support individual shops: greengrocers, fishmongers, butchers, bakers and cheese shops. They can help you to choose different varieties and can offer more local produce. I support the role of the individual shop in society; it is such a pity that the multi-nationals are putting so many of them out of business. The personal touch of the butcher who tells you which cuts of meat are particularly good, or gives you ideas as to how you can cook it, is a special part of shopping, especially if you need a little advice or inspiration, or want to know the origin of the food. Small shops are not necessarily more expensive than supermarkets, whose 'special offers' often apply only to large packs or three for the price of two deals. Another point to bear in mind is the inflated prices we pay for the so-called 'healthy options' in the supermarkets.

You can often find a range of unusual foods and spices in shops run by people of different ethnic origins. This is especially relevant when you cook dishes that are not native to Britain. When making hummus, for example, try to use the tahini from a Lebanese shop; it's much richer than the version sold in British supermarkets and makes a finer dish.

• SHOP MORE OFTEN AND BUY LESS

Try to do this if you can, as it will give you the opportunity to pick up on special offers and promotions of foods in season. Think about the amount of food you buy in supermarkets and then never get around to eating because your plans change or you forget you even bought it, it was so long ago!

• CHALLENGE THE WAY YOU THINK ABOUT FOOD

Does cheese have to be Cheddar? Why not Double Gloucester, Wensleydale or white Stilton? French Gruyère and Italian Parmesan are excellent for cooking, and there are a host of other varieties, with different textures, from cows', ewes' and goats' milk, for cooking or for nibbling.

Seek out local or organic produce. For instance, several English producers now make very good wines, as well as fantastic fruit and flower wines such as gooseberry, blackberry and elderflower. A number of small producers of specialist foods – dairies, bakeries, smokehouses – sell by mail order. This can be an excellent way of stocking up on good ingredients.

'A perfectly ripe
peach is worth
waiting for all
summer long.'
Julee Rosso and
Sheila Lukins

Think about the type of food you really love and see whether you could make it a little bit more exciting and healthier, simply by taking a fresh look.

• TRY EATING SEASONALLY

If you eat fruits and vegetables when they are in season, you will find that they have been picked at their best and not grown in glasshouses; they will have more flavour and generally have more vitamins, minerals and other nutrients than at other times of year. It is much better to look forward to tasting the first new potatoes or crisp orange pippins, rather than to eat the same boring food all year round.

Seasonal shopping can also help to keep the cost down, as prices are frequently lower when there is a deluge of produce on the market.

• START LOOKING AT RECIPE BOOKS INSTEAD OF LEAVING THEM ON THE SHELVES

You'll find ideas that will make you think about trying different ingredients. Enjoy experimenting in the kitchen and look forward to trying new flavours in your meals; this is the way to develop a healthy relationship with food.

• TRY NOT TO SHOP WHEN YOU'RE HUNGRY

This makes you dash around and make inappropriate choices. If you're tired, it may seem all too easy to grab for a shop-prepared dish, even though there are so many quick things you could cook.

• SPECIAL DIETS

If you have a special nutritional need such as diabetes, or a food intolerance, you mustn't see it as a constraint. It's not if you broaden your horizons. Food manufacturers would like you to think that you need to buy special-diet foods, but they would, wouldn't they? I frequently see diabetics who think that they need to eat diabetic jam or diabetic chocolate. They miss real foods, which is sad as it does not need to be the case. Instead of eating these specially packaged products, start thinking about all the foods that naturally don't contain a lot of sugar. For example, couverture chocolate (look in the baking section of supermarkets) isn't high in sugar and is delicious.

Women who are unable to eat gluten, instead of focusing on what they can't have, should enjoy making risotto, paella and potato bakes. Make sauces using potato flour, rather than wheat flour, or use buckwheat flour to make pancakes that you can fill with fruit or savoury fillings.

Whatever your nutritional requirement, there's always delicious normal food to be found.

BUYING AND STORING FOOD

When buying food, make sure that tins, packets and cartons are not damaged or dented, and the products have not passed their use-by date. For storing purposes, food is usually divided into three categories: the refrigerator, the larder and the food cupboard. The larder should be a cool, airy place with a temperature of about 12°C/54°F, but not many of today's homes have a cool, well-ventilated larder, so foods that should really be stored in this environment ought to be kept in the lower or salad compartments of the refrigerator. The food cupboard should be dry and cool, away from any source of heat. The coldest parts of the refrigerator are the top and middle; the door is the warmest place. Store very perishable foods in the coldest part.

• Once packets have been opened, consume the contents as soon as possible.
• If you open a tin and use only part of it, transfer the rest to a non-metallic container, cover and use within a couple of days.
• Cover all strong-smelling food in the refrigerator and do not store next to absorbent or delicate foods, such as eggs or milk.

• Meat bought wrapped in clingfilm should be re-wrapped loosely in plastic bags or greaseproof paper, or stored, covered, in a plastic box or dish.
• Store cooked meats separate from and above uncooked meats.

• FRUIT AND VEGETABLES

Buy only enough fruit for a few days, as it does not keep long at modern room temperature. It will store for a little longer in a cool, airy place: the larder or the salad box of the refrigerator.

Ideally, buy vegetables fresh as you need them for the greatest nutritional value. Salad ingredients should be stored in the box at the bottom of the refrigerator and eaten within a day or two. Other vegetables will keep for up to a week if stored in the lower section of the refrigerator or the larder.

• EGGS

Very fresh free-range eggs have the most flavour. To test the freshness of an egg, place it in a bowl of water: if it is fresh it will remain horizontal on the bottom of the bowl; slightly stale and it will tilt a little and should not be used for poaching or boiling. If it floats, it is stale – throw it out. Eggs will keep fresher for longer in the refrigerator. For cooking, eggs are best at room temperature.

• FISH

Ideally, buy fresh and eat on the day of purchase, as fish is highly perishable. However, you can keep fish overnight if you wash and dry it and store, covered, in the top part of the refrigerator.

• POULTRY

Free-range birds are well worth buying because they have much more flavour. The flavour increases with the age of the bird, but older birds may have slightly drier flesh. Poussins are the smallest, youngest and most tender chickens; the largest, oldest birds with the driest flesh are not really suitable for roasting and should be sold as boiling fowl. Chicken should be stored for no more than a couple of days. Remove from any plastic wrapping, drain off any liquid and wipe the bird. Store on a plate, covered to prevent it drying out.

• MEAT

Beef should be a plum red colour, if bright red it has not been hung properly and will not be very tasty or tender. If it is dark or sinewy, it is not a cut meant for roasting, grilling, stir-frying or other quick cooking. These cheaper cuts of beef are as nutritious as the more expensive ones, and are the best for casseroles as they tenderize with slow cooking. Beef can be kept for four days in the refrigerator. Remove any plastic wrapping, wipe and rewrap in greaseproof paper. Store, covered, on a plate.

Young lamb should be pale pink; it becomes darker with age, and the breed of sheep also affects the colour. The fat should be creamy-white. Store as for beef, although lamb does not keep quite as long.

Pork should be pale pink, with firm, white fat. Pork should be kept for no more than three days.

Bacon, gammon and ham may be smoked to enhance the flavour and keeping qualities. Store as for beef.

Kidneys, liver, heart, brain, sweetbreads and other inner organs do not keep well. Store, covered, in the refrigerator and use within a day or two.

• CHEESE

Ideally, cheese should be kept in a covered container in a cool larder. Cheese kept in the refrigerator is fine for cooking purposes, but bear in mind that cold cheese is relatively tasteless, so if you want to enjoy the flavour of the cheese you should take it out of the refrigerator about an hour before you intend to eat it.

STORING WINE

A small stock of bottles will save you having to nip down to the off-licence every day. Some wine is best drunk within a few months, other bottles need to be kept for years for their flavours to develop. This is a vast topic, which is discussed in many books about wine.

You may not have an actual cellar, but wine keeps better the more closely it approximates to cellar conditions. It should be kept at a fairly constant temperature (preferably cool, around 7–10°C/45–50°F), out of direct light and avoiding vibration. Lofts are not a good idea, because they vary enormously in temperature. The longer wine needs to be stored, the more critical the conditions become. For short periods of a week or so, don't worry unduly.

HOME FREEZING

A freezer enables you to plan well ahead, both in terms of buying in bulk and cooking. Frozen food can provide you with food that is both delicious to eat and high in vitamins and minerals. It is only when food is frozen, thawed or cooked inappropriately that it becomes significantly inferior to fresh food.

There are extremely strict regulations surrounding the production of frozen food, from the point of picking of fresh vegetables and fruits, to the production of prepared dishes. In contrast there is no legal definition of 'fresh', so food may be left sitting on the docks or in shops for days and still be called fresh. I am not advocating that we throw fresh food aside and start existing on frozen food, but I do think frozen food can be very useful in helping you to eat healthily within the constraints of a busy work and home life.

- GENERAL HINTS
- All food should be well wrapped or sealed in an airtight container to prevent ice damage ('freezer burn').
- Vegetables and fruit can be cooked from frozen. Fish,

shellfish, poultry and meat must be thawed slowly (in the refrigerator) and very thoroughly before cooking, to avoid food poisoning.

• Vegetables – freeze only young, unblemished vegetables. Blanch in boiling water, refresh in ice-cold water and drain thoroughly before packing in containers or freezer bags.

• Fruit – small berries and currants freeze most successfully: for example raspberries, gooseberries, blackberries, blackcurrants. Inspect them carefully for damaged or mouldy fruit but wash only if absolutely necessary. Apples, plums and pears freeze well; they should first be washed and dried thoroughly. Strawberries, citrus fruits, melons, mangoes and bananas don't freeze very well; they become mushy when you defrost them. The only use I have for defrosted strawberries is in pies, crumbles, jams or sauces.

• Fish – freeze as soon as possible from fresh. Remove the head and tail of large fish, and gut and descale small round fish. Interleave flat fish fillets with waxed paper. Thaw slowly and cook as soon as thawed.

• Poultry and game – freeze only young birds. Freeze giblets, liver and stuffings separately, as these keep for no longer than 1 month.

• Meat – trim excess fat. Interleave chops and cutlets with waxed paper.

• Bread – generally freezes well, either baked or part-baked. Part-baked breads can be taken straight from the freezer and baked in a hot oven. If you make your own bread you can freeze it after you have let it prove for a second time.

• GUIDE TO FREEZING PRECOOKED FOODS

One of the greatest advantages of having a freezer is that you can freeze pre-cooked dishes for later use. This can be a life-saver when you need something substantial at the end of a long day. It also means that you can have a big cooking session, eat one or two portions and then freeze the rest. You can also use your freezer to store good base ingredients: chicken portions, fish steaks or frozen vegetables.

• If you buy food that is already frozen, do not let it defrost before you freeze it. Keep it cold and out of the freezer for as short a time as possible.

• If you are going to freeze a meal that you have cooked, make sure that you begin with top-quality ingredients and that all your kitchen surfaces and equipment are clean, as freezing does not kill many food poisoning organisms.

• Season lightly; more seasoning can always be added when reheating.

• I suggest that you slightly undercook dishes, leaving about 10–15 minutes of cooking time, before you freeze them. The extra time will be made up when you reheat them, as frozen food should always be cooked so it is hot right through.

• All cooked dishes must be completely cool before packing and freezing.

• When recipes for sauces, soups, etc. use cream or egg yolks, you should not add these before freezing, as they don't freeze well. When the dish is defrosted and reheated you can add the cream or egg yolks to finish the dish.

• Dishes with a high proportion of custard, single cream or mayonnaise do not freeze successfully.

Good herb guide

Herbs, sometimes along with a little olive oil or butter to coax out the flavours, can enhance a huge variety of dishes. Grow fresh herbs in pots in the kitchen or window box, or in a corner of the garden. You can often buy packets of freshly cut herbs, but I would encourage you to grow your own. As a reserve, I suggest you stock up with a few dried herbs. Some dry more successfully than others, and I have indicated these below. You should ideally store only small amounts in dark, airtight containers. Sunlight, heat and moisture can cause flavours to fade more quickly, and even dried herbs can become mouldy. Herb racks with a dozen clear glass pots are not ideal. When you stock up, it is best to stick to a few at a time and then move on to others.

- **BASIL**

The perfect partner for tomatoes, whether in salads or sauces. Enhances the flavour of aubergines and courgettes. Delicious with garlic in Italian pesto sauce and a classic with many pasta dishes. Try it with oily fish such as mackerel; roast lamb; chicken, duck and goose. Best fresh.

- **BAY**

Tie with sprigs of parsley and thyme to make a bouquet garni, which is used to flavour soups, sauces and casseroles. Bay leaves impart flavour to pâtés and terrines; baked vegetable dishes; oily fish; goose, pork and veal. Best dried.

- **CHERVIL**

Use with delicate fish such as Dover sole and shellfish, or add to salads. Chop roughly with parsley to make a herb butter to pop on a jacket potato. A pretty herb for garnishing soups. Use fresh.

Small pots of growing herbs can be bought from the supermarket or garden centre. Try not to denude a small fragile plant of too many of its leaves before it has had a chance to bush out, otherwise it will die.

• **CHIVES**

With a mild oniony flavour, chives are classically used with potato salad, egg dishes and delicate cream or butter sauces. Use the slender leaves or pink flowers to garnish soups and salads.

• **DILL**

I use it to flavour salads, sauces, dressings and mayonnaise. It is a simple yet delicious way of accentuating the delicate flavour of poached or baked fish. The only strong-tasting fish I think it complements is smoked salmon. Use to garnish fish soups and pâtés. Best fresh.

• **FENNEL**

Three variations are available: the feathery herb, the seeds and the vegetable bulb. The feathery leaves are a lovely addition among salad leaves or with oily fish or roast lamb. The seeds are excellent with fish, chicken or roast pork.

• **GARLIC**

It has many health-giving properties, such as reducing the risk of cancer and heart disease (see page 33). I think it goes particularly well with tomato, fish, lamb and chicken dishes. Vary the taste by cooking it (for a softer flavour) or using it raw. My good friend Naji makes a pasta sauce with 20 cloves of garlic; on serving he adds raw chopped garlic for added heat! This is not ideal when you have a sensitive stomach, or you are going out! Make garlic butter for bread, baked potatoes or steaks, or use it in salad dressings.

• **MARJORAM**

Similar to but slightly milder than the oregano of the Mediterranean. Use with strongly flavoured meats such as lamb or beef, oily fish, game, chicken, tomatoes, courgettes, spinach, eggs and cheese. Good fresh or dried.

• MINT
Fresh mint sauce is traditional with roast lamb and mutton. It also enhances vegetables such as peas, broad and French beans, tomatoes and potatoes. Use whole leaves to decorate desserts, add to fruit punches and fresh fruit salads. Many varieties are available; most are best fresh.

• PARSLEY
Traditionally used with fish, in sauces and stuffings, as a garnish, and as an essential part of a bouquet garni (with bay and thyme). Boiled potatoes tossed in a little butter and finely chopped parsley are a lovely combination. Two varieties are available: the flat-leafed or Italian variety, and the curly-leafed, which does not have quite as strong a flavour. High in vitamins and minerals, so use generously. Use fresh.

• ROSEMARY
This strong herb marries well with lamb, beef and poultry. Vegetarians use it with pulse and root vegetable dishes. Fresh or dried.

• SAGE
Used with onions in stuffings for pork, duck, goose and chicken. I think it also goes well with oily fish such as herrings and mackerel. Fresh or dried.

• TARRAGON
I use this a lot: with tomatoes, beans, chicken, fish and vegetables. Quiches and other egg dishes can be greatly enhanced with tarragon. Best fresh.

• THYME
A very versatile herb. Use with pork, beef, game, chicken and oily fish, chicken and beef. Potatoes also go very well with thyme, sautéed or in a gratin. Fresh or dried.

Hot drinks

Coffee is made from the beans of a small tree which was originally found in Ethiopia. A delightful story tells of a goatherd in the remote highlands of Ethiopia, whose goats one day failed to return. After hours of searching he spied them frolicking about, and he realised that they had eaten the little red berries of a nearby shrub. He tasted some of the berries and understood what had got into his goats. History does not record how he used this knowledge, and whether he became a rich coffee trader!

Coffee and tea can be delicious drinks, but as part of a healthy lifestyle you should try to keep your intake down to two or three cups a day of either tea or coffee. This is because they contain substances that inhibit the body from absorbing the vitamins and minerals from your food. In coffee and tea, the culprits are tannins and caffeine, which is also found in cola-based and other soft drinks. In addition, caffeine acts as a mild diuretic, which means that it makes your body excrete excessive amounts of water, so you lose vitamins and minerals in your urine. Too many caffeine-containing drinks can lead to health problems such as anaemia, indigestion and lack of energy.

Rather than trying to cut them out completely, I suggest you enjoy a really good cup of well-made tea or coffee as a treat at an appropriate time; just cut out all the needless, disgusting coffee and tea drinks consumed out of habit during the day.

• COFFEE

No one knows quite who discovered that, when roasted, the raw beans of the coffee tree become appetizingly aromatic and can be ground and infused in boiling water, but coffee trees were being cultivated in Arabian countries by the sixth century AD.

The flavour of coffee is determined by where the beans are grown, the variety or combination of varieties (blend) and by the length of time the beans are roasted. As the flavour deteriorates rapidly after it is ground, many coffee-lovers prefer to grind the beans at home, just before they need them.

To make decaffeinated coffee, the green beans are processed in a bath of methylene chloride, which removes the caffeine, then steamed to remove the chloride. A newer method using steam only is felt to be more environmentally friendly.

TYPES OF TEA
ASSAM: from India;
strong, malty
and pungent.
CEYLON: medium
strength, nutty-
flavoured yet
delicate.
DARJEELING: from
India; light, with a
muscatel flavour.
EARL GREY: a blend
of Chinese teas
flavoured with oil of
bergamot (a fragrant,
sour citrus fruit).
ENGLISH BREAKFAST
TEA: a rich blend of
tea from Sri Lanka
and India.
GUNPOWDER:
Chinese green tea,
so called because
the leaves are
curled and look like
gunpowder, is a
bitter, fruity tea.
JASMINE: Chinese
tea scented with
jasmine flowers.
KEEMUN: a mellow
China tea.
LAPSANG SOUCHONG:
China tea with a
distinctive smoky
flavour.

• QUALITY COFFEE

It's surprising how much unnecessary caffeine women take in during the day, especially in an office-based job. I believe that employers hope to keep their staff on the hop by having a constant supply of coffee available! Very often it is a case of habit drinking, which if replaced by one cup of quality coffee from time to time will delight your taste buds!

To turn coffee into a treat it is worth thinking about the type of beans you buy and making it properly, whether you use a cafetière, filter machine or espresso maker.

Experiment with the many exotically named beans you will find at your local coffee shop or delicatessen, and with how strong you like your coffee. Remember that a darker roast gives a fuller flavour, but not necessarily a stronger coffee. A lighter roast is usually preferred for a breakfast coffee and a darker, richer roast for drinking after dinner in the evening.

• TEA

Tea is made from the dried leaves of an evergreen plant called *Camellia sinensis*. The leaves contain oils, which give tea its flavour, and tannin, which provides colour and pungency. Most tea drunk in Britain is black, having been fermented during the manufacturing process. The Chinese and Japanese tend to prefer their tea 'green', or unfermented. Oolong teas are partly fermented before they are dried.

The teas we buy are often blends of leaves from different regions of India, Sri Lanka and China, Chinese teas being generally gentler in flavour. Fragrant oils and flowers may be added for flavour.

• MAKING TEA

My grandfather, or Dadda as he was known, was 'the finest tea maker in Stoke on Trent'. He was never a cook but he always made the tea, in an enormous pot, which would refresh parts other teas couldn't reach! I dedicate this section of the book to him.

• The tea pot should be china or glazed earthenware. Throw the metal ones out – they don't retain the heat sufficiently.

• Fill the kettle with fresh water and bring to the boil. It is important to use fresh water and not that which has been left in the kettle. Having boiled once, it will have lost its oxygen, and the tea will not brew properly.

• Warm the pot (by filling it with hot water).

• Tip the water out and add the tea leaves (1 rounded teaspoon per person).

• As soon as the water boils, pour on to the leaves and put the lid on the pot.

• Leave the tea to infuse for 3 minutes.

• Does one put the milk or the tea into the cup first? It's up to you, but putting the milk in first protects bone china cups, which as far as I'm concerned are best for drinking tea. Of course you can have tea without milk, particularly green and jasmine teas, or with lemon.

• CAFFEINE-FREE ALTERNATIVES

I can't really recommend decaffeinated coffee and tea, because the processing often involves chemicals, whose effect on the body is unknown. However, exciting herb and fruit teas are now widely available and, after all, tea is just another herb, coffee another fruit. Alternatively, make your own teas, using fresh or dried herbs (look in health food shops for the more unusual items).

• HERB TEAS

Use a tea infuser or place the leaves in a pot or jug, pour on boiling water and leave for 10–15 minutes.

Camomile tea is traditionally relaxing, rosehips give a pretty pink drink, rosemary aids digestion of fatty foods.

• ARABIC MINT TEA

This is made by placing a bunch of fresh mint leaves in a small pot with boiling water. Leave for 5–8 minutes. Pour into a mug or glass and serve with a sprig of fresh mint. Serve hot or iced, with a little sugar or honey if liked.

• ORANGE BLOSSOM TEA

This is a perfect after-dinner drink; it cleans the palate and facilitates digestion. Pour boiling water into a mug. Add 1 teaspoon of orange blossom water and a pinch of finely ground cardamom. Sweeten with sugar or honey.

Alcohol

Alcohol, if treated with respect, can play a part in a healthy lifestyle. Alcohol has been associated with health for many centuries; medicine and drink were inextricable from the time of Hippocrates (about 400 BC) right through to the 19th century. Essences of plants, herbs and flowers were extracted, often by steeping in alcohol, sometimes by distillation, and the result was prescribed in the equivalent of a homeopathic dose.

Moderate drinking makes us feel happy, reduces stress at the end of the day, and in the case of red wine provides our body with antioxidants. In many countries wine or beer is an indispensable companion to food. However, alcohol in excess can cause liver damage and psychological problems.

• WHAT IS MODERATE DRINKING?

For practical purposes the 'unit' (8–10 grams of alcohol) has become a handy reckoning device. It is found in half a pint of beer, a small glass of wine, or a single measure of spirits. As a rough guide, the general recommendation is approximately 21 units a week for women.

Beyond this, you need to take into account such things as body size (the heavier you are, the more alcohol your body can cope with), and to note that once men reach around 50 units a week, and women 35, alarm bells should start ringing. We need to be in control, not dependent on alcohol.

I recommend that you give yourself one or two alcohol-free days a week, to cleanse the system and to remind yourself that choosing to drink is an option that you exercise.

• KEEP TRACK OF YOUR INTAKE
As far as is reasonably possible, note what you are drinking so that you can recognize roughly when you have had the appropriate two or three units. At a party it is easy to keep topping up the glass without realizing, unless you develop a 'sixth sense' about when you have reached a reasonable amount.

• AVOID NEAT SPIRITS AND OTHER HIGH-ALCOHOL DRINKS
Rather than cut them out completely, take them in dilute form, for instance, made into a long drink with ice and tonic, or take them in the tiniest quantities. Not all alcohol is equal, and the trouble with high-strength drinks is that they don't take very long to consume and their effect on the body is quite swift. That is why many people find the proportion of alcohol to the total volume of liquid just right in wine.

• EVEN WITH WINE, IT IS BEST TO DRINK SLOWLY
If you are really thirsty, have a glass of water first. Use wine for sipping and savouring, don't just glug it back and hope to feel refreshed.

If you think you are beginning to drink more than usual and find that you need five or six glasses to make you as happy as everyone else's one or two, do be careful. It is much easier to deal with any problems of over-indulgence if they are caught sooner rather than later. Wine is to be enjoyed. Don't spoil years of future enjoyment with excess now.

Smoking

Smoking has profound effects on your body's ability to derive all the goodness from a well-balanced diet. Cigarette smoke adversely affects the nutritional status not only of women who smoke, but also those who passively inhale. As part of your positive health plan it really is important to try to give up. Smoking cigarettes increases your requirement for most vitamins and minerals, particularly vitamin C. If you smoke, you lose more vitamin C from your tissues and blood. Your body therefore needs more vitamin C, to counteract the damage inflicted on your cells.

Unfortunately, cigarette smokers often eat fewer vitamin C rich foods, as they tend to smoke rather than have a piece of fresh fruit in between or after meals. Since vitamin C is one of the major antioxidants, which have been linked to the prevention of cancer, cigarette smokers are at a much greater risk of developing cancer as a result of poor antioxidant intake and damage to the cells inflicted by the smoke. The main organs to be affected are the lungs, breasts and cervix.

In order to counteract the disturbance in vitamin C metabolism, a smoker's requirement for vitamin C increases to approximately 2,000 milligrams a day. (See page 22 for foods rich in vitamin C.) If you cannot give up, it is even more important for you to make sure your diet is exceedingly well balanced, containing all the nutrients outlined in the section on What your body needs and 2000 mg of vitamin C. It is difficult to take in 2000 mg from food alone, but I suggest you eat as many vitamin C rich foods as you can and also take a daily supplement of 2000 mg, to try to prevent your body suffering more than it has to.

• WEIGHT GAIN

If you manage to give up smoking, you should be aware that your metabolic rate decreases very slightly. This may cause your weight to increase by a few pounds only, not stones, as many women believe. The main reason for gaining weight when you give up smoking is that you put food in your mouth on occasions when you would normally smoke a cigarette. Food provides oral satisfaction.

If you are worried about gaining weight, I suggest you read the chapter on weight loss and also the section on the appetite mechanism. Remember that if you can resist unnecessary eating, your weight will not increase more than about a kilogram (two to three pounds).

• GIVING UP

As soon as you give up, concentrate on eating healthily and getting your body feeling fit; you should find this helps distract you from smoking. If you need help in giving up, I suggest you discuss it with your doctor, who may advise nicotine patches or chewing gum, or may be able to offer other ideas.

Although you can't see the damage you're doing to your heart and lungs, don't forget that smoking can cause eye problems, stained teeth and premature skin ageing (wrinkles!).

1 Weekend cleansing programme

Every now and then, ideally once every four to six weeks, it is a good idea to devote a whole weekend to yourself. Tell partners and friends that you are otherwise engaged, or ask your husband or a friend to look after the children. If you feel you cannot spare a whole weekend, at least try to get a full day. Giving time to yourself should be an empowering experience, but it may feel strange at first.

The aim of this programme is to enable you to take stock of your body. Women who visit me feeling run down and stressed out frequently use this programme to reacquaint themselves with healthy eating and to give their bodies and minds the incentive to continue through the following few weeks. You could use the weekend to lose a little weight, to detoxify your body of needless substances, or simply to re-establish a balance in your life. Don't expect to feel totally different after one weekend; this is just one small positive step.

If you suffer from any medical conditions such as diabetes or cancer or regularly take any medication, you should check with your doctor before you engage on a cleansing programme, as you may need to modify it slightly to accommodate your specific needs.

PLANNING YOUR TIME

• BOOK A BEAUTY TREATMENT

The first stage, a week or two ahead, is to book a massage, facial or pedicure, either at a local salon or, if possible, by a beautician who will visit your house. In some areas there are companies who will come to your home and give you a 'health farm'-style beauty, exercise and food routine. However, if you are not used to it, you will probably find that one pampering treatment is enough. You may like to consider asking a friend to join you, either for your beauty treatments or for the day, but make sure she is someone you can relax with.

• INDULGE YOURSELF

Stock up with new magazines, one or two books and your favourite music, so that you can lie back in the comfort of your own home and completely indulge yourself.

Treat yourself to some new beauty products: for the bath or shower, for your hair, nails or skin. If you are going to try the natural face packs I have suggested (page 76), don't forget to include the ingredients on your shopping list.

• SHOPPING

The day before, go to the shops or markets and buy plenty of fresh vegetables and fruits. Make sure that your refrigerator and cupboards are well stocked, so that you can easily prepare food that is both appetizing and healthy, such as a fruit shake or vegetable soup. As well as the fruits and vegetables I suggest you buy bunches of fresh herbs and plenty of limes and lemons, as these will help to make your salads and cooked vegetable dishes even more delicious. Also make sure you have a good-quality virgin olive oil, mustard, salt and pepper to make dressings for your salads.

• EXERCISE IS OPTIONAL

Some of you may like to combine the cleansing weekend with visits to your local gym. This would be excellent, but is not essential as the aim of this programme is to get you to feel energized by food.

GENERAL GUIDELINES

• EAT REGULARLY
Even though you will be eating different types of
food during this weekend, it is important for you to
eat regularly. This will help to protect your gut from
stomach acids and keep a steady flow of food through
your bowel muscles. Also, if you let yourself get too
hungry, you are likely to give in to a craving for something less healthy.

• PREPARE DELICIOUS FOOD
Devoting time to making something delicious for only
yourself to enjoy should be a major priority. This weekend there is no need to worry about other people's
needs, but many women feel that it is not worth
the effort of preparing something special just for
themselves. This shouldn't be so – you're worth a lot.
Think of cooking or preparing delicious vegetable and
fruit dishes as an empowering activity.

• ENJOY YOUR MEALS
Think about the presentation of the meals and take time
to enjoy them. In the summer you might like to take
your food outside and sit in the garden or a park.
In winter, make sure the house is warm enough for you
to relax without having to have lots of clothes on.

• AVOID HIGH-PROTEIN FOODS AND CARBOHYDRATE
Just for two days, try to keep off protein-rich foods such
as meat, game, chicken, fish, shellfish, eggs, cheese,
dried beans and lentils and nuts (although a few nuts
will not hurt), and carbohydrate foods such as bread,
potatoes, rice and pasta. Of course they have their place
in a balanced diet, but two days of not eating these
foods will not harm you. You will be amazed how
well you feel after two days of eating just fruits
and vegetables – flavoured with honey or sugar, and
delicious oils and vinegars.

• **AVOID CAFFEINE**

Caffeine prevents your body from absorbing many vitamins and minerals from the fruits and vegetables you will be eating. Since the aim of this weekend is to boost your health and energy, it would be better to avoid tea, coffee, hot chocolate and cola-based drinks. I should warn you that if you have been a heavy caffeine drinker you may suffer from a mild headache for a couple of hours when you stop drinking it. I wouldn't recommend that you drink decaffeinated tea or coffee as these frequently contain chemicals, which not only make the drink taste strange, but their effect in the body is not fully known. Instead drink plenty of water, herb teas, fresh fruit or vegetable juices.

• **AVOID ALCOHOL**

Alcohol isn't bad for you, but in a weekend where we are trying to get you to feel full of energy, I suggest you avoid it. This will give your liver a rest as well as enable your body to regain its natural energy balance.

It is fine to use alcohol to poach fruits, or to splash into vegetable soups, as long as it boils for at least a minute or two: the alcohol evaporates off, leaving its lovely flavours in the food.

• **MAKE A HEALTH PLAN**

Take this opportunity to plan how you can keep the next few weeks healthy and less stressed. Making lists of things to do, blocking out time for yourself and organizing the shopping so your cupboards are stocked with good foods, can all help keep you on the straight and narrow.

Remember to examine your body regularly. Get advice on how to examine your breasts and do this at least once a week. Don't just rely on your doctor to pick up problems: you know your body better than anyone, so keep in contact and you will notice if things are changing. Report any changes or worries to your doctor.

FRUIT SHAKE

This energizing drink is a great way to boost your vitality. I recommend it to help many conditions, including anaemia, diabetes and hypoglycaemia, eating disorders and fatigue. In some circumstances you may like to add a little icing sugar or sugar syrup, but the type of fruit you use dictates the level of sweetness: a mango, banana and strawberry shake would be sweeter than an apple and orange shake. If you use dried fruits they provide a lovely concentrated 'tart' flavour.

Take a selection of fresh and soaked dried fruits such as pears, apricots, peaches, pineapple, grapes, bananas, strawberries, oranges, apples, melon, kiwi fruit, mango. Cut them into pieces and blend them together using a hand blender or liquidizer. You probably will need to add a little water. Use ice and milk or yoghurt instead of water to give a creamier taste.

EATING PLAN

• Drink at least two litres (four pints) of water every day. Drink it plain or add a small amount of elderflower, ginger or lime cordial. See page 62 for other caffeine-free drinks.

• Include a small pot of 'live' yoghurt every day. Ideally it should contain bifidus and acidophilus, the bacteria that help boost the immune system and keep the gut healthy (see page 34 for more information). If you cannot get hold of these, other 'live' (unpasteurized) yoghurts contain lactobacillus, another bacterium that has proved beneficial. You can eat the yoghurt on its own, serve it with compotes or fruit salads, add it to fruit shakes or use it in savoury salad dressings.

• Eat as many vegetables and fruits as you fancy.

• **FRUIT**

Think beyond your everyday apple, banana or orange. There are many exciting fruits to choose from, so seize the opportunity to experiment with new varieties. Buy just one or two of each fruit, so you can enjoy a really good selection. Remember, the more visual appeal and variety in texture and taste, the greater the degree of satiety you will experience (see page 6). Use fruit to make fruit shakes (see margin), or in any number of dishes, cool and refreshing or warm and satisfying.

• Fruit salads are traditional in summer, when strawberries, melons and peaches are in abundance; one of my favourites is a simple bowl of fresh strawberries dressed with a few drops of elderflower cordial. But at any time of year you can make a delicious cocktail of succulent imported fruit such as pineapples, oranges, kiwi fruits or lychees. In winter, use dried fruits such as peaches, apricots or prunes, which have been soaked in a little water, elderflower cordial or fresh orange juice, and mix them with sliced apples, tangerines, bananas and grapes.

- Baked fruits are more of a winter treat. Try Bramley apples stuffed with chopped figs and raisins or with sultanas, dried apricots and cinnamon.
- Poached fruits, such as pears flavoured with ginger or peaches with vanilla, can be served hot or cold, with damson or raspberry purée.
- Stewed fruits are good at any time of year, from rhubarb with ginger or strawberries in spring and early summer, to autumn and winter's plums, blackberries and apples.

All these ideas are extra luxurious with a spoonful of fromage frais or 'live' natural yoghurt.

• VEGETABLES

Eat as many vegetables as you like – they are rich in vitamins, minerals and fibre and low in fat, protein and carbohydrates. They help the body to produce therapeutic substances that may protect it against heart disease and cancer. Vegetables also stimulate the body to excrete waste products and are perfect body cleansing material, as long as there is enough water around to enable the fibre to swell and do its work. Vegetables can be prepared in many ways.

- Soups such as parsnip and apple or pea and mint.
- Salads are usually associated with health, but they need never be boring. We are lucky in having a vast choice of vegetables, lettuces and herbs to make salads not only taste good, but also look extremely attractive. Be adventurous and mix fruits with savoury tastes: tomato and orange is a favourite of mine, or try pear and watercress or strawberries and avocado.

Make a simple vinaigrette dressing with salt, pepper, mustard, lemon or lime juice and a good olive oil, and flavour it with freshly chopped garlic or herbs (see page 57 for ideas on matching herbs with vegetables). Dress salads lightly, just before serving, so they don't become soggy.

- Chargrilled vegetables can be served hot or chilled. Good vegetables for this method include peppers, aubergines, chicory, shallots, tomatoes, courgettes, artichoke hearts and asparagus. You can buy special ridged chargrilling pans, but I also use a normal grill pan, covered with aluminium foil. Slice the vegetables, drizzle with a little olive oil and place under a hot grill. Grill until golden brown and slightly charred at the edges. They are lovely eaten hot, just as they are, or you could drizzle them lightly with a vinaigrette dressing made with garlic or herbs such as mint, parsley or dill.

• Roasting produces a similar effect to chargrilling, but the vegetables are kept whole or cut into large chunks. Parsnips, baby turnips, courgettes and peppers are all excellent when roasted in a hot oven with a little olive oil. I love the flavour of a whole aubergine that has been lightly pricked with a fork and roasted until it collapses completely, which usually takes about 20–30 minutes. Once it has collapsed, scrape the flesh out of the skin and mix with a little olive oil, lemon juice and seasoning. Alternatively, mix with yoghurt to make moutabel. This makes a delicious snack or accompaniment to other roasted or chargrilled vegetables.

• Stir-fries are fantastic made with ginger, garlic, spring onion and vegetables such as mangetout, baby corn, baby aubergines and baby cauliflowers. The secret is to make sure that the oil is hot and to fry the vegetables quickly over a high heat, stirring frequently so they cook evenly and do not stick. If the heat is low the vegetables steam rather than fry and therefore they become soggy. Season vegetables with soy sauce and a few drops of sesame oil and serve at once.

• Hot pots are very good in winter, with root vegetables such as carrots, parsnips, swede and turnip. Other good vegetables for hot pots include cauliflower, courgettes, pumpkin and leeks; these cook more quickly and you may like to add them half way through the cooking time. Begin with a base of onions fried in a little olive oil, then add roughly chopped garlic, a bay leaf, some sprigs of thyme and roughly chopped tomatoes if you wish. If you prepare a hot pot early in the day you can leave it to cook gently for two to three hours while you pamper yourself or go out for some exercise. Slow cookers are excellent for this, or you can use a moderately low oven. A further advantage of vegetable hot pots is that any leftovers can be made into a soup the following day, by adding some vegetable stock or a little wine.

BEAUTY TREATMENTS

Taking the time to cleanse, exfoliate, tone and moisturize your body and deep-cleanse your face will make you feel relaxed and pampered. You may choose to luxuriate in a long bath or step under an invigorating shower, where it is easier to exfoliate.

There are so many skin products on the market today that it is difficult to know which to choose. Why not try making your own natural face pack?

First prepare your face by thoroughly cleansing the skin and if possible using a gentle exfoliator, such as washing grains, to slough away any rough skin. The skin will also benefit more if the pack is applied after the face is steamed. You will need a large bowl and a towel large enough cover your head and leave a good curtain around the sides. Fill the bowl with boiling water, place your face over the bowl and completely cover your head with the towel, so that the steam is held inside. Leave your face to steam for 5–10 minutes.

After steaming, apply the face pack. Most packs should be left on the skin for about 10–15 minutes, but remove straight away if you feel any discomfort, such as stinging or itching. Lie down, relax and let the face pack do its work. Remove the pack with warm water, tone the skin with a suitable tonic and moisturize with your favourite cream, to seal in the moisture derived from the mask.

• HONEY AND YOGHURT
Good for dry and tired skins. Mix a small pot of live yoghurt with an equal quantity of clear honey. Spread over the face, avoiding the eye area. Leave for 15 minutes.

• EGG WHITES AND ALMONDS

Suitable for all skin types, unless you have an egg allergy. Good for refining and tightening the pores. Whip the whites of 2 eggs until stiff and gently stir in 2 teaspoons of ground almonds. Spread over the face, avoiding the eye area. Leave for 15 minutes.

• AVOCADO AND WHEATGERM

Good for dry and stressed skins. If your skin is particularly sensitive or you are allergic to wheat you may like to omit the wheatgerm. Mash an avocado and mix with 1 teaspoon of lemon juice and 2 teaspoons of wheatgerm. Spread over the face, avoiding the eye area. Leave for 10 minutes.

• CUCUMBER AND GREEK YOGHURT

Good for revitalizing oily skins. Grate half a cucumber and mix with 2 tablespoons of Greek yoghurt and 1 teaspoon of lemon juice. Spread over the face, avoiding the eye area. Leave for 10–15 minutes.

• FRESH FRUIT AND VEGETABLE RECIPES

Chilled mint and cucumber soup
Parsnip and apple soup
Pea, mint and lettuce soup
Carrot and orange soup

Guacamole
Tomato and tarragon vinaigrette
Radicchio and grape salad
Pear and walnut salad
  with watercress
Artichoke and avocado salad
Grilled vegetable salad

Broccoli with roasted tomatoes
Spiced red cabbage with apples
Gado gado

Fruit compote
Tropical dried fruit salad
Oranges in caramel
Poached pears with ginger
Vanilla poached peaches
Cinnamon apples and plums
Chilled gingered rhubarb

2 Allergies

More and more women consider themselves to be allergic to some food or other. Although specialists differentiate between food allergy and food intolerance, both represent an over-sensitive reaction to food and the guidelines for their nutritional management are very similar. In my experience the following are the most common food sensitivities:

- Milk
- Egg
- Wheat and gluten
- Additives

Candida, while not a food allergy or intolerance, is treated by excluding food and drinks that cause an unpleasant reaction in the body.

• SYMPTOMS OF FOOD SENSITIVITIES

If you suffer from symptoms such as diarrhoea, constipation, bloating of the stomach, eczema or other skin conditions, migraine, irritability or extreme tiredness, it is possible you have a food sensitivity. Other less common symptoms include asthma, recurrent ear infections, urticaria (itchy red or whitish raised patches, also known as hives or nettle rash), swelling of the lips, mouth and tongue. Seek immediate attention in cases of swelling of the throat, as this can cause breathing problems and is extremely serious.

I suggest that you consult your doctor in any case, so that he or she can examine you and rule out any non-food cause. Once you have established that you don't have anything more serious wrong with you, you can start looking at the foods you eat. Bear in mind that any major dietary change, such as eliminating all wheat, sugar and yeast products on a long-term basis, needs professional guidance, but in the short term you can explore your diet on your own.

Some patients ask whether you naturally dislike the food that you shouldn't have. For instance, some women who don't like milky products are diagnosed as being intolerant of lactose (found in milky foods). Others find the opposite: they crave the thing that they are sensitive to; the body can be cruel at times. In cases of suspected food sensitivities, I look for any out-of-the-ordinary food likes or dislikes, as these may provide clues. My view of food sensitivities is that as long as you gain relief from your distressing symptoms and do not compromise yourself nutritionally or psychologically, there is no harm in avoiding certain foods.

• SOCIAL IMPLICATIONS

One of the often-ignored aspects of a diagnosis of food sensitivity or allergy is the social and psychological implications. People are sometimes told to avoid as many as 20 different foods, but frequently are not told what they can eat. This is very destructive and it can be difficult to put into practice, because it is hard to know what foods are free from the allergens (the substances capable of inducing the allergy). Some women end up avoiding so much that they become malnourished, which of course makes them feel unwell. There is always something you can eat that will provide you with the nourishment and enjoyment food deserves. The simpler and fresher your diet and the less you rely on ready-made foods, the fewer potential unknown quantities you will consume.

There is no need to suffer in dietary isolation, unable to share dishes with other people or to go out for meals. Food is more than just a physiological requirement: we also use it in our society to acknowledge the receiving and giving of affection. It is a form of communication, and if you take that away from someone you withdraw something very important from their life, not just food. While food sensitivity should be treated seriously, it is important to keep it in perspective in life; becoming obsessive about what you eat will not help you.

• EATING OUT

Eating out may be a problem for people with food sensitivities, as it is difficult to know what has gone into the dishes. Firstly remember that simple, good-quality food such as fish, free-range meat and poultry, fruit, vegetables and rice is less likely to contain a lot of additives. Also, if you stick to simple foods you should be able to spot any ingredient to which you are sensitive. Try to choose restaurants where the food is prepared fresh and not somewhere where you can have a meal in two minutes. The food in fast-food restaurants is far more likely to have a lot of hidden ingredients and additives, and these restaurants don't have the staff or time to provide an individual service. Never be afraid to ask how things are cooked and tell staff that you are allergic to something. If you mention it in good time, the chef may be able to make you a sauce without cream, for instance, if you are milk-sensitive. Most good restaurants will take your requests seriously: they certainly don't want to be sued for making you ill!

• DO YOU HAVE AN ALLERGY OR AN INTOLERANCE?

It is interesting to understand the difference between an allergy and an intolerance. The term 'food intolerance' is used when a specific food or food ingredient causes an unpleasant reaction such as mild diarrhoea, tiredness, mild eczema or constipation. Some women just seem to feel unwell when they eat the offending food, without suffering any particular symptoms. A 'food allergy' is a form of intolerance in which a food causes an abnormal, unpleasant, measurable immunological reaction. This can be detected in blood tests carried out by a gastroenterologist or immunologist. Your doctor can arrange this for you. Symptoms of an allergy range from stomach discomfort to severe pain, violent sickness, diarrhoea and swelling of the lips, tongue and throat.

Some women have a mild food sensitivity and can eat a small amount of the offending item without experiencing any symptoms, whereas others with an extreme sensitivity need to remove the offending item completely from their diet in order to avoid serious symptoms. Some people choose to put up with the symptoms produced by an occasional lapse. Others decide it is not worth the discomfort or risk of any severe reactions.

CAUSES

Your body's reaction to an unwanted food has three likely causes:

- ### THE RELEASE OF HISTAMINE
This substance is over-produced by the body when it is faced with foods that are rich in certain unwanted nutrients. Shellfish, for example, contain substances that some women's bodies cannot tolerate, causing them to become violently sick. This severe histamine reaction normally occurs with food allergies, rather than intolerances.

- ### AN ENZYME DEFECT
This is when the body does not produce sufficient enzymes, substances which enable the body to break down and make use of various nutrients. For example, a deficiency in the enzyme lactase means that lactose (the sugar found in milk and milk products) is not broken down. This causes an abnormal build-up of lactose in the gut, which may result in pain, sickness and diarrhoea. Some women completely lack a particular enzyme, while others have a small amount. This accounts for why some are occasionally able to eat a small amount of the offending food.

- ### IRRITANT EFFECT
The gut can become irritated by certain food ingredients. Common irritants are chillies, some spices and monosodium glutamate (MSG), a flavour 'enhancer' found in many processed foods.

ARE FOOD SENSITIVITIES INCREASING?

The more conventional or cynical members of society mutter that food allergies are not more common, it's just that we are becoming more aware of our bodies and how we perceive they should function. Sometimes we notice things that, not so many years ago, would have been ignored or considered normal. This increased awareness of our bodies is on the whole healthy, although it may be taken to extremes, and some women worry far too much. We are all susceptible to the odd 'off' day, when we might be a little constipated or bloated. Also, as some women grow older their digestive system becomes poorer at dealing with certain foods. However, if you have an 'off' day more than occasionally, you are right to look for a cause and solution.

Theories vary as to why so many women appear to be suffering with food sensitivities. One or more of the following factors may tip the body into food sensitivity.

• PESTICIDES
Some people believe sensitivity results from increasing quantities of pesticides and chemicals used in the production of our food. Our guts are being exposed to so many unnatural substances that some women are starting to reject even the most straightforward, unprocessed foods. A food sensitivity may be a result of the accumulation of foods or toxins, which the body rejects once a specific threshold is reached.

• STRESS
The digestive system is a collection of muscles and glands and it is sensitive to stress. A food sensitivity may be the way in which the body shows it cannot cope with a certain level of stress.

• HORMONAL CHANGES

For some women, age-related hormonal changes drastically affect the bowel; others just don't react well to artificial hormones. Since so many women are undergoing Hormone Replacement Therapy and taking other hormone-based drugs, this could account for some of the sensitivity cases. Women who believe that we should grow old without taking HRT and should not chemically prevent pregnancies strongly support this theory. In some cases, stopping these drugs can eliminate the food sensitivity. However, in other women, hormones can improve the way in which the bowel works. It's very much a personal issue, but one that is worth exploring with your doctor.

• ANTIBIOTICS

Both short and long courses of antibiotics can render the gut temporarily or permanently intolerant to a particular food. The gut normally contains a collection of flora and bacteria, which produce energy, vitamins and other substances that are beneficial to the body. When you take antibiotics these beneficial flora are killed and bad, pathogenic bacteria grow in their place. The presence of bad bacteria may cause some women to develop food sensitivities. Some people believe that the use of antibiotics in the production of meat, poultry and vegetables may cause the gut to become 'florally unbalanced'. So whether the antibiotics are taken as tablets or unconsciously in our foods, we need to look at ways of minimizing their damage if we are to prevent or cure food sensitivities. Looking after your body and eating healthily so that you don't render yourself susceptible to bacterial infections, and eating fresh, preferably organic produce, are two positive steps you could take.

IDENTIFYING A FOOD SENSITIVITY

CHOCOLATE
CRISPY CAKES

Simply melt a good-quality chocolate (one with no milk powder) in a bowl over a pan of simmering water. Stir until it is smooth, then stir in rice crispies, adding just enough to get them all coated in chocolate. Spoon the mixture on to a piece of nonstick baking paper or into small cake cases and leave to set.

It is important to understand how your body reacts to foods. Once you have grasped how to reduce or eliminate symptoms of sensitivity, you will be able to make adjustments in your diet and get on with your life. The difficult part can be finding out what you're sensitive to. Seek the advice of a doctor or dietitian before starting this means of investigation.

Remove the suspected item from your diet for approximately one to two weeks. If your symptoms disappear, you can probably assume that you have a sensitivity related to this food. If they continue, seek professional advice before proceeding any further, as once you start removing more than one food, things can become complicated.

Once you have found that you are sensitive to a particular food, make sure that your body is not going to become malnourished by removing it. Find other foods that provide the same beneficial nutrients (see What your body needs in Part One) without the offending ingredients. Seek the advice of a dietitian who will check whether your body requires any extra vitamin or mineral supplements. Psychologically you also need to ensure that you are not going to spend the rest of your days feeling deprived.

Beware of self-diagnosis. I see many cases of women who wrongly diagnose their sensitivity and proceed to exclude far too many products from their diets on a long-term basis. This can lead to a number of problems, including severe lethargy, depression and malnutrition. Some women follow this sort of exclusion diet when they are suffering from a serious eating disorder such as anorexia or bulimia. Focusing on any eating plan that 'allows' you to cut out foods can mask a more serious problem.

MILK SENSITIVITY

There are two main types: lactose intolerance and cows' milk protein sensitivity. Both may cause diarrhoea, sickness, stomach and abdominal cramps and headaches, and may aggravate skin complaints such as eczema. Some scientists believe that half of the world's population is unable to tolerate cows' milk.

Lactose sensitivity is mainly due to a deficiency in the body's production of lactase, the enzyme that breaks down lactose, the natural sugar found in all animal milk products. Without sufficient lactase, lactose cannot be broken down and absorbed by the body and therefore there is a build-up of undigested lactose in the gut.

If you are lactose sensitive you should avoid all milk products other than soya milk. This includes cows', goats' and ewes' milk, cream, yoghurt, butter, cheese, skimmed milk powder, lactose, casein and whey, which are present in many baked and processed foods. Food products that contain monosodium glutamate also frequently contain lactose.

Children are quite commonly lactose sensitive until their gut becomes more mature, usually around two years old. Always consult a doctor or dietitian if you suspect that your child is lactose sensitive, as it is vital that you do not deprive the body of essential nutrients such as calcium and protein.

Cows' milk protein sensitivity is slightly less common than lactose sensitivity; it can occur at any age. Although the body is unable to tolerate any form of cows' milk, it may be able to tolerate sheep's or goats' milk, and cheeses and yoghurts made from them. Some women unfortunately seem unable to tolerate milk products from any source.

SCONES

Sift 225 g/8 oz self-raising flour and 1/2 teaspoon bicarbonate of soda into a bowl. Using your fingertips, lightly rub in 50 g/2 oz butter. Add about 150 ml/1/4 pint milk to make a soft, but not wet, dough. Roll out about 2.5 cm/1 inch thick, cut into rounds and brush the tops lightly with milk. Bake in a preheated oven at 200°C/400° F/Gas 6 for 10 minutes or until golden. To vary the recipe you could add 50 g/2 oz sultanas and a large pinch of cinnamon, or 50 g/2 oz chopped dates and the grated zest of an orange.

• CALCIUM INTAKE

Milk and its derivatives provide a rich source of calcium in most women's diets; once you remove it it is most important that you do not become calcium-deficient. You can buy calcium-enriched soya milk and margarine. You should eat plenty of other calcium-rich foods and will probably need to take a calcium supplement; consult your doctor or dietitian, and read the section on calcium in What your body needs, in Part One.

A word of warning. If you take a calcium supplement it is vital that you don't choose calcium lactate, as this is derived from lactose. There are other types, such as calcium oxalate; ask your dietitian or pharmacist for advice.

• WHAT YOU CAN EAT IF YOU'RE SENSITIVE TO MILK

Many food manufacturers label products that contain neither cows' milk protein nor lactose as 'milk-free'; these should be suitable for both types of milk sensitivity. There are a few margarines that contain no whey, casein or other milk derivatives; you will have to spend a few minutes reading labels to find out which these are, but you will then be able to use them all the time. Soya milk, soya yoghurt and soya cheese can directly replace the dairy versions in most recipes. Also remember that if you suffer from cows' milk protein intolerance you can still enjoy a wide range of sheep's and goats' milk cheeses and yoghurts. Milk-free biscuits and cakes are hard to find, but you can make your own by replacing the butter with milk-free margarine in many recipes. One quick and easy idea is that old childhood favourite, chocolate crispy cakes (see page 83). The recipes I have given for barabrith and carrot cake are also suitable. Fruit desserts are fine; instead of cream or yoghurt, use a fruit coulis as a sauce: rub strawberries or raspberries through a sieve and add icing sugar or lemon juice to your taste (make plenty in the summer and freeze). Remember that Chinese and Malaysian food use little or no milk products, so these are good choices when eating out.

EGG SENSITIVITY

Egg sensitivity is slightly less common than milk sensitivities, but it is usually associated with quite severe symptoms. The women I see frequently suffer from very unpleasant bouts of diarrhoea, which may be the chief gut symptom. Others suffer from acute and chronic episodes of constipation and stomach cramps or find that it can aggravate eczema, affect their moods and even disturb their sleep.

If you suspect that you have an egg sensitivity, you need to avoid eggs and foods containing whole egg, egg yolk, albumin, egg lecithin and dried egg. Some women may be sensitive to either egg yolk or egg white but not both. I suggest that you avoid both for a trial period of one or two weeks. Then, if eggs seem to be causing your problems, you can reintroduce either yolks or whites and see what happens. You should not experiment with a food allergen if your symptoms are very severe. Always seek professional advice. Equally, if you suspect your child has an allergy, don't tackle it alone.

• **WHAT YOU CAN EAT IF YOU'RE SENSITIVE TO EGGS**
Avoiding egg and its derivatives is relatively straightforward as long as you steer clear of bought biscuits, cakes, meringues, mayonnaise, egg pasta and other manufactured foods containing albumin, lecithin and dried egg. If in doubt, read the label, as some cakes and biscuits are free of egg products; flapjacks and shortbread, for example. Some chocolate contains lecithin, so avoid this or look for soya lecithin. There are some egg replicas for use in cooking, but they may change the consistency of the finished product and are an unnecessary reminder that you are being marginalized by your condition. You can enjoy most fruit desserts, crumbles and tarts, as long as the pastry does not use egg in any way. Filo pastries such as baklava and apple strudel should be egg-free. Scones are simple to make and do not use eggs (see p. 85).

WHEAT AND GLUTEN SENSITIVITY

The severity and symptoms of these sensitivities vary greatly: some women feel that simply by avoiding the ingredient they feel more energized, less bloated and suffer less pain with rheumatoid arthritis; others need to eliminate the offending foods to avoid being completely incapacitated with severe pain, profuse diarrhoea or internal bleeding. At this end of the spectrum, some people are diagnosed as having a condition resulting from a severe intolerance to gluten, known as coeliac disease.

The first step in managing a wheat or gluten intolerance is to establish whether your sensitivity is to wheat or gluten. Wheat is a grain, whereas gluten is a protein that is found in wheat, oats, rye and barley. If you are just sensitive to wheat you may be able to eat oats, rye and barley. However, if gluten is the offender you must avoid all sources of gluten.

There are various theories as to why so many people seem to be sensitive to wheat and gluten. It may be environmental, genetic or simply that there is an increased awareness about wheat and its effect on the body. Women in the past may have had to cope with the symptoms that are now associated with wheat or gluten intolerance. Nowadays, thankfully, it's a matter of knowing how to treat them.

If wheat sensitivity is your problem, you can follow the nutritional guidelines for gluten intolerance (below) and can also include rye bread, oatcakes and oat-topped crumbles. Gluten intolerance and coeliac disease can be very different in severity, but have the same nutritional treatment: avoid gluten-containing foods.

• COELIAC DISEASE
This is an immunological condition that can be diagnosed only by a surgeon taking a small 'nip' of the lining of the intestine and studying it under a microscope.

If coeliacs eat gluten their intestine becomes inflamed, which results in pain, diarrhoea and in some cases severe problems with malabsorption of nutrients. The good news is that once you remove gluten from the diet the gut frequently returns to behaving normally. It is generally necessary to avoid all forms of gluten for life, but some women may be able to tolerate some oat or rye-based products. The gluten content of these is a lot lower than wheat, but you should seek professional guidance before you experiment.

• HOW DO I AVOID GLUTEN-CONTAINING FOODS?

Primarily you need to avoid wheat, barley, oats and rye, and products containing them, including beer and whisky. You additionally have to avoid food starch (edible or modified starch), unless the product clearly states that it is gluten-free. In practice this means avoiding bread, crackers, biscuits, cakes, pasta and sauces containing flour. You need to look at packets to see whether bread is used as a 'filler'. Sausages, salamis, pâtés and other meat products commonly fall into this group. You must also check baking powder, mustard powder, white pepper and gravy thickening as these sometimes contain gluten. Soya sauce contains wheat, but tamari, which is very similar, does not. The Coeliac Society, whose address is given at the end of the book, produces a list of manufactured products that are free from gluten. It is useful to have this as a source of reference.

Don't feel, however, that you need to spend your life eating specially prepared gluten-free products. Women frequently come to see me suffering from 'food fatigue'. This is a psychological condition that is caused by focusing on foods they can't have and special products. As with any other nutrient constraint, you need to broaden your horizons. Start thinking about all the foods which naturally don't contain gluten and how you can use them to make exciting dishes. For example paella, risotto, rice and potato bakes, buck-wheat pancakes, sauces using potato flour or cornflour.

It's just a question of changing your outlook, which of course takes time and effort, but once you've cracked it, a gluten-free lifestyle can be just as delicious and varied as any other healthy eating pattern.

- **WHICH OTHER STAPLE FOODS CAN I EAT?**

Rice, potatoes, polenta (corn or maize meal), millet, buckwheat.

- **HOW DO I MAKE A SAUCE IF I CANNOT USE NORMAL FLOUR?**

You can use potato flour as a direct replacement for wheat flour. Potato flour is a little more inclined to thicken in lumps, especially if the heat is too high. Use an electric hand blender in the pan or whisk vigorously using a balloon whisk over a low heat. A little cornflour can be used to thicken sauces; follow the packet instructions.

Alternatively you can use the reduction method. This means simmering meat, chicken, vegetable or fish stock until it reduces to a thick syrup. It should be done over a low heat and may take up to 30 minutes to reduce 250 ml/8 fl oz of liquid down to a richly flavoured syrup. You could begin with the meat juices in a roasting tin or frying pan and stir in a splash of wine and some good-quality stock. Just before serving you could add some chopped fresh herbs: dill, parsley, coriander or basil. For a luxurious finish, whisk in a little cream or some cubes of chilled butter.

For a sweet sauce reduce some orange, apple or strawberry juice to a syrupy consistency. At the last minute, whisk in some cream, yoghurt or Cointreau.

- **CAN I MAKE MY OWN BREAD?**

Yes, of course you can, but don't expect it to look or taste like bread made with wheat flour, because it is the gluten that allows bread to rise and stay risen when baked. Enjoy it as a different product with its own taste and texture. Be aware of the difference between yeast-free bread and gluten-free bread. The yeast-free bread sold in health food shops very often contains gluten or wheat. You can buy gluten-free breads, but it is hard to find good ones. Try to spare the time to make your own: gluten-free bread is best eaten fresh and hot. It freezes very well, so freeze it in slices and then make it into toast straight from the freezer.

The secret to making delicious gluten-free bread is to use a wide variety of sources of starch; most of them should be available from health food shops. Millet and sorghum flours are good for baking, especially when combined with rice or gram (pea) flour. Sweet chestnut flour (sometimes sold in Italian shops) is one of my favourites for making a light, soft, sweet bread. Mix it with sorghum flour for particularly good bread and cakes. Buckwheat flour bakes well but it has a stronger flavour.

ADDITIVE SENSITIVITY

We in the densely populated, so-called 'developed' countries could not survive without some food additives. They serve valuable functions as food preservatives, keeping food spoilage organisms at bay, and play a major role in the enhancement of the flavour, texture and colour of our food. The down-side of the mass production of food and the heavy use of additives is that many people have become so used to eating foods with lots of additives that they have forgotten how good fresh food looks and tastes.

While most food additives are not associated with food sensitivities, some people are extremely sensitive to a few of them. Symptoms range from hyperactivity in children, headaches, hives and other skin complaints, to mood swings and depression. Some women are sensitive to many additives, but the most common culprits are the sulphating agents sulphur dioxide, sodium metabisulphite and potassium metabisulphite (used as preservatives), yellow azo dyes and monosodium glutamate or MSG (used as a stabilizer). All of these additives have to be declared on food labels either under their chemical name or as an E number, which means they have been recognized and classified by the European Union. Numbers E100–E180 are colouring agents, E200–E290 are preservatives, E300–E322 are antioxidants, E400–E495 are emulsifiers and stabilizers; E420 and E421 are sweeteners.

If you suspect that you have an additive sensitivity you just need to read labels. While this takes time to begin with you will soon become familiar with the foods you can and cannot have. Remember, the simpler and fresher you keep your diet and the less you rely on made-up processed foods the fewer additives you will consume.

• SULPHATING AGENTS

In America sulphites have been banned for use on fruits and vegetables, but in Europe this legislation is still going through. If you suspect that you have a sensitivity or intolerance to a sulphite, look carefully at the following list of foods, which frequently contain sulphites.
• Wines, cider and beers
• Dried potatoes, including crisps and other savoury snacks
• Dried fruits
• Dried vegetables
• Canned soups and sauces and all processed foods and ready-made meals
• Canned and bottled soft drinks
There is a huge lobby for many foods to be spared the sulphating process and an increasing number of foods, such as dried apricots, are now available without sulphites.

• TARTRAZINE

One of the commonest additives to upset children is tartrazine (E102), a colouring agent. It is used in many foods, but you can avoid the majority of sources by checking the packets. Common foods containing tartrazine include orange-coloured drinks, jelly, red or dark yellow cheese, cheese-containing meals and snacks and lemon-flavoured sweets and dessert mixes. Instead, choose natural fruit juices and naturally produced, freshly cut cheeses. You can easily make your own jelly using fruit juice and gelatine.

CANDIDIASIS

Everyone's gut contains some Candida albicans, a yeast which, along with several thousands of other bacteria in the gut, produces energy, vitamin K and other beneficial substances such as anti-cancer compounds. Many women occasionally suffer from a slight over-growth of Candida albicans, which manifests itself as vaginal or oral thrush. This is especially common when taking antibiotics, eating a lot of dairy products, or generally feeling run down. Some people believe that more serious symptoms, ranging from extreme tired-ness, headaches, joint pain, indigestion and irritable bowels to skin complaints and rashes, can be put down to an overgrowth of Candida albicans throughout the body. This condition is known as Candidiasis. Candidiasis is not technically a food allergy or intoler-ance, but it does require dietary management.

I am extremely sceptical about the widespread diag-nosis of Candidiasis, for various reasons. While this book encourages women to tackle their symptoms and use food to help them, I do not advocate self-diagnosis. Equally, beware of any health practitioner who makes this diagnosis without laboratory tests, then tells you to follow an 'anti-candida' diet without ruling out any other cause of your symptoms or giving you any posi-tive advice about what you should eat. The anti-candida diet excludes many foods, and without specialist advice it may lead to other problems such as malnutrition, severe lethargy and depression. I sometimes see women who have other minor or more serious medical or psychological problems which have been missed because they have been told to go away and follow the anti-candida diet.

A bout of vaginal or oral thrush should always be checked out by your doctor, who can identify the specific offending organism by taking blood tests and swabs. After laboratory analysis, the results should enable your doctor to treat you appropriately. Not all thrush is a result of Candidiasis: there are plenty of other bacterial and viral causes and it is very often aggravated or caused by anaemia, depression or a more serious bowel problem. If the results of laboratory tests show that you have an overgrowth of Candida albicans you can then treat it nutritionally, as outlined below.

• FIRST STEPS IN MANAGING CANDIDA
Eat some live (unpasteurized) yoghurt containing bifidus and acidophilus every day. This should help replenish the gut with beneficial bacteria, which in turn reduces the amount of undesirable bacteria such as Candida albicans.

Reduce the quantity of yeast-containing and yeast-producing foods, for no longer than two weeks at first. These take many forms. Excessive amounts of these foods may aggravate the situation at times when you have a lot of Candida in your body. You should therefore avoid the following:
• All breads containing yeast, including pittas and naan bread.
• Bread-containing foods, including taramasalata, sausages and bread-crumbed foods such as croquettes.
• Fermented dairy products. These include cheese, most yoghurt, buttermilk and soured cream. Fresh milk should be fine as it has not undergone any fermentation process. Fermentation usually involves the addition of yeast.
• Yeast extracts such as Marmite.
• Dried fruits, over-ripe or mouldy fruits, grapes and

mushrooms. These are all likely to contain a large number of yeast cells. You should also avoid fruit juices, unless they are drunk immediately after they have been squeezed. Fresh fruits, other than grapes, are absolutely fine. Wash them first, and avoid fruits with a 'bloomy' coating, as this may mean that they contain lots of yeast.

• Sugary and treacly foods. Although these do not contain yeast, they feed the yeasts, including Candida, that are in your body. You should avoid all sweet things, whether they are made from white or brown sugar, honey, treacle or even fructose (fruit sugars); any of these can feed the yeasts. However, you do not need to start looking at food labels for these ingredients, because most foods, even savoury ones, contain some sugar. Just avoid sweet-tasting foods.

• Brewer's yeast, which is used in the fermentation of alcoholic drinks. I advise that you avoid all alcoholic drinks at first. However, some women may find that they can drink clear alcohols such as gin or vodka without any ill effects.

• MAKE SURE THAT YOUR DIET IS WELL BALANCED
Read the chapter on What your body needs, in Part One.

• WHAT YOU CAN EAT TO AVOID EATING YEAST
There are some excellent yeast-free breads, including Irish soda bread, chapatis, matzos and other yeast-free crackers and crispbreads. The recipes I have created for wheat-free diets are also yeast-free. Remember all the other starch providers: pasta, potatoes, corn, oats, cracked wheat (bulgar wheat), the many varieties of rice and beans, lentils and other pulses.

Fish, poultry and meat, fresh fruits (except grapes) and vegetables. Choose organic if possible.

Some women find that they can manage small amounts of some cheeses, for example white rather than blue cheeses. Blue cheeses are particularly high in yeast. Others find that pasteurized cheeses suit them better than unpasteurized varieties, as the pasteurization

process decreases the yeast and general bacterial population in cheese. Take the time to experiment, as it
would be a pity to miss out on all cheeses when you may
find that some suit you well.

If after two weeks you find that your symptoms have
lessened or disappeared, see your doctor or dietitian
to find out how you can manage this sort of diet in the
long term. If you restrict dairy products you must ask
whether you need to take a calcium supplement.

MULTIPLE FOOD SENSITIVITIES

If, after reading this chapter, you feel you are sensitive
to more than one food you should seek professional
advice. Your dietitian will be able to advise how to
identify the culprits safely and help you put together
a practical and well-balanced eating plan. I don't
recommend that you follow some of the extreme exclusion diets that take out more than one food at a time, as
you may end up confused and wondering whether you
are feeling tired or unwell from a lack or excess of a
particular food.

If you don't feel that any of the sensitivities I
have discussed in this chapter applies to you, consider
excluding the following foods for a week or two;
they are known to produce sensitivity in some people:
apples, apricots, melons, nuts (especially peanuts),
oranges, pears, pineapple and tomatoes.

3 Anaemia

Anaemia affects many women at some time in their lives, but it is most common in women who smoke, have heavy periods or an eating disorder such as anorexia. It is defined in medical textbooks as a reduction below the acceptable norm of the concentration in the blood of a protein called haemoglobin. Haemoglobin gives red blood cells their characteristic colour and, more importantly, enables them to carry oxygen around the body.

There are many forms of anaemia, including folate deficiency and pernicious anaemia, but the most common form of anaemia is iron deficiency anaemia. It is believed to affect between 15 and 20% of women, mainly those in their childbearing years, and young children.

Symptoms of anaemia include tiredness, irritability, loss of appetite, pallor and a general feeling of being 'run down'. Severe iron deficiency anaemia can lead to breathlessness, headaches and an inability to complete even the simplest of tasks. If you have any of these symptoms it is wise to go to your doctor in order that he or she can check the cause. It is very important to establish which sort of anaemia you have before you embark on any self-help programme, so don't just diagnose yourself. Iron deficiency anaemia is relatively easy to correct through changing the foods you eat and your general lifestyle, but the other sorts of anaemia are a little trickier and you should consult your doctor or dietitian for more specific advice.

CAUSES OF IRON DEFICIENCY ANAEMIA

There are six main causes of iron deficiency anaemia. One or more may apply in your particular case, and it is important to look at the whole picture.

• INCREASED DEMAND FOR IRON

Your body may at certain times start to require a little more iron than it previously needed. This may be as a result of a growth spurt, where the tissues within the body are rapidly dividing, athletic training, where your muscles, heart and lungs are put under greater strain, or when you are pregnant or breast-feeding. Between 500 and 600 mg of iron are needed in total for each pregnancy, to satisfy the baby's growth requirements and the blood loss experienced at childbirth.

• LOSS OF BLOOD

For many women this occurs when they are experiencing heavy or lengthy menstrual periods. Between 15 and 30 mg of iron are lost each month through menstruation, so it can be quite easy to become a little anaemic if you're not careful about replenishing these losses.

• INSUFFICIENT IRON

Even if the body does not have any increase in iron requirements, some women become anaemic because their diet is just not rich enough in the essential nutrients, perhaps because they don't like many of the iron and crucial nutrient-rich foods, or they see red meats and offal as bad for them, or for moral reasons they have decided not to eat red meat.

I see this more and more frequently in young women who have decided to follow some sort of unusual diet. Equally, iron deficiency anaemia can be one of the first clinical signs to appear in a young woman who has an eating disorder such as anorexia or bulimia.

• INHIBITED IRON ABSORPTION

Several substances common in the Western diet are known to inhibit the body's absorption of iron and other vitamins and minerals from your food. The chief culprits are tannins and caffeine, found chiefly in coffee, tea and cola-based drinks. I sometimes see women who are anaemic not only because they have a low iron intake but because they drink a lot of coffee and tea.

• INSUFFICIENT VITAMIN C

Vitamin C helps your body absorb iron from food. If you don't have enough vitamin C in your diet the iron will stay in the gut and won't be absorbed; a useless situation. Women who either don't eat many fruits or vegetables that contain vitamin C or who smoke are particularly susceptible to developing iron deficiency anaemia as a result of a poor vitamin C intake.

• PROBLEMS WITH IRON ABSORPTION

As with all nutrients within the diet, iron relies on a healthy gut to absorb it. Some women with digestive problems such as irritable bowel syndrome or chronic constipation can have slightly disrupted iron absorption. If you have a specific bowel problem see your dietitian or doctor for advice.

CORRECTING THE BALANCE

For the majority of women, iron deficiency anaemia is a simple matter of a negative iron and vitamin C balance; you retain less iron than you need, partly because of natural loss through menstruation and partly because of taking inhibitors such as tannins and caffeine. This negative balance means that your body does not have enough iron to form sufficient haemoglobin to carry the oxygen needed for energy creation, tissue formation and repair.

The good news is that it is not difficult to redress this balance by making a few changes in your diet and lifestyle. It usually takes three to four weeks for the body to benefit from these changes, so give it time.

It is very important once you have embarked on an anaemia-correcting eating plan to keep in touch with your doctor. He or she will be able to tell you how effective your new diet is and whether or not you need any additional supplements.

The two most important nutrients involved in iron deficiency anaemia are iron and vitamin C.

• IRON

There are two sorts of iron in food. Haem iron (from the Greek word haema, blood), found in animal foods such as lean red meat and offal, is easily absorbed by the body. Non-haem iron, derived from 'bloodless' foods such as plants and grains is absorbed less efficiently because of various 'salts' (oxalates and phytates) found in these foods. You therefore need to eat a lot more of these foods to obtain sufficient iron. Eggs also contain substances that decrease the amount of iron the body can absorb and are considered in the same way as vegetable sources.

• VITAMIN C

In addition to looking at the iron content of foods it is also important to address the vitamin C issue. Vitamin C helps your body to absorb iron. You therefore need to concentrate on having plenty of citrus fruits, kiwi fruits, strawberries, blackcurrants, cranberries and other 'tangy' fruits. Potatoes, red and green peppers and green vegetables also supply vitamin C in the diet.

DIETARY GUIDELINES

• EAT FRESH FRUIT OR DRINK FRUIT JUICE EVERY DAY

The ideal is to have a small glass of juice or a fruit shake (page 54) before or after every meal, as this will help the body absorb the iron from your food. Freshly squeezed fruit and vegetable juices contain large amounts of vitamin C and other natural nutrients, but some carton juices can also have a high vitamin C content: cranberry juice has one of the highest.

Drinks that are labelled 'orange (or other fruit) flavoured' rarely contain significant amounts as they are not closely related to fresh fruit. Some, however, have artificial vitamin C (ascorbic acid) added. There is no difference between having a drink with a vitamin or mineral added and taking a tablet. Both can be useful on occasions, but look to the natural food first.

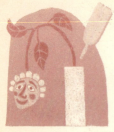

If you feel that citrus fruits are a little acid, have another fruit, such as strawberries, after your meal as a dessert.

Keep your vitamin C topped up by including some dark green leafy vegetables with each of your main meals. This could be a soup, a salad, or perhaps steamed broccoli tossed in a light olive oil with freshly chopped root ginger.

Champagne is relatively high in iron because of the effect of the limestone soil in the Champagne region of France. Some English wines grown in the southern limestone soils are high in iron for the same reason.

Full-bodied red wines have an even higher iron content, particularly those from the Graves and Médoc regions of Bordeaux, the Napa Valley in California, and Cabernet Sauvignon and Shiraz-based wines from Coonawarra or the Hunter Valley in Australia.

• **EAT ONE OF THE RICH SOURCES OF IRON TWO TO THREE TIMES A WEEK**

If you eat meat this could be either lean red meat, game or offal such as liver, kidney, oxtail. Many women are turned off by the idea of a slab of red meat on a plate, but think about the many delicious ways in which meat or offal could be easily incorporated in your diet. Tender calves' liver on a bed of caramelized onions; a casserole of minty meatballs in a yoghurt sauce; black pudding with sautéed potatoes and apple; chunks of fresh baguette spread with chicken liver and sherry pâté; or a slice of homemade meat and potato pie, served with lashings of pickle!

Remember that the body absorbs 20–40% of the iron available in meat sources, but only 5–20% of the iron from vegetable sources and eggs. If we eat a mixed diet including fruits, vegetables, meat and fish we are thought to absorb approximately 15–20% of the iron in the food.

• **EAT PLENTY OF NON-HAEM SOURCES OF IRON MOST DAYS**

This means eggs, green leafy vegetables such as spinach, Savoy cabbage, curly kale, watercress, broccoli, baked beans, soya beans and other pulses, black treacle, nuts and dried fruit (especially apricots). Vegetarians and vegans, who eat very few or no animal products, should include a rich source of non-haem iron every day.

It is especially important for vegetarians and vegans to have a glass of freshly squeezed fruit juice with each meal, as you really need the vitamin C to help your body absorb the iron. Some vegetarians may need to take an iron supplement if they cannot get enough iron from your diet. An additional – if occasional – source of iron is Champagne!

It is a myth that stout is high in iron; there is ten times as much iron in a pint of Champagne as in a pint of stout. Obviously we don't drink pints of Champagne every day, but it's nice to know that something so enjoyable has this nutritional benefit. Some red wines contain more than twice as much iron as Champagne, but since red wines tend to be high in tannins, the absorption of iron is less efficient. However, in fuller-bodied wines that have aged in the bottle for a few years the tannins will have softened considerably.

- AVOID HAVING EXCESSIVE AMOUNTS OF FOODS AND DRINKS THAT INHIBIT IRON ABSORPTION
Coffee, tea and cola-based drinks will prevent the body from absorbing iron effectively because they contain tannins and caffeine. You should keep your tea and coffee intake down to a maximum of two to three cups a day and allow at least one hour between drinking tea or coffee before or after a meal, to give your gut a chance to absorb the iron from the food. Anaemic women should make a real effort to cut out the excessive, needless consumption of these drinks; it is far better to make a really good cup of coffee or tea and enjoy it at a suitable time of day. Other hot drinks to try include herbal or fruit teas, mugs of warm milk mixed with malted powders or just hot water with slices of lemon or drops of orange blossom water.

Remember that chocolate, although it contains iron, also contains substances that prevent efficient iron absorption, so don't over-indulge, even though you may feel as if you need an energy boost; chocolate is not the answer. Choose a zingy piece of fresh citrus fruit or a glass of mango juice instead. A particular favourite of mine are the Persian sweet lemons available from Iranian shops and some of the larger supermarkets. They really give you a burst of energy, as well as containing lots of vitamin C...they're fantastic.

- **KEEP THE BULK DOWN**

While you are trying to boost your iron and vitamin C intakes, try to keep the amount of cereal fibre such as wholegrain cereals and wholegrain bread low. Not only does high-fibre food contain 'salts' (oxalates and phytates) that inhibit the absorption of iron, it also acts as a buffer, itself absorbing some of the iron. I don't mean that you should cut out fibre completely, but try not to hide the red meat or vegetable source of iron in mounds of cereal fibre. Cook fragrant basmati or creamy arborio rice rather than brown rice, and choose white rather than wholewheat pasta. If you eat a lot of wholegrain bread, swap a little of it for white baguettes or tomato or olive focaccia.

GENERAL LIFESTYLE TIPS

- **REST**

Try to make sure that you have plenty of rest and don't allow yourself to become psychologically run down by putting unrealistic demands on your time. It amazes me to hear women complain of extreme tiredness, which may be partially attributable to anaemia, but is just as likely to be the result of being driven to do too much! If necessary, start time management strategies so that you don't end up running round inefficiently. If your lifestyle normally demands a lot of physical exertion you should try to cut this down, as you will be putting your body under too much physical stress.

It is far too easy to go to the doctor, receive the diagnosis of iron-deficiency anaemia, take an iron supplement and expect your body to recover overnight. It cannot happen this way. Three to four weeks is far more realistic: your body needs time to recover and the time has to come from somewhere.

• CUT DOWN ON STRENUOUS EXERCISE

Although it is good to include some regular gentle cardiovascular exercise such as swimming or dancing to help the body tick over, I offer a word of warning for those of you who are following intensive training programmes. When you are anaemic you should just concentrate on the gentler exercises, rather than the full training schedule. Remember that the major function of haemoglobin is to carry oxygen around the body, so if you're anaemic you may find it difficult to exercise to your usual degree. Take things easy and don't place unrealistic strains on your body. It is not, as some of my determined athletes think, just a case of mind over matter. Your body is below par and therefore needs to be treated with care.

• IRON SUPPLEMENTS

Many women think of anaemia as something that just requires an iron supplement, without really looking to see why it occurs and how to use foods to correct and prevent it from reappearing. Supplements have their place, but only after other issues have been explored.

Don't forget the above food and lifestyle advice, but if you are unable to eat as much iron as your body requires, either because you do not like the appropriate foods or because your iron status is a little too low to be corrected by diet alone, you may need to take an iron supplement.

There is little to distinguish between the many supplements on the market, apart from the fact that some contain just iron, whereas others contain iron with vitamin C. It is generally a good idea to choose a supplement that incorporates some vitamin C with the iron. A supplement that provides a daily 12 mg of iron with 500–1000 mg of vitamin C should be adequate for most women, but if you are unsure about the dose ask your doctor or dietitian.

A number of herbal iron supplements are available in most good health food stores. These contain herbal sourced iron, which, unlike other plant sources of non-haem iron, the body seems to be able to absorb quite efficiently. For advice as to which particular one you should take, ask your doctor, dietitian or a pharmacist – someone who doesn't have a financial incentive to sell a particular brand.

Some iron supplements can cause a little indigestion, diarrhoea or constipation. Try to avoid taking them on an empty stomach as this can make the problem of indigestion worse; the information in the chapter on indigestion may help. If the symptoms persist, see your doctor or pharmacist about changing the supplement. Some forms of iron and vitamin C supplements are better tolerated than others – it's just a question of trial and error.

OTHER FORMS OF ANAEMIA

When you are tested for anaemia you should be told whether your anaemia is due to iron deficiency alone, or is related to a lack of vitamin B12 or folic acid, two nutrients from the vitamin B complex. Both these nutrients help the body absorb iron, but also, in their own right, help to produce healthy red blood cells. Inadequate intakes of these vitamins can not only aggravate iron deficiency anaemia, they can also cause other forms of anaemia.

• PERNICIOUS ANAEMIA
Lack of vitamin B12 can cause pernicious anaemia. The symptoms of lethargy, depression, extreme tiredness and paleness are virtually identical to iron deficiency anaemia, and a vitamin B12 deficiency can mask iron deficiency anaemia and vice versa. Vitamin B12 deficiency may be caused either by a poor intake of foods rich in the vitamin, or by the lack of a substance known as 'intrinsic factor'. This substance is present in the digestive juices produced by the glands surrounding your stomach and is needed for the body to be able to use vitamin B12.

Your body needs only a very small amount of vitamin B12, which is found in foods of animal origin – meat, poultry, fish, dairy products – and yeast extract. Vegetarians and vegans may need to take a supplement of B12, best incorporated in a general B complex supplement, as all the B vitamins help each other to be absorbed. You can also buy soya milk fortified with vitamin B12. Pernicious anaemia is most commonly due to a lack of intrinsic factor in the body. Unfortunately you cannot increase your intrinsic factor through eating any particular food or taking a tablet; instead you will need a course of vitamin B12 injections, as this delivers the B12 directly into the blood, bypassing the intestine. However, in addition to the injections it is important to maintain a good dietary intake of vitamin B12.

• FOLATE DEFICIENCY ANAEMIA

Folic acid is found naturally in many foods in the form of folate. Unfortunately it is easily lost in cooking and storage time and in processing. In addition, various medications such as aspirin and contraceptive pills hinder the absorption of folic acid. Since folic acid is needed by the body for the absorption of iron, a deficiency of this vitamin may result in anaemia. The major sources of folic acid are vegetables such as asparagus, Savoy cabbage, Brussels sprouts, curly kale, spinach, fresh oranges and wheat germ, which is found in wholemeal bread and cereals. Various breakfast cereals are fortified with folic acid, but the naturally occurring folic acid is absorbed more effectively. In order to keep the level of folic acid as high as possible you should steam or lightly boil foods rather than boil them for long periods, and eat them as soon as possible after they are cooked.

In order to prevent or correct a deficiency of folic acid try to eat two to three servings of fresh vegetables every day, as part of a good, well-balanced diet.

• RECIPES TO CORRECT ANAEMIA

Chicken liver and tagliatelle soup

Spinach borscht

Carrot and orange soup

Leek and potato soup

Smoked mackerel pâté

Chicken liver pâté

Broccoli with roasted tomatoes

Christmas salad

Eggs Benedict

Cheese fluff

Spinach and goats' cheese soufflé

Spinach and watercress roulade

Somerset cider and steak pie

Minted meatballs with
  yoghurt sauce

Blackberry and ricotta pancakes

Mixed fruit with
  butterscotch sauce

Mixed berries in Grand Marnier

Oranges in caramel

Fresh figs filled with almond cream

Cinnamon apples and plums

Fig and ginger parkin

4 Arthritis

Arthritis (inflammation of a joint or joints) is the largest cause of disability in Britain. There are several types, including alkylosing spondilytis, psoriatic and crystal arthritis (gout), but the most common in women are rheumatoid arthritis and osteoarthritis. Women may look to nutritional advice either as a last resort, after they have tried every 'conventional' therapy, or to avoid relying solely on conventional medicines, using food as a 'natural' therapy.

Nutrition can bring tremendous relief to many arthritis sufferers, but it usually takes a little time to fathom out your body's individual reaction and how it can be helped by food. I see some women who are sadly suffering more than they have to with their arthritis as a result of following various extreme exclusion diets, frequently upon the advice of other professionals. Such diets hinder the body's ability to cope with the arthritis and in some cases may cause more serious problems. This chapter shows how food can most positively be used to help women who suffer from rheumatoid arthritis and osteoarthritis.

RHEUMATOID ARTHRITIS

More than a million people in Britain suffer from rheumatoid arthritis, with women affected more than men. It is thought to be a disease of the body's immune system. It generally begins with a feeling of swelling or pain and stiffness in the joints, which is usually worse in the morning. The joints most commonly affected are the wrists, hands and feet.

As time goes by, the chronic pain and more general physical and emotional strain make the task of dealing with arthritis more difficult. Many women end up suffering from some degree of disability and some may even develop lung, skin, liver and kidney problems directly connected to severe arthritis.

A good diet can be designed to eliminate or reduce symptoms and avoid any long-term complications that may arise as a result of either the arthritis or the steroids that many take to control inflammation and pain. There are lots of remedies around, including those encouraging you to put yourself on exclusion diets or to use enemas. But in order for nutrition to help rather than hinder, your nutritional plan has to be carefully executed. You could become severely malnourished if you just start eliminating foods. Malnutrition may cause more serious problems both in the short and long term. This chapter outlines the advice that I frequently give to my patients. If you feel you need more detailed advice, do consult a dietitian.

First of all, there are a few general guidelines.

GENERAL ADVICE

• TRY GENTLE EXERCISES TO KEEP YOUR JOINTS MOBILE AND LESS PAINFUL

Generally the less pain you experience, the less the degree of disability you may experience at a later stage. Ask your doctor to refer you to a physiotherapist, who can teach you how to do stretching and strengthening exercises, and may also be able to arrange for you to exercise in water of the appropriate temperature. Many women find it easier to exercise in water as the buoyancy and warmth of the water helps your body move with less pain. Perhaps your local hospital has a hydrotherapy pool or there may be a special class that will help you feel at ease in the water. Follow the instructions of a professional physiotherapist, as he or she will be able to tell you which exercises can help your body; the wrong sort can put strain on your joints and damage them further.

• REST YOUR JOINTS REGULARLY

This is particularly important when your arthritis is flaring up badly. Remember, though, that too much rest will cause your joints to seize up, so it's a question of getting the balance right.

• TRY TO GET THE MOST FROM YOUR PERIODS OF REST

Feeling stressed and tense will aggravate your symptoms. Listening to relaxing music, soaking in a warm bath or having a remedial massage can work wonders. Aromatherapy oils can be marvellous. Aromatherapists particularly recommend benzoin, which gives a lovely, lazy, warm sensation, marjoram, which helps you to switch off, and vetiver, for tranquillity.

• WATCH YOUR WEIGHT

There are a number of reasons why women with arthritis are prone to weight gain (see page 117). However, excess weight puts added pressure on the joints. Remember it's much easier to stop weight piling on in the first place, by being aware of what you eat, than to try to lose it later. See the chapter on Weight loss for more advice.

• TAKE YOUR PAINKILLERS WITH OR AFTER FOOD

This helps prevent any gastro-intestinal discomfort. Have a chat with your doctor if you feel you're not getting the right sort of pain relief, as there are plenty of options available.

• LISTEN TO HOW YOUR BODY IS FEELING

On occasions when you feel sensitive or vulnerable, try not to push yourself or expose yourself to anything that you feel may upset you. I especially encourage women who suffer from food intolerance-related symptoms not to have any food that they feel may aggravate their symptoms. This may sound obvious, but some women crave the thing that they know or suspect they shouldn't have when their system is vulnerable.

Most arthritis sufferers go through good and not-so-good periods. Try to organize your schedule so that when you're feeling good, you stock up the freezer and cupboards, then when you're not feeling so good you have everything at your disposal.

NUTRITIONAL MANAGEMENT OF RHEUMATOID ARTHRITIS

There are several alterations you can make to your diet to help reduce symptoms of rheumatoid arthritis, and I shall discuss these further on the following pages, but if any dietary modification is going to work, you need to have firm foundations on which to build and execute the changes. For further information, read the sections on What your body needs and Healthy eating for life, in Part One.

• EAT A WELL-BALANCED DIET
This means eating small meals at least three times a day, which should provide carbohydrate, fibre, protein and plenty of fresh fruits and vegetables.

• CHOOSE FOODS AND A STYLE OF EATING THAT HELP KEEP YOUR WEIGHT WITHIN THE IDEAL RANGE
See page 46 for your ideal weight range. Excess weight causes more pain and discomfort. Make sure that your food doesn't rely too heavily on convenience foods, which tend to contain a lot of fat and sugar, making it far too easy to pile on excess weight.

Too low a body weight may be a sign that you are not receiving the necessary quantities of nutrients. If you are worried about your weight being too low, I suggest you first follow all the advice in this chapter and then if you're still worried consult a dietitian.

• MAKE SURE THAT YOUR DIET IS RICH IN VITAMINS AND MINERALS

The general vitamin and mineral intakes of many of my female patients with rheumatoid arthritis are frequently rather poor. This may be as a result of having a poor appetite, especially during times when energy levels are low and pain levels high, or because conventional 'convenience' foods, which may be all you feel you can cope with, are generally not particularly rich in vitamins and minerals.

With patients taking medication such as steroids, there is the added problem that the medication may interfere with the metabolism of vitamins and minerals – folic acid, vitamin E, pyridoxine (vitamin B6), zinc and magnesium seem to be particularly badly affected – and may cause malabsorption, so your body doesn't absorb as many nutrients. Taking steroids also increases the amount of zinc, calcium and protein the body excretes. The lack of these nutrients may have a detrimental effect on your immune response, so it is very important for you to make sure that you eat a well-balanced diet, with plenty of fresh fruits and vegetables. If you feel that you need a vitamin or mineral supplement I suggest that you consult your doctor or dietitian.

• CHOOSE YOUR YOGHURTS CAREFULLY

Acidophilus and bifidus cultures may cause your arthritis symptoms to flare up. Despite the fact that these cultures have been found to help many health problems and should generally be included as part of a well-balanced diet, they are not always helpful to arthritis sufferers. Other yoghurts, including 'live' (unpasteurized) ones containing lactobacillus, should be fine, as lactobacillus does not seem to affect arthritis.

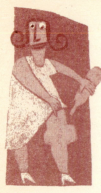

As a grape ripens, the sun causes the level of acidity in the grape to decrease and the sweetness to increase.

Different grape varieties have different patterns of ripening, but usually wines from southern Europe and the Mediterranean are less acidic than the crisp northern European wines. Wines from Italy are typically low in acidity. However, even if a wine tastes sweet, it doesn't necessarily mean that it contains less acid, it could just be that your perception of acidity is masked by the sweetness.

A good soft red would be a wine made from the Merlot grape, as it tends to have low tannin and acidity levels.

- **DO NOT DRINK MORE THAN TWO TO THREE CUPS OF COFFEE, TEA OR COLA-BASED DRINKS A DAY**
These drinks contain caffeine and tannins which inhibit the absorption of vitamins and minerals from the gut. (See page 60 for more information and other drinks to try.)

- **WATCH YOUR ALCOHOL INTAKE**
While alcohol isn't bad for you, many women with rheumatoid arthritis find that wines with a high level of acidity may aggravate their symptoms.

- **EAT ORGANIC PRODUCE WHENEVER POSSIBLE**
Although the evidence is not beyond question, a lot of my patients find that they feel a lot better if they avoid foods high in additives (most convenience and fast foods). This may be because highly processed foods often contain a lot of salt, which may lead to the body becoming dehydrated, or as a result of the chemicals and hormones that are present in non-organic produce. Dehydration may aggravate both pain and feelings of weakness, so drink at least two litres (four pints) of water every day to avoid becoming dehydrated.

- **CHOOSE DISHES THAT INCORPORATE PLENTY OF GOOD INGREDIENTS**
This leaves less room in your diet for high-fat and high-sugar ingredients. Combinations of fish, shellfish, rice and vegetables are perfect. Mediterranean-style dishes such as risotto, pasta or paella are all good examples.

DIETARY MODIFICATIONS

Whether dietary modifications such as avoiding red meat or citrus fruits have been scientifically proven or not, they can give you the feeling of being in control. Control over your destiny is a very important part of anyone's life, especially if you are unwell and having to receive help from professionals. The modifications that have gained the most acclaim involve fish oils, the oil of evening primrose and food intolerances.

Science cannot explain why these work for some women and not others. Just as everyone's metabolism responds differently to the hormones and chemicals released during severe episodes of arthritis, similarly food affects people in various ways. It may well be that the intake of different substances benefits the immune system. Sometimes these changes encourage weight loss, which alleviates your symptoms. As long as you feel that the diet is helping, the power of your mind often means that you feel less pain and stiffness.

Whatever the reason, while it is always important to feel that you are doing what you can to help yourself, don't compromise your overall health by eliminating foods without thinking about the overall balance of your diet. It is to some extent trial and error, but any changes must be treated seriously and conducted with care. Check your nutritional intake by consulting a dietitian; if he or she is happy that you can do yourself no harm by following a particular dietary regime, go ahead, but listen to their suggestions if they feel there are areas of concern.

• FOOD INTOLERANCES

There is a great deal of controversy over the role that food intolerance plays in rheumatoid arthritis. Many doctors dismiss the food intolerance theory, but I have seen miraculous results in patients who had either given up hope with conventional treatments or who have decided they want to do something other than taking drugs or simply putting up with pain.

The range of unproven diets covers excluding all meat, eating no cooked foods or grains, excluding citrus fruits, excluding diary products or drinking whole milk before meals. The respective theories being that meat causes arthritis, raw foods, especially vegetables, cleanse the body, citrus fruits contain too much acid, dairy foods aggravate arthritis or, alternatively, milk helps to lubricate the joints. Although I don't hold any of these theories myself, I feel they are worth a try, as long as your diet remains well balanced after you have excluded items to reduce your symptoms.

Rather than cutting out a food completely, I think it is a good idea just to reduce the quantity of the particular food you eat in one go, as it could be that your body doesn't react as badly if the quantity decreases.

If you then feel that you want to experiment with excluding the food completely for a trial period, do it for no longer than two weeks, but do it thoroughly, avoiding all products containing the food.

Red meat Many women find that avoiding red meat and offal reduces their symptoms. It is relatively easy to do this, since there are so many other protein providers, such as chicken, fish, pulses and grains. However, you should be aware that meat provides women with a very valuable source of iron, so if anaemia is an area of concern, I suggest you read the chapter on anaemia for other iron providers.

Dairy products I suggest that you firstly avoid having large amounts of milk, cheese, butter or yoghurt in the same meal. Spread your intake of these foods evenly through a daily healthy eating pattern. For instance don't have a cheese sandwich followed by a yoghurt. If you decide to exclude dairy products from your diet you need to avoid milk, cheese, butter and yoghurt, and all foods containing milk products, such as pastries containing butter, cream sauces and many cakes and biscuits. See the chapter on allergies for more details. If you avoid dairy products you should take a 500 mg calcium supplement every day, to help maintain calcium levels in your bones.

Citrus fruits A lot of women find that their symptoms improve when they avoid citrus fruits: oranges, lemons, grapefruits etc. You should, however, make sure that your vitamin C intake is satisfactory by eating plenty of green leafy vegetables, kiwi fruits, blackcurrants and other foods rich in vitamin C. See What your body needs in Part One.

The anchovy, a
member of the
herring family, is
native to the English
Channel and the
Mediterranean.
The best are said to
come from the area
between Nice in
southeastern France
and Catalonia in
northeastern Spain.
They are usually sold
as fillets, preserved in
brine or oil, and used
as a topping for
pizzas and canapés,
or as a flavouring in
salads such as salade
niçoise. However, you
can occasionally buy
them fresh, which is
my favourite way to
eat them, grilled or
used in risotto.

Coffee and tea Most women can easily cut down the amount of tea and coffee they drink. See page 46 for alternative drinks.

Convenience/highly processed foods I believe everyone, not just arthritis sufferers, should keep their intake of these foods to a minimum. They are generally high in additives and salt, which in some people can cause allergic reactions and dehydration. Instead we should base our eating patterns around fresh foods, preferably organic produce, reserving convenience foods for occasions when we can't get fresh produce.

• FISH OILS

Many women with rheumatoid arthritis find that a diet rich in oily fish helps reduce the amount of pain, discomfort and overall disability. This occurs as a result of the presence of certain types of omega-3 fatty acids, which significantly reduce the inflammatory process. The fish that are highest in this type of fatty acid include mackerel, herrings and kippers, sardines, pilchards, salmon, anchovies, mullet, trout and tuna. I would therefore encourage you to try to eat an oily fish dish three to four times a week. The tangy, sharp flavours of lemon, garlic, spinach, watercress and rocket complement oily fish recipes.

If you do not eat fish, either for moral reasons or because you dislike it, then take a fish oil supplement. The correct dosage would be 600 mg of omega-3 fatty acids per day. You should find this concentration of omega-3 fatty acids in a carefully prepared supplement, but it is very important to make sure that it has this level of omega-3 oil and not just any fish oil. The equivalent dosage is found in approximately 50 g/2 oz of herring or 300 g/11 oz of cod.

• EVENING PRIMROSE OIL

Some people find that evening primrose oil has a similar beneficial effect to the omega-3 fatty acids. Evening primrose oil contains gamma linoleic acid (GLA), which seems to have the effect of reducing the inflammation process and resulting pain. You can get GLA only from evening primrose oil tablets, as there does not appear to be any equivalent dietary source of GLA. The current recommended dosage of evening primrose oil is 2000–4000 mg per day, usually taken in 500 mg tablets.

• KEEP YOUR SATURATED FAT INTAKE DOWN

One important point is to remember to keep your saturated fat intake low when taking evening primrose oil or eating a diet high in omega-3 fatty acid. Some of the fatty acids in animal fats, such as butter, cream, cheese and fatty meat, compete with the omega-3 fatty acids and the GLA inside the body. If you have too much animal fat in the diet, the beneficial fatty acids cannot work effectively, therefore their potential healing power is lost. However, a generally healthy eating pattern should already be low in saturated fats.

I must point out that the evidence supporting oily fish and evening primrose oil is not conclusive; ultimately, the choice is yours.

• OTHER SUPPLEMENTS

There is quite a lot of ongoing research into the role of copper, zinc and nicotinamide supplements, but I am not convinced of their efficacy or safety. Many people believe that wearing a copper bracelet can alleviate arthritis symptoms, and it doesn't seem to harm anyone. It may be that a small amount of copper seeps through the skin and in some way reduces the inflammatory response of the body.

TROUBLESHOOTING

• ANAEMIA

Anaemia is quite common in women who suffer from rheumatoid arthritis. This may be a result of a poor dietary intake of iron or folic acid, two important nutrients needed to keep the blood healthy. If you find that you are anaemic then I suggest you boost your intake of iron, folic acid and vitamin C and follow the advice given in the chapter on anaemia.

Anaemia may also result from gastro-intestinal bleeding that may occur when you take a lot of non-steroidal painkillers. Unfortunately these drugs irritate the stomach lining and in some cases may cause it to bleed. To reduce this you should always eat something before taking any painkillers.

Sometimes when your body is generally inflamed, as is frequently the case with rheumatoid arthritis, your production of haemoglobin, the substance in the blood that carries oxygen, may be rather low. This can cause anaemia, but you need specific advice from your doctor as to how to tackle this, as it is a little more complicated than just boosting your intake of certain foods.

• EXCESSIVE WEIGHT GAIN

Excessive weight may be one of the most difficult problems to tackle when you have rheumatoid arthritis. Steroidal medication is frequently used for women with either acute episodes or a chronic level of pain and inflammation. Steroids help to reduce the inflammation but unfortunately they may also cause your appetite to increase and in some people may cause fluid retention. The weight can creep on before you have really noticed. Frequently pain relief is the major thing on your mind and a little bit of excess weight is low down on your priorities. Unfortunately, once the weight has crept on, it is very difficult to get rid of. With pain and disability, you can easily get into the vicious circle of being unable to get around a lot to burn off the calories, which in turn causes depression. All of these can make you more inclined to indulge in comfort eating. It's much easier to stop your weight from creeping on, simply by being aware of what you eat, than to try to lose weight later. Look at the chapter on Weight loss for tips as to how to reduce your weight gradually and how food can be delicious without being high in calories.

• **STEROIDS AND DIABETES**

Taking steroids may also cause a few problems with the control of your blood sugar level. This may result in your becoming diabetic. If you find this is the case look at the chapter on diabetes to see how you can minimize the problems. In general terms it just means that you have to be extra diligent in eating a healthy, well-balanced diet.

OSTEOARTHRITIS

Osteoarthritis is the most common form of arthritis in Britain. It is a degenerative condition that seems to be more common as you get older, but it is by no means just a disease affecting the elderly. Other factors which are thought to play a role in the onset of osteoarthritis are climate, heredity and other metabolic conditions in the body.

Osteoarthritis occurs as the cartilage in the joints wears away and in its place new bone material grows beneath the worn cartilage. This then leads to abnormal bone formations, which may cause pain when moving the joint. With the growth of the bone tissue, the joints may become twisted and generally deformed. This in turn places stresses and strains on muscles and nervous tissue, leaving you with problems moving around or in considerable pain at times.

GENERAL ADVICE

• **ASK YOUR DOCTOR TO DISCUSS GOOD PAINKILLERS**

Remember that there are many excellent drugs on the market, so if you're not happy with the degree of pain you're suffering, ask for advice. Don't assume that nothing can help.

● **USE HEAT, COLD OR SOUND WAVES TO HELP REDUCE THE PAIN**

This may be as simple as taking warm baths or applying hot water bottles or ice packs (or the good old bag of frozen peas) to the joints. You can also get special sound wave machines that help your body to produce natural painkilling substances. Ask your doctor or local physiotherapist to find a suitable supplier.

● **ASK YOUR DOCTOR OR DIETITIAN TO REFER YOU FOR SPECIALIST ADVICE FROM A PHYSIOTHERAPIST OR OCCUPATIONAL THERAPIST**

They can both help make your life a lot easier to manage by giving you advice about exercises to do, and equipment you can buy that is specially designed to aid everyday tasks. There are some fantastic gadgets available, including specially adapted cutlery, saucepans and cooking equipment, plugs and adaptations on telephones.

● **DIET AND OSTEOARTHRITIS**

There is unfortunately no special diet that will cure osteoarthritis, but I would recommend that you read the advice for rheumatoid arthritis to help you establish a well-organized pattern of eating.

The fish oil and evening primrose oil supplemented diets which some rheumatoid arthritis sufferers find helpful do not seem to benefit osteoarthritis sufferers so much. However, some of my patients find that a diet rich in oily fish helps reduce their symptoms. There is no physiological reason for this, but it may be that there is a little bit of inflammation around your joints or more likely it is the fact that you are doing something to help yourself. Being stressed about being unable to do anything for yourself doesn't help anyone to feel well, so if you would like to try this, then go ahead.

Some women also find that wearing a copper bracelet helps reduce osteoarthritis symptoms.

There is no evidence to support any food exclusion diets in the cure or relief of osteoarthritis, but there has been some encouraging research into the green-lipped mussel from New Zealand; the results are not yet conclusive.

Although, sadly, food can do little to help osteoarthritis, there are certain problems that can be addressed through the foods you eat.

• WEIGHT GAIN

Women with osteoarthritis may find that their weight increases quite significantly, partly as a result of not being able to move around easily, and also because if you have problems preparing meals you may well be eating more biscuits, cakes, crisps, take-aways and convenience foods, which tend to be rather high in fats and sugars and low in other important nutrients.

Because osteoarthritis commonly affects your 'load-bearing' joints, the knees and hips, if you do carry excess weight you will place an enormous strain on these joints. You can reduce the stress and consequent pain and maintain your mobility by ensuring that you don't gain excess weight; and if you have, you should do as much as you can to lose it.

Many surgeons advise patients who need surgery to replace knee or hip joints to reduce their body weight before undergoing surgery. Losing weight increases the success rate and also reduces the risks associated with a general anaesthetic.

Please don't think that you can go on a 'crash diet' to lose the weight. They don't work in the long run and it is especially important not to try them when you need all your strength to keep your joints mobile. Instead, read the chapter on Weight loss and then if you need more advice see a dietitian. There are so many delicious dishes that contain all of the nutrients you need without exceeding your body's requirements.

Above all, keep in touch with your doctor and dietitian. We much prefer to know about the little things that are concerning you than to sort out huge problems, which could have been avoided or at least minimized had we had a little more warning.

• RECIPES TO RELIEVE ARTHRITIS

Carrot and orange soup

Spinach borscht

Pea, mint and lettuce soup

Sorrel soup

Smoked salmon ramekins

Smoked mackerel pâté

Apple, dolcelatte and walnut strudel

Spinach and goats' cheese soufflé

Spinach and watercress roulade

Tomatoes stuffed with olives, garlic and parsley

Broccoli with roasted tomatoes

Tabbouleh

Chicken with melon, grapes and asparagus

Smoked cheese olive pasta

Monkfish and mussel paella

Salmon and asparagus risotto

Smoked mackerel and spinach fishcakes

Salmon and celery kedgeree

Salmon and lemon lasagne

Chicken stroganoff with tarragon

Coconut chicken

Garlic and herb chicken

Fruit compote

Lemon syllabub

Oranges in caramel

Blackberry and raspberry fool

Fig and ginger parkin

Flapjacks

5 Cancer

Cancer is a big subject: not for nothing is it called
The Big C. For most people who have not encountered
it close to, it is one of the most sensitive illnesses to
discuss and one that is so loaded with fear and other
issues that it is difficult to address the subject with ease.

However, as with most things that worry us, the
more the topic is discussed and out in the open, the
more the fear of it dissipates. Very often, women who
come to see me having recently learnt that they have
cancer are surprised to find that they are one of many
who have also had it at some time. There is an increasing
number of women who have survived cancer of all types
and degrees, or who are learning to live with it. Equally
important, there are those who are learning how to care
for cancer sufferers on a daily basis.

I believe that the speed with which a return to health
is achieved is greatly affected not only by which foods
are eaten, but how they are eaten. In this chapter I want
to instil you with confidence as to how to use food to its
best advantage. There are many delicious dishes and combinations of foods that will boost your nutritional status
and in consequence your immune system. Most importantly, this can be achieved in a way that offers culinary
excitement and prevents the cancer patient from becoming the socially isolated sufferer, the spectator at the feast.

Eating the right foods improves the body's immune
system and its ability to fight off cancerous cells. In
simple terms eating more or less of certain foods may
help prevent certain cancers.

The right food will also help stabilize you and
energize you if you have to undergo surgery or toxic
therapies, radiotherapy or chemotherapy. If a cancer
patient, particularly when undergoing toxic therapy, is
inspired by the food that is prepared for them, if they
look forward to their next meal, however small, if every
dish that they are served is a delight to the eye as well as
the palate, they are more likely to survive.

'What some call
health, if purchased
by perpetual anxiety
about diet, isn't
much better than
tedious disease'.
George Dennison
Prentice (1860)

Most importantly, remember that if you are suffering from a condition where chemotherapy and surgery dominate, food can be used as an empowering tool. Here is an area where you can make a decision over what you feel would be good to eat, to help yourself. You shouldn't feel as if you have to eat something that is prescribed and alien to what you fancy. Obviously there are certain foods that with my experience I can encourage you to eat to help the situation, but you should always use food positively and not let it become a negative, eat this or die, situation.

In this chapter I shall address the nutritional guidelines that can be helpful in preventing cancer. I will then discuss the problems that may occur for those who have been diagnosed as having cancer and are undergoing treatment, and how the problems can be helped and even redressed by what they eat.

• **GENERAL GUIDELINES**
Before I look at the food issues, I feel it is important to give a few general guidelines that may help reduce your chance of developing cancer. Don't just focus on one point and hope that this will be enough; look at how your whole life shapes up. Food, marvellous as it is, cannot work well for you unless you allow it to, by setting the scene both psychologically and physically.
• If you are a smoker, get on a programme to help you stop.
• Try to avoid areas where you could be exposed to passive smoking.
• Always wash fresh fruit and vegetables before eating, as nitrites and nitrates used in fertilizers, chemicals from vehicles and industrial pollution can build up on the skins and become carcinogenic. I would encourage you to eat organic produce if possible, as it is grown without artificial fertilizers. Environmental toxins (including those from cigarette smoke) are believed to be a major cause of free-radical damage within the body. Free radicals are highly reactive molecules that attach themselves to cells within the body, causing them to behave

abnormally, which may manifest itself as premature ageing or in the formation of cancerous cells.

• Take regular aerobic exercise (brisk walking, running, swimming) at least three times a week.

• Check your body regularly so that you can monitor any changes; after all, you know your own body better than anyone. Look out for any lumps, particularly in the breasts. The majority of lumps found in the breasts are non-cancerous, but it is a good habit to check the breasts and surrounding area once a month, after your period.

• Above all, respect your body and the food you put in it, but do not let what you eat become an obsession.

FOOD AND CANCER PREVENTION

Professional opinion throughout the world strongly supports the role of nutrition in helping to prevent major diseases such as cancer. There is a definite correlation between what you eat, your general state of health and your ability to resist disease. With regard to cancer, there are many forms and types, some more prevalent in certain parts of the world, some linked to genetic inclination. Whether or not you have a family history of the disease, what you eat still has a most important part to play in your ability to resist it. No single food will prevent all cancers, but particular foods and eating patterns can certainly help ensure that your chance of developing a malignant tumour is reduced. I suggest you follow the healthy eating principles of a low-fat, high-fibre diet featured in Part One, with emphasis on the following points:

• EAT FOODS RICH IN FIBRE

This means eating plenty of fresh vegetables and fruit, pulses and wholegrain breakfast cereals, oats, wholegrain breads, wholewheat pasta and brown rice. A diet rich in fibre has many health advantages, one of which is its ability to help the body to eliminate free radicals (see General guidelines, above).

Lentils, chickpeas and the huge variety of dried and canned beans that are now available can be served as side dishes or salads, in soups and many excellent vegetarian dishes.

Most importantly, you should include at least one portion of fresh vegetable or fruit in every meal and try to have a total of five servings of fruits or vegetables every day. This sounds a lot, but get into the routine of doing it. Enjoy choosing from all the different varieties in the shops throughout the seasons and eat them raw or cooked, preferably as lightly as possible. If you are eating out, be sure to order some fruit or vegetable as a side dish.

Fresh fruit and vegetables are important providers of both fibre and the antioxidant vitamins A (as beta-carotene) and C. For beta-carotene, look to dark green, orange and yellow vegetables and fruit such as carrots, peppers, melons, apricots, spinach, watercress and parsley. Rich sources of vitamin C include citrus fruits, blackcurrants, strawberries, cranberries, kiwi fruits, peppers, cabbage, spinach and watercress.

• INCLUDE PLENTY OF GARLIC

Garlic has very special nutritional qualities, discussed in more detail on page 33. It has powerful anti-cancer properties, which are shared to a lesser extent by other members of the Allium family such as onions and leeks. Apart from its use as a flavour enhancer, it can be enjoyed as a vegetable in its own right, in soups or roasted and spread on bread.

• VARY YOUR PROTEINS

There have been a few studies that have linked diets high in red meat with an increased risk of cancer. Although the evidence is not conclusive, I feel that all women, and especially those with cancer, should try not to have red meat more than three times a week. This is not to say that meat is bad for you, as it is a good source of many minerals and vitamins, but it should form just a part of your diet rather than being a dominant factor.

Other good sources of protein are chicken and other poultry, game, fish and shellfish, eggs and pulses.

There is another advantage of eating a lot of fish rather than meat. Fish oils, particularly those found in oily fish such as mackerel, herrings, tuna and salmon, are rich in omega-3 fatty acids and omega-6 fatty acids. These are thought to have a powerful 'cancer-slowing' action, as well as being helpful in the relief of arthritis (see separate chapter) and in cleansing the blood of unwanted cholesterol (see the chapter on high blood cholesterol).

• ENSURE YOUR DIET IS LOW IN ANIMAL FATS
Animal fats, when consumed in large quantities, have been shown to be linked to the development of various cancers, including those of the breast and the colon. Breast cancer is thought to be more prevalent in women who have a diet high in animal fats and low in fibre.

The artificial hormones used to promote rapid growth in the production of many of our animal foods are also starting to cause concern. Try to buy organically reared animal products whenever possible, as they don't use artificial hormones or any of the other chemicals whose effects on the body are highly questionable.

• CHOOSE FOODS THAT ARE NATURALLY LOW IN FAT
Avoid fatty meats, oily and fried foods and those coated in copious amounts of creamy, cheesy or oily sauces. This does not mean trying to eat only fat-free products, as these are often tasteless and it is in any case unnecessary and virtually impossible to do. Just keep the amount of fats low, particularly animal fats such as butter, cheese and cream. However, I don't suggest that you replace butter with a hard margarine or low-fat spread. These may contain high levels of trans-fatty acids, which if eaten in large quantities may lead to an increased risk of some cancers. Instead, use small amounts of natural oils such as olive, sunflower and safflower.

- **ENSURE YOUR DIET IS LOW IN SUGAR AND SWEETENERS**
It has been implied that if you eat a lot of products that contain artificial sweeteners such as aspartame and saccharine you may be at an increased risk of developing cancer. I recommend that you use only small amounts of products that contain the 'naturally occurring' sugars: glucose, fructose and sucrose, rather than artificially sweetened foods. For a sweet taste, eat sweet ripe fruits as snacks or use a small amount of fruit sugar to provide the sweetness you want in dishes. For instance, purée mango, sweet English apples, apricots or pears and add to natural yoghurt, rather than choosing an artificially sweetened yoghurt or one with a ladle of honey added. Most of us have become accustomed, through eating junk food and sweetened drinks, to a much higher level of sweetness than is natural. You will do well to wean yourself off the sweet taste as often the more you have the more you want. You will be surprised how quickly you can get used to less sugar.

- **DRINK PLENTY OF WATER**
You should aim to drink at least two litres (four pints) every day. This has many health advantages and is essential for the fibre in your diet to work effectively.

- **KEEP YOUR INTAKE OF TEA, COFFEE, HOT CHOCOLATE AND COLA-BASED DRINKS LOW**
These all contain caffeine, which inhibits the body from absorbing the nutrients from the food you eat. Stick to a maximum of two or three cups a day of caffeine-containing drinks. See page 62 for more information and alternative drinks.

- **EAT A SMALL POT OF 'LIVE' YOGHURT CONTAINING ACIDOPHILUS AND BIFIDUS EVERY DAY**
These organisms occur naturally in the gut and are believed to reduce the likelihood of developing cancer, either through the production of anti-cancer substances or more generally through the boosting of the immune system. By taking additional acidophilus and bifidus

you will encourage the growth of the good bacteria in your gut. If you can't eat yoghurt you could ask your dietitian to suggest another source.

However, people who have a sensitive immune system or gut, including those with irritable bowel syndrome, Crohn's disease or arthritis, should seek advice before taking these flora as they could potentially irritate their gut and immune system.

FOOD'S LINK WITH CANCER

There has been much research over the past few decades that has strongly and not so strongly linked certain foods with the development of various forms of cancer. There are frequently a number of other contributing factors, and it should not be thought that a certain food directly causes cancer, but there are a few points worth noting.

• BOWEL CANCER

Fat in the diet has a direct connection with cancer. In particular there is an increased risk of developing bowel cancer if you have a diet that is high in fat and low in fibre. The presence of fibre helps the body to produce beneficial anti-cancer substances and to break down harmful cancer producers.

• STOMACH CANCER

Research in countries such as Japan and Sweden, where there is a high consumption of salty foods such as smoked fish and pickled vegetables, has suggested that excess salt may put you at an increased risk of developing stomach cancer. However, it is not as simple as the salt causing cancer; a contributory factor is that in these countries there is also a lack of fresh fruits and vegetables. Fruit and vegetables provide fibre and beneficial vitamins such as vitamin C; if these are lacking in the diet and there is a high salt intake, there is a potential risk of stomach cancer. You do not need to avoid salty foods completely, but you should make sure that you eat plenty of fibre, such as fresh fruits, vegetables, wholegrain cereals and breads, to cushion the potential cancer-causing effect created by the salt.

• MOUTH, THROAT AND LIVER CANCER

There is a link between a high consumption of alcohol and cancer of the mouth, throat and liver. This is particularly significant in countries where the consumption of alcohol is high, such as France, but we should all keep our alcohol intake down to the recommended 21 units a week for women (see page 64). You are also at greater risk if you smoke.

• BREAST CANCER

Breast cancer has some connection with a diet high in animal fats. It is thought that the reason for this lies in the relationship between oestrogen, the female sex hormone, and fat. Oestrogen may be produced in greater quantities or reabsorbed in greater quantities by women used to a diet high in animal fats. High oestrogen levels have been associated with an increased risk of breast cancer. Keeping your saturated fat intake low can protect your body against many ills, including cancer and heart disease.

There is also a link between fibre and breast cancer. If your fibre intake is low you are at greater risk. The presence of plenty of fibre in the diet not only helps to eliminate cancer-related toxins, it can also produce cancer-fighting substances in the body.

IF CANCER HAS BEEN DIAGNOSED

The last thing you will probably want to do at this time is eat. All during the period from first knowing that there is something not quite right to being told the awful truth, fear is the uppermost emotion in everyone. Fear is always there, just below the surface, ready to undermine the strongest and most determined of characters. With fear comes the nausea, the feeling of not being able to touch a thing, except maybe the bottle or the sleeping pills, in order to block it all out. During this time most of all, you need help and understanding from those around you. I often find that recently diagnosed cancer patients, even if they are not in a life-threatening situation, will lose an inordinate amount of weight in a short time, largely because the fear, worry and stress renders them unable to eat properly. It is at this time of course that you most need to keep your strength up, as you embark on surgery and/or a course of chemo- or radiotherapy.

FINDING AN EATING PLAN

Once the initial period is over and you can face up to what is happening to you, you will want to find out what you can do to help you through the treatment and stop the cancer spreading. You will probably start to think about what it was you did and what you were eating that caused all this. As far as food is concerned, there are many, often conflicting, ideas and research findings which may or may not help you to fathom it all out. The truth is, no one can be certain why cancer starts and there may be a multiplicity of triggers that turn some cells carcinogenic. Many people feel better if they can do something about it, once it has been diagnosed, and doing something about your diet is the most obvious place to start.

• RADICAL DIETS

Many people feel that they want to cleanse their system and start afresh. There are numerous books on the subject that suggest grapes only, caffeine only and other radical diets. Many medical professionals advocate a fruit and vegetable only diet, or advise a macrobiotic diet of whole grains such as brown rice, pulses, vegetables and seaweed. Though the need to cleanse is perfectly understandable, there is no need to go to such lengths. If you want to try it, it will do no harm just for a few days, except perhaps to your taste buds. However, I believe that such a dramatic change from your regular diet will not support your return to health and good spirits and may even be psychologically damaging. I would encourage you to eat plenty of fresh fruit and vegetables, as this is always a vital part of a good eating plan, but by all means augment this with whole grains, cereals, pulses, lean meat and other animal proteins, especially fish. You can eat healthily and still eat well!

• SOURCES OF NUTRIENTS

If you decide to go on a strict fruit and vegetable diet, there is a potential problem in getting all the nutrients you need. Although they are high in vitamins and minerals, with pulses, grains and nuts providing other valuable nutrients, including protein, some of these nutrients are not as easily absorbed by the body as those found in animal products. This means that you would have to eat a good deal more fruit and vegetables to obtain the same amount of nutrition. This can be difficult when you are feeling low and not inclined to eat very much. At these times it is quality, not necessarily quantity, that counts: little and often is a good maxim to follow. Without realizing it, you could become malnourished, simply because you have drastically reduced the concentrated sources of nutrients in your diet.

It is most important to ensure that your energy and protein intake is high. Not only can some of the treatments for cancer put you off your food and reduce your desire to eat, they can also increase your need for certain important nutrients. You need to ensure that your body has the resources with which to fight the cancerous cells and any other infections that may beset you when your defences are low. On good days you need to build up a reserve to sustain you on the days when you really cannot face any food at all. So my advice is to keep eating a well-balanced healthy diet, but make a special effort to include some of the concentrated sources of protein such as meat, chicken, fish, cheese, as well as some vegetables, pulses and fruits, with additional sources of concentrated energy as reserves to help you keep going through the low times. Examples of high-energy foods include cheese, lean meat, poultry and fish, milk, cream and thick creamy yoghurt, natural sugars from fruit and honey, and even small amounts of chocolate.

• AVOID ANY RISK OF FOOD POISONING

When you have cancer it is important to realize that your system is taking quite a battering and you should think twice before you eat anything that could be a little risky. After all, even when we are healthy, fighting a bout of food poisoning takes quite a lot out of our system. I suggest that you read the section on food poisoning in the chapter on pregnancy. Be particularly aware of the following:
• Never eat food from tins that are damaged or 'blown' at the ends.
• Rice in restaurants is sometimes cooked and then left in a warmish environment, where bacteria may develop. Always make sure that any rice dish is really hot, as these bacteria are killed by thorough reheating.
• Uncooked eggs and poultry that is not thoroughly thawed or cooked may cause salmonella poisoning. Mayonnaise and some sauces should be avoided.
• You need to be careful at parties, where food is often left in warm rooms, encouraging the growth of bacteria in rice, eggs, soft cheeses and chicken.

TROUBLESHOOTING

• LACK OF APPETITE

Please do not worry if you have the odd day when you cannot manage to eat as much as you feel you should. This does not necessarily mean that your prognosis is worse. Take things easy and treat yourself to something different, refreshing and light. It is more than likely that you will feel a little stronger and more inclined to eat the following day. However, if you find that you are going for a few days without feeling like eating, you must seek medical advice.

Be easy on yourself, do not overface yourself with food. Do not even try to keep to the routine of three good meals a day; little and often is the way to keep your strength up. If you have a large serving and cannot eat it, you are reinforcing the sense of negative achievement. Go for a variety of tasty little dishes that are prettily presented, and if you find you can easily get through a small portion you can always have seconds!

Go ahead and spoil yourself. At this of all times, don't hold back, except perhaps on too much alcohol! Imagine you are convalescing from a tummy upset and make a list of the things that you might find tempting or comforting; it could be scrambled eggs, poached eggs on toast, poached white fish, creamy mashed potato, or tasty little crispbreads with caviar. Then add something that lifts your favourite food out of the everyday. For example, you could make scrambled eggs into a treat by adding flaked smoked salmon. Turn poached eggs into gourmet Eggs Benedict by serving them on a slice of ham with a little hollandaise sauce. Buy a piece of delicate sea bass or salmon and poach it in white wine with a slice of lemon. Make those mashed potatoes extra creamy and add a spoonful of double cream or sour cream to your caviar. By doing this, you are making your favourite dishes more nutritious, so that even though you don't feel like eating very much, the nutritious value of each mouthful is increased.

Plan to stimulate your appetite. If catering just for yourself, in fact particularly if you are eating on your own, make a special effort to plan. Try to avoid finding yourself with the cupboard bare and only a box of cereal staring bleakly at you! You will be surprised how much more appetizing your food will seem if you have thought through what you are going to prepare, looked at recipes and listed some ideas. Going to the shops to buy some fruit, browsing the counters to see what unusual things you could try, even dipping into the ready-prepared chilled meals section, will stimulate your taste buds before you eat the dish itself. If you are preparing food for someone else, discuss recipes together, bring home a selection of things that have caught your eye and talk about what you can prepare with what you have found.

Plan for variety in the day. Keep your taste buds on their toes with plenty of variety during the day in terms of colour, taste, temperature, texture and tantalizing smells. Buy a selection of breads and rolls, with nuts, herbs, olives, sun-dried tomatoes, cheese or spices. Store them in small portions in the freezer and take them out when you fancy one, perhaps to accompany a compatible dish, for example a walnut roll with a cheese soufflé. Warm bread and rolls before serving to bring out tempting aromas and subtle flavours.

Try serving a selection of dishes to make a meal, perhaps by giving two or three tartlets different fillings or by putting together lots of little samples of cheeses, vegetables or dips.

Use those moments when you are peckish. Keep little bowls of nibbles around the house or on your desk at work. This will stimulate the appetite, and tempt the eye and the taste buds. If you have little cheesy biscuits, dried apricots or raisins, roasted almonds, tasty crisps, filled dates, crystallized fruits or chocolate truffles readily available and at your fingertips, you will be surprised how you will graze your way through quite a lot without realizing!

Have some unusual fruit sliced and arranged in a small bowl. Keep it covered or chilled in the refrigerator ready for you to pick at. Similarly have some raw vegetables such as sticks of carrot or celery, strips of peppers or cauliflower florets together with a dip of soy sauce in a small ramekin dish. Make up some canapés such as cheese-filled celery sticks or little chicken satay sticks. Keep a supply of little treats such as tasty creamy cheeses, smoked salmon, pastrami, delicate pâté, potted

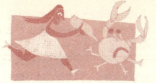

shrimps or potted Stilton and a pot of caviar (or lumpfish roe). Remember to respect food hygiene. Enjoy browsing the delicatessen for your treats, you deserve them!

To stimulate your appetite, share a half bottle of sparkling wine between two of you or have a glass of dry sherry or Montilla. Exploring sherries can be fun as there are many different styles: a fino sherry is lighter than an amontillado, and the fullest dry style is oloroso. It is worth paying a little extra for a good dry sherry. Always buy from a shop which has a rapid turnover of sherry, as they don't store for ages. It is also a good idea to buy a half bottle, as fino in particular should be drunk within a week or two of opening. Serve lightly chilled.

You could also try some of the unusual fruit wines such as elderflower, gooseberry, plum, blackberry, or a glass of sparkling elderflower water.

• CHANGING TASTE BUDS

When undergoing drug treatment or radiotherapy your taste buds may change. See this as a journey of discovery and don't despair. Enjoy experimenting with different flavours and spices.
• If you feel your food lacks flavour, try marinating meat or fish in wine, vinegar, rosemary or a similar robust herb before cooking.
• Some strongly flavoured foods such as red meat may start to taste unpleasant. If this happens, choose alternative protein dishes based on cheese, fish or egg.
• Drinks such as tea or coffee may also taste unpleasant, which is particularly frustrating if you are in the habit of having them at certain times of the day. Search around for alternatives, try different herbal hot drinks until you find one that works for you. Orange blossom essence or elderflower cordial are particularly refreshing either hot or cold, perhaps diluted with sparkling water. A glass of freshly boiled water with a slice of lemon or lime cleanses the palate and provides the comfort you want from sipping a hot drink.

• ALCOHOL?

Check with your doctor first and if he or she approves, have a tipple when you feel like it. Alcohol may help increase your appetite. Take a little time to choose a nice wine or aperitif before your evening meal. Choosing the wine will help stimulate your taste buds, but do not overdo the consumption, as you want to stimulate your appetite, not drown it!

• FEELING PERMANENTLY FULL

This feeling may occur even when you have had nothing at all to eat. It is most uncomfortable as the feeling of being already full and bloated conflicts with the guilt of feeling you should be eating to keep up your strength. It is most frequently associated with radiotherapy to the stomach or following surgery to have part of the stomach removed.

• Make a point of sitting down to eat all your food and laying a place and taking time to eat your main meals. Do not rush eating and try not to take your evening meal on your knee while watching television. Rushing food may mean gulping and taking in unnecessary air, which contributes to bloatedness.

• Resist drinking while you are eating. Drinks fill your stomach with fluid rather than valuable nutrients. Leave half an hour after you have eaten before you have a drink; by then the stomach will have more space available. If you find it hard to swallow food without a drink, try taking small mouthfuls and choose food with a sauce.

• Break up the day by having more than three meals. At any time of day delve into appetizing snacks that are small but concentrated in nourishment.

• SORE OR SENSITIVE STOMACH

If you are being prescribed non-steroidal or other strong painkillers, you may find that your stomach has become slightly sensitive and rather sore. I suggest you also read the chapter on indigestion.

• Always take something to eat at the same time as your medication.

• Try to eat a little something every three to four hours, to line your stomach.

• Choose food that is quite bland, not too highly spiced. Many soups come into this category: French onion soup with Gruyère cheese-topped croûtons would be a good choice. Alternatively try eggs baked in little ramekin dishes, perhaps with a little flaked salmon trout and chopped dill.

• Avoid the temptation to drink milk. Although this gives you an initial cooling effect, it makes your stomach secrete more acid in the long run. Instead try Arabic mint tea or orange blossom tea (see page 62).

• STOMACH AND BOWEL UPSET

If you tend to suffer from constipation, whether infrequently or more permanently as a result of treatment, the chapter on constipation will help you. If diarrhoea is the problem, keep to lower-fat, non-spicy dishes that are not too high in vegetable fibre. Avoid fried foods and instead choose dishes based on pulses, pasta, potatoes or eggs. Avoid having too much dairy food in one go. Sometimes the concentration of lactose (milk and sugar) can upset the stomach. Instead of a glass of milk or a tub of yoghurt, use these ingredients combined with others in a recipe.

• DRY OR SORE MOUTH

This uncomfortable state can arise if you have had radiotherapy, especially to the mouth or throat. It can also happen if you are undergoing chemotherapy, because the cocktail of strong drugs kills many of the good cells as well as the cancerous ones. Chemotherapy can also affect the rapidly proliferating cells in the mouth and stomach which in turn can affect the natural process of salivation.

• Have on hand plenty of refreshing, tangy juices and drink these throughout the day. Homemade lemonade, mango juice, freshly squeezed lemon or grapefruit juice may seem rather a chore to prepare, but a jug full of juice chilled with plenty of crushed ice is a real pleasure to pour out. Add a sprig of fresh mint and you'll be surprised at the delicious flavour it brings out. Another favourite from summer days in France is mint or grenadine syrup (or even – occasionally – crème de menthe) filled up with sparkling lemonade.

• Sorbet or ice cream, bought or homemade, can be very mouthwatering.

• Instead of grills, roasts and fries, or very hot or spicy foods, choose casseroles of lean meat, or fish poached or baked in a wine or cream sauce.

• If you find vegetables such as carrots or broccoli difficult, try them puréed in a food processor with a little cream.

• SWALLOWING DIFFICULTIES

Many women undergoing cancer treatment have difficulty in swallowing (dysphagia), but their tolerance to the type and consistency of food varies considerably. Some may have trouble managing pieces of meat or crispy bread or crackers, whereas others may be able to take only liquid foods.

• Choose something you really feel like eating and do not feel you have to liquidize everything. An interesting recipe will encourage you to eat with your family or your companion, not become isolated with a dish of 'slop' food.

• If you can face only soft food, think of soups, soufflés and mousses.

• Sometimes a chilled drink will help the action of swallowing. Take small sips while you eat, as this can help ease the food down. If your doctor approves, sip something alcoholic. Otherwise have a pure fruit juice or chilled water.

• SICKNESS AND NAUSEA

If you are feeling sick the last thing you will want to do is to eat, but a little nourishment, however small, is very beneficial.

• If you have someone to help you cook, let them do it when you are not feeling well. Staying away from the kitchen helps as cooking smells can sometimes put you off your food.

• While food is being prepared, go for a little stroll or a longer walk if you are up to it. Not only will the fresh air perk up your appetite, it will also reduce the stale feeling of sickness.

• If you are not quite well enough, simply sit outside or by an open window. Breathe in the air and fill your lungs; you will feel more lively and more keen for your meal.

• If you are eating alone, settle for cold dishes, which can be more appealing when you are feeling sick. Try something flavoursome such as smoked salmon with dill and cherry tomatoes, a small bunch of chilled grapes, some fresh figs. Warmed walnut bread or olive bread is delicious with a slice of cheese.

COOKING AHEAD

Keep stores of favourite things in your freezer for days when you do not feel up to much else or are coming back from hospital. On a happier note, you might also like to keep some food ready for having friends round or days when you want to take advantage of the weather and go out for a picnic.

Take the opportunity to stock up your freezer when you are having a good day, or put some time aside with a friend or your partner to prepare a quantity of food for the freezer.

• FOODS TO SOOTHE AND HEAL

Garlic bean soup

French onion soup

Pea, mint and lettuce soup

Leek and potato soup

Carrot and orange soup

Chilled mint and cucumber soup

Baked garlic bruschetta

Guacamole

Aubergines au gratin

Smoked salmon ramekins

Smoked mackerel pâté

Eggs Benedict

Tomato, pesto and olive omelette

Spinach and goats' cheese soufflé

Warm goats' cheese salad

Grilled vegetable salad

Chicken with melon, grapes and
  asparagus

Smoked haddock spinach pasta

Pasta with wild mushrooms

Smoked fish casserole

Salmon and lemon lasagne

Salmon and asparagus risotto

Garlic and herb chicken

Winter vegetable and oxtail pie

Sausage, tomato and potato pie

Coconut ice cream

Brown bread ice cream

Praline ice cream

Apricot filo tart

Boston brownies

Lemon cake

Banana cake

Carrot cake

6 Constipation

Ask any health practitioner what is the most common bodily preoccupation of the majority of women and they will answer, the bowels. Constipation is for many women a distressing problem that can amount to a fixation. For decades, women have worried about flushing food through their system every day, hence the widespread use of laxatives and enemas. Young women obsessed about their body weights frequently come to see me, worried that they will get fatter if they don't empty their bowels at least once a day. They don't realize that chronic constipation is often a result of abnormal eating habits and a negative relationship with food.

The majority of women feel that their bowels just won't work properly or are lazy. Many refer to themselves as being constipated if they don't empty their bowels every day. While it is not a good idea to go for days without having emptied the bowel, studies in recent years have lent much support to the theory that not everyone needs to have a bowel movement every single day. For many, every other day is perfectly normal. While the symptoms and 'clogged-up' feelings are not pleasant, the odd day of not going to the loo will not harm either your bowel or the rest of your body.

If you know your own habits, the rhythms of your body, you will know whether your system is running smoothly. If you know that you tend to get a little constipated when you are abroad or feeling stressed, you can treat yourself, but if your bowels are causing you pain, discomfort or distress of any sort, or your regular habits change significantly, then you should visit your doctor. Otherwise, constipation is one complaint that you can do quite a lot about.

• WHAT EXACTLY IS THE BOWEL AND HOW DOES IT BECOME CONSTIPATED?

The bowel is the part of the intestine that retains waste matter prior to expelling it from the body. It is a large muscle which contracts and relaxes in ripple-like waves, a motion known as peristalsis, causing the food to be squeezed through, from top to bottom. The dictionary definition of constipation is 'difficulty or infrequency in evacuating the bowels'. If faeces or waste remains for too long in the bowel, too much water is absorbed from it so it dries and hardens, making the faeces more difficult to expel.

When the bowel is continually overloaded in this way the bowel muscles lose their tone and constipation becomes chronic. If you have to strain all the time when you go to the loo, the blood vessels around the bottom of the bowel can become irritated and swollen. This leads to haemorrhoids or piles. Once you have piles and constipation you are likely to suffer from a great deal of discomfort, and you can also lose blood.

Constipation may be a symptom of an underlying disorder, such as an obstruction of the bowel by a tumour or structural deformity. However, it is more likely that the problem is caused by several other more minor conditions, which cause bowel muscles to lose their normal ripple-like, propulsive ability.

NUTRITIONAL CAUSES

• LACK OF FIBRE

The most common cause of constipation is lack of fibre in the diet. Fibre works by absorbing water as it passes through the digestive system, allowing the bowel to form a soft stool which it can expel easily and without strain. It is this straining that can lead to piles and start off another cycle of problems and remedies. Excess pressure can cause weakening of the bowel lining or the small blood vessels in the bowel to burst, causing small amounts of bleeding. The presence of a soft stool stimulates the bowel into action.

Fibre in the diet comes from the cell walls of plant foods: fruits, vegetables, grains and pulses. In order to gain maximum benefit from the fibre, the cell walls need to be intact. For this reason the highest fibre foods are those that have not been heavily processed. For example, wholemeal bread has more fibre than white bread. In white bread, as with other white flour products such as pasta or pastry, the outside of the wheat grain has been removed to give a fine-textured flour. The fibre content is therefore low.

High-fibre foods include fruits and vegetables, wholemeal bread, whole-grain cereals, pulses, nuts and seeds (pumpkin, sesame, sunflower). There are plenty of sources of dietary fibre beyond the traditional plain bran cereals.

If fibre is the answer to preventing or curing your constipation, it clearly must form part of your daily eating plan. Our mothers, and their mothers before them, understood the need to include ingredients that are naturally high in fibre in the family diet. It is worth the effort to re-establish this habit, and there are tips on how to do this on pages 146–147.

• LACK OF WATER

The other most common cause of constipation is lack of water. Many women eat fibre, particularly in the form of wholemeal bread, but they just don't drink enough water to enable the fibre to swell within the gut, form a soft stool and stimulate the bowel into moving. If you feel that your fibre intake is high and yet you still don't seem to be able to go, I suggest you drink at least two litres (four pints or eight to ten large tumblers) of water every day. Tap water is fine, although you may prefer still or sparkling mineral water; add a slice of lemon or lime or a few drops of elderflower syrup or orange blossom water for variety.

In these days of central heating and air conditioning, the body loses a lot of water. Constipation is one of the first signs of an imbalance in the amount of water in the body. Keep some water on your desk at work or on the side at home, so you don't have to venture far to get it.

Once you get into the habit you will be amazed how great you feel. Some women worry that this will make them bloated, but in fact increasing the amount of water you drink can greatly reduce the feeling of being bloated, full and 'stuck'.

Although coffee can help correct constipation in the short term, by causing the smooth muscles in the bowel to relax, it also contains caffeine, which is a diuretic. Diuretics make your body lose water and hence aggravate constipation. Try to have no more than two or three cups a day of coffee, tea or cola-based drinks, all of which contain caffeine.

• INTOLERANCES

The term irritable bowel, which so many women seem to suffer from, encompasses episodes of constipation. Some women become constipated as a result of food intolerances, for example to eggs, wheat or lactose. Eliminating the offending food can cure the constipation, but these conditions are more unusual and are dealt with in the chapter on allergies.

NON-NUTRITIONAL CAUSES

• EMOTIONAL AND PHYSICAL TENSION

While constipation is more often than not caused by a diet lacking in fibre and water, many women are troubled by a stress-related type of constipation, which seems to occur when they are very stressed, tense or emotionally upset. Since the bowel is a muscle, it is very receptive to the stress hormones such as adrenaline. Fluctuations in the levels of stress hormones can upset your normal bowel function. Some women find that when their level of stress rises their bowel goes into 'shut down' and they become constipated. However, others find that stress has the opposite effect; it can cause their bowel to relax or go into spasms which expel the waste matter. While nutritional advice can minimize adverse effects, the underlying stress needs to be addressed.

• OVERUSE OR INAPPROPRIATE USE OF LAXATIVES

Many women fail to realize that laxatives, designed to relax the bowel, can have the opposite effect. Laxatives should never be taken on a daily basis. Only if all avenues of the diet have been explored should one turn to laxatives, and this should be done with medical approval.

There are three types of laxatives:

• Bulking agents, which contain gels that swell within the gut. Their action is very similar to the way in which fibre works within the bowel, in that they swell and help form a soft stool. An example is Fibrogel. These are the most gentle kind of laxatives.

• Irritant-based laxatives such as Sennacot, which irritate the bowel and make it expel the waste matter.

• Propulsive laxatives, which affect the muscle function within the bowel. They cause the muscles to contract and relax, like normal peristalsis.

The choice of laxative is very important, as an inappropriate choice can potentially aggravate rather than help. Much depends on the cause of your constipation and your general diet. Some women are unable to eat a diet rich in fibre, for instance if they have a gut problem or an intolerance to a type of food. For these women the bulking laxatives can be very useful. Other women have a mechanically based constipation problem rather than a lack of fibre. In these cases the irritant or propulsive-based preparations are more appropriate. You should always consult your doctor before you start taking a laxative, as he or she will be able to assess your specific needs.

Nutrition should always be addressed as part of your treatment plan. I often see women who take a lot of laxatives rather than look to foods to help them. There are several problems with taking too many laxatives, which includes the so-called natural plant or fruit-based preparations sold in health food shops:

• Your gut can become lazy. The bowel can start to rely on the laxative to stimulate it into action, rather than trying to work itself.

• The irritant laxatives can cause your bowel to become very sensitive and sore. This can lead to piles and bleeding.

• You could lose food too quickly. This usually occurs only with the propulsive or irritant types, and it is very important not to overdose on them, as you could end up with chronic diarrhoea.

• Your body can become nutritionally depleted. Your bowel contains beneficial bacteria which provide the body with vitamins, notably vitamin K, and other anti-cancer substances, which are very important in reducing the risk of bowel cancer. If you overuse laxatives the bowel will flush out these bacteria, along with vitamins and minerals such as potassium and sodium, and disturb their natural healthy balance in your body.

• IGNORING YOUR URGES

As with any other muscle in the body, it is important to train the bowel and listen to the signals it gives you. Keep your bowel muscles strong by allowing them to empty when they give you the signal. Don't 'hold on' too long, as this can cause increased pressure in the lower bowel and rectum. If you get into this habit, in the long run you could suffer from incontinence or piles. If you are holding on because it is painful to empty your bowel, do see your doctor as you may have an underlying problem.

SOLUTIONS

If you are inclined to be constipated you should persevere with re-educating yourself to eat more fibre, especially fresh vegetables and fruits. Browse the vegetable sections in supermarkets and market stalls regularly. Be open to the possibilities of what you see and be adventurous in your cooking. Don't be afraid to ask for extra portions of vegetables in restaurants.

In addition you should include some form of exercise as part of your weekly routine. Thirty to forty minutes of aerobic exercise three days a week must be considered the minimum, four or even five days would be ideal. The easiest form of exercise to plan into your day is a 'power walk', brisk walking in appropriate footwear and comfortable clothing, unless you can discipline yourself to run or can afford go to a gym or health club regularly.

• NUTRITIONAL TIPS

Try to have some fibre provider five times a day. The following tips give you ideas as to how you can easily and deliciously achieve this by including fruit and vegetables throughout the day. High-fibre foods also include wholegrain bread and cereals. Wholemeal bread need not be dry, heavy and boring: there are now many fantastic varieties in the shops.

A word of warning. Food manufacturers have realized that we should be looking for high-fibre foods and they label their products accordingly. Unfortunately, they very often mix a lot of sugar and salt in with the high-fibre cereals. So while they are high enough in fibre they are not altogether 'healthy'. While the sugar and salt levels in high-fibre breakfast cereals are not a problem for some people, they can be for others, including women who are trying to lose weight. You will generally get just as much fibre and less sugar and salt in a couple of slices of wholegrain bread as in a bowl of high-fibre breakfast cereal. I recommend that you stick to one of the non-deluxe cereals and add your own sweet touch with some chopped fresh fruit. Wholegrain rolls with butter and a pure fruit spread or a slice of lean ham can also make a delicious high-fibre start to the day.

• Keep a compote of fresh and/or soaked dried fruit in your refrigerator to serve over cereal in the morning or to snack on in the evening.

• Turn a simple piece of fruit into a more stimulating snack by chilling it slightly and slicing it on to a plate. Give it visual appeal by arranging it in a fan or perhaps by adding a couple of strawberries or a few slices of kiwi fruit.

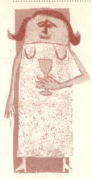

There are a few wines that taste like the good old-fashioned remedy for constipation: syrup of figs. Liqueur Muscat and liqueur Tokay from Australia are known as 'stickies', because they are very thick and sweet, oozing with fig, date and Christmas pudding flavours. Commandaria, the sweet tawny wine from Cyprus, also tastes of figs.

A glass of Madeira may also get things moving. The four main types – Sercial, Verdelho, Bual and Malmsey – are usually sold as dry, medium-dry, medium-sweet and sweet Madeira.

• Grilled or baked vegetables, plain or scented with herbs such as rosemary, thyme or basil, with a good-quality olive oil drizzled over the top, are quick, easy and delicious. Cut a variety of vegetables – aubergines, peppers, courgettes – into chunks and grill or barbecue them.

• Puréed vegetables, steamed or lightly boiled then whizzed in a blender, are remarkably easy to prepare, keep well and can be prepared in advance, which is helpful for those out at work all day. However, do not keep them in the refrigerator for more than a couple of days, as the vegetables tend to oxidize and lose their colour, going slightly brown. Vitamins, particularly folic acid, are also lost in storage.

• Puréed vegetables can be put together in intriguing and delicious combinations. A purée of parsnips and Bramley apples, for instance, is wonderful served with a flavoursome oily fish such as grilled or poached mackerel.

• Puréed vegetables look particularly appetizing when served in little scoops, made using an ice-cream scoop. Try this at a dinner party with different coloured vegetables such as carrot, parsnip and spinach.

• **SHORT-TERM NUTRITIONAL MEASURES**

If you have a day when you feel a little shock treatment is needed, a cup of good coffee and a bowl of stewed prunes should produce quick results! Many people find that coffee, with or without the prunes, helps to get the bowel going in the morning, as caffeine is a smooth muscle relaxant. As long as you do not have in excess of two to three cups a day, this should do no harm. However, large amounts of coffee can have adverse side effects, which are discussed in more detail on page 60.

Prunes are one of the well-known traditional remedies for constipation – and they really work! Here are some ideas for featuring prunes in your eating plan.

• Buy a jar of prune butter or make it yourself by puréeing pitted prunes (canned, ready-to-eat or soaked dried prunes) in a blender. You can spread this on wholegrain bread for breakfast.

- Top your morning breakfast cereal with chilled cooked prunes and a spoonful of natural yoghurt.
- Add prunes to a casserole, such as chicken, rabbit, beef or oxtail.
- Stuff tenderloin of pork with pears and prunes.
- Add chopped prunes to cock-a-leekie soup.
- Chop prunes into pickled red cabbage.
- Soak a bowl of prunes in Armagnac and serve with vanilla ice cream.
- Rub plump prunes with Kirsch and serve with dark or white chocolate sauce.
- Dip brandy-marinated prunes in melted chocolate, allow to harden and serve with cinnamon-flavoured sauce.
- Prune and chocolate tart.

• WATCH YOUR BODY WEIGHT

For some women, a side effect of having a high-fibre diet is that they lose weight. By boosting their intake of fibre-rich foods, which are bulky and generally relatively low in calories, they may lower their calorie intake. This can be helpful for women who need to lose weight, but for others it can be a problem. If you find you are losing weight and don't want to, I suggest you enhance your high-fibre meals with cream, butter or cheese, or serve custard or thick yoghurt with sweet foods. It's easy to increase your calorie intake, for instance by grating fresh Parmesan cheese over a ratatouille dish, or serving scoop of real dairy ice cream with your bowl of fruit compote.

• BALANCE YOUR DIET

Foods that contain fibre also contain substances such as phytates and oxalates that bind vitamins and minerals in the gut and therefore reduce their absorption. It is very important to make sure that you eat a wide range of foods, as outlined in the section What your body needs, to help minimize this effect. Consult your dietitian if you're worried.

• COLONIC IRRIGATION

Fans of colonic irrigation believe in the use of enemas to relieve constipation and other health problems. While enemas can be useful in extreme cases, I do not recommend them, certainly not without medical supervision. Injecting large amounts of water or potions such as coffee or camomile juice into your bowel causes irritation and pressure in an area that is very sensitive. It was not designed for this. Overuse of enemas, whether natural or drug-based, frequently leads to more serious health problems such as incontinence and piles. Always look to food first.

• RECIPES TO GET YOU GOING

Hummus

Goats' cheese and aubergine crostini

Baked garlic bruschetta

Minestrone soup

Lentil soup

Carrot and orange soup

French onion soup

Chicken with melon, grapes and
   asparagus

Pear and walnut salad with
   watercress

Warm salad of spinach, French
   beans and pancetta

Grilled vegetable salad

Gado gado

Vegetarian chilli

Yam biryani

Baked pasta with ratatouille sauce

Prawn curry

Smoked mackerel and spinach
   fishcakes

Garlic and herb chicken

Winter vegetable and oxtail pie

Tropical dried fruit salad

Fruit compote

Mixed fruit with butterscotch
   sauce

Fresh figs filled with almond cream

Blackberry and raspberry fool

Apple and fig crumble

Prune and bitter chocolate tart

Fruit cake

Date and walnut cake

Banana cake

Carrot cake

Flapjacks

7 Depression and feeling down

Everyone feels down on occasions, but depression can range from normal feelings of being fed up and low to more serious feelings of utter hopelessness, which may escalate into suicidal thoughts or actions. While food alone cannot cure clinical depressions, all of us at some time turn to food for comfort.

We each have our own individual perception of comfort foods, the foods that, in one way or another, make us feel happier. Many of the foods we use to cheer us up are connected with our childhood, when sugary foods were frequently given as treats and rewards. As adults we can, when we feel down, remember good feelings by eating the foods associated with those occasions.

In this chapter I explore the physiological reasons why particular foods make us feel happier, why bad eating habits and some foods make us depressed and how drugs we use to relieve depression affect our eating habits. I will help you to choose foods to make your life happier. Some of you will be just going through a low period and need a nutritional overhaul to make sure that you come out of your blue feeling as soon as possible. Others with acute or chronic depression may find the lightness of the general tips a little inappropriate, but I suggest you read the whole chapter in case there is be something to be gleaned. Depression is not something you can just snap out of. There are many factors involved, physical, genetic, emotional and social, some of which may require professional help to manage.

HOW CAN FOOD AFFECT YOUR MOOD?

Within the brain, chemicals help transmit messages from one nerve cell to another. There are two such substances, known as endorphins, that seem to affect our moods: serotonin and norepinephrine. The body makes these particular endorphins from the food we eat and therefore we can, to a certain extent, raise the level of these substances in the brain by eating specific foods. Scientifically, food has been shown to have a significant effect on raising the mood only if the level of serotonin or norepinephrine is low before you eat. It is not a question of the more you eat the happier you become ad infinitum, but more a question of helping to reverse a negative feeling that has been induced by a low serotonin or norepinephrine level.

• THE SUGAR 'HIGH'

The main source of these endorphins is sugary and carbohydrate-rich foods. This is why some women seem to feel happier after they have eaten sweets, cakes, biscuits or chocolate. They would get the same effect from honey, jam, soft drinks, sugary breakfast cereals, white bread, white rice and pasta.

The problem with eating these foods to pick you up is that sugary foods are very rapidly absorbed into the blood. The sudden influx of sugar causes a serotonin rush, but unfortunately a secondary effect is a rapid production of insulin. Insulin is a hormone that breaks down sugar so the body can absorb it. If there is a sudden rise in the sugar level in the blood the insulin quickly breaks it down, leading to a drop in both sugar and endorphin levels. This leaves you feeling even lower than you were before.

Some women seem to be particularly sensitive to this effect and experience extreme reactions. The swings in endorphins make them agitated, moody and aggressive. These women should therefore avoid very sugary foods. Some even have to avoid all sugar-containing foods, but this is an extreme precaution.

For the majority of women, I suggest you either have a meal as soon as possible after you eat the sugary food or choose to get your sugar/endorphin 'fix' from a more slowly absorbed carbohydrate. Good examples include a wholemeal biscuit or a piece of wholegrain bread, with or without a topping of fresh fruit or low-sugar fruit spread. Having a little fibre intertwined with the sugar in these foods helps to lift a low, but not too fast. You are therefore much more likely to stay happy for longer.

Serotonin and norepinephrine are not only made by sugary and starchy foods. They are also made from tryptophan and L-phenyl alanine, amino acids present in certain protein foods. It has been suggested that people with low intakes of these amino acids are more likely to feel down, or even suicidal. However, this finding is not that easy to act upon. Even if you increase your consumption of the relevant protein foods, your brain can only use a certain amount of the amino acids. Some scientists suggest that we might take a supplement of tryptophan and L-phenyl alanine. I do not advocate this, as the supplements may cause stomach upset and diarrhoea. Instead, I suggest that you make sure that you are having a healthy, varied, balanced diet, to avoid exposing your body to a lack of serotonin or norepinephrine.

VITAMIN AND MINERAL DEFICIENCIES AND DEPRESSION

Feeling happy is not just a matter of including serotonin- and norepinephrine-producing foods in your eating plan. There are also important links between vitamins, minerals and depression. Certain vitamin and mineral deficiencies may cause you to feel low or aggravate depression. In addition, if you are depressed and not eating properly, your body may become deficient in various nutrients, setting up a vicious circle which should be broken. Certain situations make you more prone to develop a nutrient deficiency. Do any of the following apply to you?

REHYDRATION
DRINK
This is a lot cheaper
than buying
commercial drinks.
The salt and sugar
help the body
to balance the
potassium level.
Take ½–1 teaspoon
of glucose and a
pinch of salt and
dissolve them in
100 ml/3½ fl oz
of hot water.

• you haven't been eating properly, either as a result of too much work or generally not feeling like eating
• you've been feeling unwell or just 'not yourself'
• you take drugs, whether as regular medication or a short course of antibiotics
• you feel stressed
• you've been drinking copious amounts of alcohol or drinks such as coffee and tea, which can cause your body to excrete more nutrients
• you've had a particularly heavy menstrual period.

If you are worried that your depression may be a result of a deficiency, you should ask your doctor to arrange a few simple blood tests. Deficiencies of the B vitamins and vitamin C are most commonly associated with feeling depressed. This happens mostly with people who have been depressed for some other reason and as a result neglected their diet. What your body needs, in Part One of this book, lists good sources of these vitamins. The two mineral deficiencies most likely to cause depression and generally feeling run down are iron and potassium. If you suspect you have iron deficiency anaemia, consult your doctor and see the chapter on anaemia.

• POTASSIUM DEFICIENCY
This mineral deficiency often follows a period of being sick or suffering from diarrhoea. It can be corrected or prevented by having small sips of clear liquids while you are suffering, or by taking rehydration fluids. You can buy these from a pharmacist or make them yourself (see margin).

You should not take any supplementary source of potassium except under the guidance of your doctor. If you are recovering from a bout of sickness and diarrhoea, the first step once your body can tolerate food should be to include lots of green leafy vegetables and fresh fruits. If you can't quite manage a meal, have a banana, a glass of tomato juice or freshly squeezed fruit juice. All of these foods are rich in potassium.

• POOR APPETITE

The 'catch 22' situation is the fact that depression may put you off your food. Over time this may cause your body to become deficient in vitamins and minerals, which in turn makes you feel even more depressed. This is not an easy thing to overcome, as very often the last thing you feel like doing when you're depressed is to go out shopping to buy fresh foods which need assembling into a meal. If you have been depressed for quite a long time and know that you haven't been eating properly, this is one occasion when I feel it is a good idea to take a vitamin and mineral supplement. But remember that your body absorbs vitamins and minerals most efficiently from a varied and balanced diet, so don't see the supplement as an alternative, just as a short term extra. Equally, don't think about 'mega-dosing' in the hope of curing depression; it won't work and could cause serious problems. Seek the advice of your dietitian or doctor.

ACTION PLAN TO HELP YOU GET OUT OF A 'LOW'

• TREAT YOURSELF WELL AND CHOOSE YOUR FAVOURITE FOODS

A low time is not always the best time to start a weight-reducing programme. Have a deliberately indulgent day and then see how you feel tomorrow. However, some women would feel happier if they lost a little weight or cleansed their bodies of 'junk'. If this applies to you, use this time to begin a programme of weight loss or detoxification. You may like to start with the weekend cleansing programme in this book. Whether you are aiming to lose weight, detoxify or simply turn over a healthy new leaf, your primary goal is to enjoy your food. Never punish yourself for indulgences.

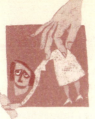

A glass of sparkling wine is a perfect pick-me-up. It doesn't have to be Champagne; there are plenty of other excellent sparkling wines at around half the price. Those made in California, Australia and New Zealand are particularly good, or try sparkling Saumur or Blanquette de Limoux from France or Cava from Spain.

If you think of port as a particular treat, you might like to try the 'weighty' wines from northern Italy, called Recioto or Amarone della Valpolicella.

- **TRY TO MAKE SURE THAT YOUR MEALS ARE NUTRITIOUS**

Look at food as an empowering tool and eat a well-balanced diet, including plenty of fresh vegetables and fruits, wholegrain cereal foods, some lean meat, fish, chicken and dairy products. A delicious and healthy eating pattern will help you both physiologically and psychologically.

- **DON'T WORRY IF YOU FEEL YOU NEED A SHORT BURST OF 'HAPPINESS'**

An occasional sweet, cake, chocolate or piece of lovely fresh bread won't hurt; a helping of a delicious pudding such as sherry trifle, treacle tart, chocolate pudding or ice cream can really cheer you up. However, remember that very sugary foods will give you a mood crash if you don't follow them with some fibre. Better still, eat something that is both sweet and high in fibre. Fruit – fresh, dried or compote – or oat biscuits are good mood boosters.

- **KEEP YOUR MEALS SIMPLE**

Luckily, some of the most comforting foods are the simplest to prepare, such as soups, bangers and mash (but make them good-quality sausages and luxurious creamy or buttery mashed potatoes), omelettes, tomatoes and cheese on toast (try walnut, olive or onion bread). But don't feel guilty if you choose a ready-prepared meal. It's much better to have something easy and hassle-free than to slave over the stove and end up feeling tired and potentially more depressed.

- **MAKE EATING A PLEASURABLE EXPERIENCE**

Try to include a variety of fresh, colourful and tasty ingredients in your meals. Explore food markets and look at magazines and cookery books for inspiration. Eating out with a friend in a relaxed restaurant or in the fresh air in a beautiful spot can also help lift your mood.

• ENJOY A LITTLE ALCOHOL

A glass or two of delicious wine, a long, cool gin and tonic, a good whisky or brandy may be just what you fancy, so go ahead. You must watch that you don't consume too much alcohol, however, as the problems don't go away. They'll still be around in the morning, along with a hangover. Try not to get into the habit of turning to alcohol as the only thing to promote relaxation or happiness. Don't cut yourself off from all of life's other enjoyable experiences: music, exercise, books, plays, films. There is no need to feel guilty about having a tipple, though, and in addition, alcohol can help to give you an appetite, which could help if you are feeling too low to be bothered to eat.

• AVOID LARGE AMOUNTS OF COFFEE AND TEA

One really good cup of tea or coffee may be just what you need, but that doesn't mean that two or three cups will be better. The caffeine in these drinks can cause some people to become agitated or even cause a headache. Caffeine also increases the excretion of vitamins and minerals from the body, which doesn't help in times of stress and feeling low.

• TRY REGULAR EXERCISE

Exercise can help you to feel happier as it causes your body to produce endorphins such as serotonin (see page 151). It can also act as a step to help you out of the situation that is making you feel down. Bringing you into contact with other people can help on occasions. You may feel a further benefit of exercise if you're worried about excess weight gain, which may happen if you are taking anti-depressants (see below). Exercising gives you an opportunity to burn up some calories and can distract you from comfort over-eating. In a situation when you feel hopeless and helpless, exercise can be an empowering activity.

If you have followed all of the advice given in this chapter and still don't feel any happier do consult your doctor. He or she will be able to put you in touch with professionals trained to help you conquer the depression or may suggest that you take an anti-depressant drug.

ANTI-DEPRESSANTS

There are many different types of anti-depressants. The ones that most commonly affect your food intake and nutritional status are the tricyclics (such as Amytryptaline), chlorpromazine (Largactil), lithium, Prozac and amphetamines.

These drugs have various side effects and you will find that your metabolism changes because of the interactions between foods and the drug. Many women find that their appetite is affected: they may feel permanently hungry and unable to acknowledge the usual satiety feelings (see the section on the appetite mechanism). Others complain of huge sugar cravings or an increase in fluid retention. As you will appreciate, these side effects may lead to escalating weight. This may make you feel even more depressed. On the other hand some women lose too much weight when they are depressed, and do not take in enough nutrients; by taking anti-depressants they can reverse a negative nutritional balance. Other women feel slightly nauseous when taking anti-depressants and may therefore decrease their food intake. Whichever category you fall into, try to keep an eye on what you are eating and how your body seems to change. You may find it helpful to consult other chapters in this book to help you manage any unwanted side effects.

• FOODS TO LIFT YOUR MOOD

Pea, mint and lettuce soup

Parsnip and apple soup

Leek and potato soup

Carrot and orange soup

Cheese fluff

Tomato, pesto and olive omelette

Warm goats' cheese salad

Tomato and tarragon vinaigrette

Chicken with melon, grapes and asparagus

Warm duck breast and apricot salad

Smoked cheese and olive pasta

Pasta bows with courgettes

Oysters with cream and Parmesan

Salmon and lemon lasagne

Salmon and celery kedgeree

Spicy fish kebabs

Prawn curry

Coconut chicken

Somerset steak and cider pie

Sausage and bean casserole

Brown bread ice cream

Lemon syllabub

Mixed fruit with butterscotch sauce

Bread and butter pudding

Apple and fig (or other fruit) crumble

Apricot filo tart

Boston brownies

Flapjacks

Date and walnut cake

Banana cake

Lemon cake

8 Diabetes

There are two main types of diabetes: diabetes mellitus and diabetes insipidus. Diabetes mellitus is the most common form and this is the one I shall cover in this chapter. Those of you with diabetes insipidus should see your doctor and dietitian for more specific advice.

People who are suffering from undiagnosed diabetes frequently complain of an excessive, unquenchable thirst, the continual, very often nocturnal, passing of urine, tiredness, headaches and nausea.

As soon as you're diagnosed with diabetes, you will most likely hear all sorts of stories about restricted lifestyles, injections and gangrenous legs. You can ignore the horror stories. In this chapter I aim to show how to minimize the restrictions on your lifestyle by looking after yourself sensibly; much of this advice applies to all women, not just diabetics.

• WHAT IS DIABETES?

Diabetes mellitus is a condition characterized by an excess of glucose (sugar) in the blood. This happens because the body is not producing enough insulin, the hormone it needs to break down sugar. Normally, after you have eaten foods containing sugar, your blood sugar level rises, whereupon the pancreas releases insulin to help the cells absorb and use the sugar. The blood sugar level should then return to normal. With diabetes there simply is not enough insulin in the body to help the cells absorb the sugar. Some people refer to diabetics 'starving in a sea of sugar'. The sugar is present, but the body cannot use it. The most effective way for the body to get rid of unwanted sugar is by producing urine. To do this effectively, it needs a large supply of water, which is why continual thirst is one of the symptoms of undiagnosed diabetes.

The reason diabetes needs controlling is that abnormally high quantities of sugar in the blood can cause potentially serious problems. If blood sugar levels continually run high, a state which is called hypergly-caemia, in the long term several tissues in the body start to suffer, especially the eyes, kidneys and blood vessels leading to the arms and legs. However, once the sugar level is corrected and well controlled, diabetics can lead normal lives.

• UNDERSTANDING DIABETES

You need to establish which form of diabetes you have. Diabetics fall into three medication categories: those who require insulin injections, those who need tablets to stimulate the body produce to produce more insulin and those who are able to control their diabetes by monitoring their diet and don't need any medication. Experiences and challenges differ, depending on your age and the severity of diabetes, but once your doctor explains which category you fall into, you should be able to lead a perfectly happy and healthy life.

In some people the pancreas is incapable of producing any insulin, which may be diagnosed in childhood or may appear later, usually under the age of forty. In these cases, injections of insulin are necessary. This is referred to as insulin-dependent diabetes (mellitus) or IDDM. In other cases the pancreas can produce some insulin, but not sufficient for the body's needs. This type, non-insulin-dependent diabetes mellitus (NIDDM), is more common in older women, especially those who are over-weight. It may be that the pancreas gets tired or that the body's cells, particularly the fat cells, seem unable to take up the sugar. Some diabetics in this category who manage to lose excess weight (in particular, fat) find they no longer suffer from any further symptoms. In a few cases the pancreas needs a 'kick start' from tablets that stimulate the pancreas into producing more insulin. Others simply have to monitor their food intake and activity levels and balance it with the amount of insulin in their body.

Now you have seen how the metabolism of a diabetic is different from normal you can begin to understand how you can get food to work for your body.

MANAGING YOUR DIABETES

The management of diabetes has changed profoundly in recent years. Diabetics have benefited from major advances in the refinement of medication: there are better tablets to encourage the pancreas to produce more insulin and, perhaps even more importantly for women who need insulin injections, the invention of short-acting insulin.

Some insulin can provide the body with a small amount of insulin over a long period of time, usually a few hours, and is hence called 'long-acting' insulin. 'Short-acting' insulin provides a concentrated dose with a faster action in the body. Most diabetics who require insulin use a combination of the two types: a dose of a long-acting at night topped up with three doses of short-acting before meals. Women can inject themselves through their clothes using pen-like needles, which can be done sitting at the table; very few have to roll up their sleeves or retreat to the ladies' room. An exciting area of research which is currently being perfected is the invention of insulin patches. Maybe one day we'll say 'goodbye' to needles.

Whichever situation you're in, gone are the days when you had to measure fastidiously the amounts of food eaten, avoid absolutely everything containing sugar and stick to extremely rigid meal times. It's now more a question of understanding how your body and medication reacts to food and building a general healthy lifestyle around this. A good diabetic diet is high in fibre, low in fat and low in refined sugars; in other words a normal healthy diet. It just needs to be finely tuned and executed.

CONTROLLING AND MONITORING YOUR SUGAR LEVELS

The name of the game is to keep your blood sugar level constantly within the acceptable range; your doctor will discuss the ideal range for you. Many of you who control your diabetes through diet only or take tablets such as Metaclopramide or Glibenclamide won't need to take regular blood sugar measurements. You will possibly be asked to monitor your urine, which indicates levels of sugar in your blood. Insulin-dependent diabetics are often encouraged to monitor their blood sugar level regularly, by taking small samples of blood from a pin prick to the thumb. Accurate machines offer precise blood sugar level information and can assist in making appropriate adjustments to the insulin or diet. However, this should be overseen by your doctor and dietitian. Only when you are experienced at managing your insulin levels and meals should you alter either of them without professional supervision. I always encourage my female patients to keep in touch with the experts, rather than run into problems on their own.

Things can go wrong in one of two ways. Your sugar level may go too low because there is either too much insulin around in the body and/or too little sugar, a condition called hypoglycaemia. Alternatively the sugar level goes too high, because there is too little insulin and too much sugar; this is referred to as hyperglycaemia.

HYPOGLYCAEMIA

Hypoglycaemia, usually known as a 'hypo', occurs when your blood sugar drops too low. The symptoms you may experience include dizziness, headache, extreme hunger, blurred vision, sweating, pins and needles, trembling, paleness, or odd behaviour such as crying. The thing to remember is that the symptoms can come on quickly, but they are easy to correct.

They can arise for various reasons, chiefly when you

haven't eaten enough carbohydrate – bread, potatoes, rice, pasta – or you've left too long a gap between your injection of insulin and eating. (Non-insulin-dependent diabetics should not have hypos.) Your doctor should explain what to do on these occasions, but generally you should:

- **HAVE SOMETHING VERY SWEET AS QUICKLY AS POSSIBLE**

To stop a little 'hypo' from escalating into a big one (you will soon learn to identify the early symptoms), always carry a sugary snack around with you. This could be a couple of flapjacks, a piece of shortbread, fruit cake or malt loaf. Or if you don't have a sugary snack available have a drink such as fresh orange juice, a glass of milk or a full-calorie fizzy drink. Not a 'diet' drink as this doesn't contain the right sort of sugar. Forget your weight; at this particular moment, the most important issue is your blood sugar level. Recently I've seen some young insulin-dependent women who are more concerned about their weight and body image than their diabetes. This state of mind needs careful counselling, but it is important to realize that 'diet' drinks are not appropriate when you have a 'hypo'.

- **FOLLOW YOUR SUGARY SNACK WITH A NOURISHING MEAL**

As soon as it's feasible to do so, eat a good meal containing some high-fibre carbohydrate. You should contact your doctor immediately if you don't feel any better.

- **TRY TO MAKE SURE THAT SOMEONE WITH YOU KNOWS THAT YOU ARE DIABETIC**

I am not suggesting that you should make a big issue of it, but tell your friends and close work colleagues, just in case you get into difficulties. Make sure that they know the basic things to do to treat a 'hypo'. It may prevent an unnecessary and sometimes embarrassing situation or visit to casualty. If you're treating a friend whose blood sugar has dropped so low that she has lost consciousness you should:

• Turn her on to her left side.
• Make sure that her airway is clear by tilting the chin up slightly. Look to see that the tongue hasn't rolled back as this could obstruct the throat.
• Once you've done this you should call the doctor or ambulance.
• Never give someone anything to eat or drink if they are not fully conscious.

Once you've worked out how your body responds to exercise and how much carbohydrate you need to get through the day, hypos shouldn't occur. I occasionally see diabetics who live in fear of having a hypo. I try to reassure them that it shouldn't happen, provided they look after themselves and are able to get used to how their body feels and respond accordingly. If you are having frequent hypos and you've checked that you are taking the correct dosage of medication and eating properly, consult your doctor. If you often feel 'hypo-ish', see your doctor for advice, as your symptoms may indicate something else.

HYPERGLYCAEMIA

Hyperglycaemia is commonly experienced when you have either not taken enough insulin or have eaten something too high in sugar. It can also occur when you have not done as much physical activity as usual, so have used less sugar. Mild hyperglycaemia, which you detect by testing your urine or taking a blood sample, is easily corrected by avoiding very sugary foods and taking the correct amount of insulin on time.

Sometimes diabetics may have severe hypergly-caemic attacks. This could be when you're ill or unable to take your insulin. The symptoms are very similar to those you experienced before you were diagnosed, i.e. extreme tiredness, thirst and frequent urination. These are quite different to 'hypo' symptoms, so it is important to not have sugary foods as these make the sugar level go higher and the situation worse. Get in touch with a doctor as quickly as possible so that you can be treated appropriately.

If you have just the occasional episode of hyperglycaemia, you should make sure that you are doing everything possible in terms of eating the correct foods, exercising the same amount and taking your insulin appropriately. If you then do not seem able to correct it, you should seek advice. It may be that your body has changed a little and you need a slight adjustment in your diet or insulin levels. Your doctor would much rather hear from you than have you 'soldier on' and then end up in a more serious condition. However, as with hypoglycaemia, it shouldn't happen if you are paying attention to your body.

EXERCISE

As with non-diabetic women, you should include some aerobic exercise in your daily routine. Exercise helps keep the body tissues supplied with oxygen, the muscles toned, the heart healthy and the mind content. Exercise produces substances called endorphins, which create a feeling of well-being and act as an excellent stress reliever. If you don't want to participate in a regular aerobic class or work-out in a gym, you could take a more gentle form of aerobic exercise such as swimming, jogging, cycling or brisk walking. You should aim to take at least a good brisk walk, ideally lasting at least 20 minutes, every day.

A word of warning. Exercise lowers your blood sugar level, as the muscles use glucose (the sugar in the blood) as a form of fuel. You therefore need to make sure that you have enough carbohydrate to regulate your sugar level. Insulin-dependent diabetics should have a sugary snack (a handful of dried apricots or dates, some fresh fruit with yoghurt and honey, a fruity or nutty cake or biscuit) before any strenuous exercise. Some people find that delaying taking their insulin can help, but you should discuss this with your doctor before you change your routine.

FOOD GUIDELINES

There are two important targets:
• To achieve and maintain control of your blood sugar level
• To regulate your body weight within the ideal range (see the chart on page 46)
I feel it is important to point out that diabetic women should be able to join in with all 'foody' occasions. There is no need to be reminded that you are different, and indeed this is psychologically damaging. It's especially important not to isolate a diabetic child. The less fuss made, the better.

• DIABETIC PRODUCTS
There is really no need for special 'diabetic foods'. Many of them taste very unlike their non-diabetic equivalents and contain unnecessary substances. For example, many diabetic products contain a substance that can have a laxative effect. Their calorie content is sometimes higher than the non-diabetic products and this can lead to weight gain, or make it more difficult to lose weight. The weight issue exists throughout society, but for diabetic women it is slightly more complicated to keep their weight under control or to lose it safely.

Of course the food manufacturers want you to think that you are different to others and require special, expensive products, but this is not true. The majority of the nutritional and lifestyle principles for a diabetic woman are exactly the same for healthy women looking after their present and future health, set out in the sections on What your body needs and Healthy eating for life in Part One.

HEALTHY EATING FOR DIABETICS

Your daily eating pattern should consist of about three regular small meals, and plenty of water. To summarize, the meals should contain: high-fibre carbohydrate, fresh vegetables and fruit, a portion of lean protein, a small amount of dairy produce. The 'watch points', particularly important for diabetics, are: saturated/animal fats, sugary, low-fibre foods and alcohol.

• YOU NEED A REGULAR AMOUNT OF HIGH-FIBRE CARBOHYDRATE

Carbohydrates are broken down by the body to provide sugar in the form it needs to give you energy. For a diabetic, it is particularly important to choose high-fibre versions of carbohydrate foods, such as wholemeal bread or brown rice. Physiologically this is because the thick plant cell walls in these foods take longer to break down, allowing a steady release of sugar into the blood. This makes it easier to keep the blood sugar level within the desirable range. The high-fibre carbohydrates also have a greater satiety value, in other words they keep you satisfied for longer, making it less likely that you will over-indulge in inappropriate foods. (See The appetite mechanism on page 6).

Try to keep to roughly the same amount of carbohydrate in each of your meals. For both insulin-dependent and non-insulin-dependent diabetics you should work out how much carbohydrate you need, firstly to maintain good sugar levels and energy levels and secondly to maintain your weight at the level at which you feel comfortable. It will be a matter of trial and error to begin with, but should be quite easy with the supervision of your doctor and dietitian. For the majority of women it will be roughly the same size portion as you would choose had you not been told that you were diabetic.

The modern diet offers a wide variety of high-fibre, 'slow release' carbohydrate-rich foods. Think of whole-wheat breads with added grains and seeds, wholemeal

Irish soda bread, rye breads, oats for porridge or muesli, wholewheat pasta and buckwheat noodles, millet bakes, brown rice, potatoes. Don't stick to just one source of carbohydrate, but keep the quantity constant.

If you positively don't like the high-fibre versions of some foods, you should regulate your portion size of the lower fibre food and boost the fibre content of your meals with vegetables, pulses or fruits. There are no more carbohydrates or calories in white bread or white rice, it's just that the release of the sugar into the blood is quicker than in the wholegrain version. This can cause the blood sugar level to rise too high as the body is unable to meet the intake of sugar with the correct level of insulin.

• AIM TO HAVE FIVE PORTIONS OF VEGETABLES OR FRUITS EVERY DAY

A diet high in fruits and vegetables not only helps you regulate your blood sugar levels, it also has other advantages.

• It can help to prevent cholesterol from depositing in the blood vessels, which reduces the risk of heart disease and strokes. This is particularly important for diabetics, as it has been found that diabetics are slightly more prone to 'furred up' arteries. You should not worry about this, but you should be aware of it. (Note that garlic has similar benefits in keeping your arteries free of unwanted cholesterol deposits.)

• It can reduce the risk of certain cancers.

• It can reduce the signs of ageing. Research is still in its early stages, but it is apparent that a healthy, well-balanced diet that is rich in vitamins C and E (found in vegetables, fruits, grains, nuts and seeds, as well as in vegetable oil and eggs) helps keep the body, and especially the skin, looking and feeling younger.

Some people think that fresh fruit is too high in sugar for diabetics to enjoy, but this is not the case. Fruits do contain sugar, but the fibre in the fruit helps to slow down the release of the sugar. It's therefore good to get into the habit of having a portion of fruit after and in between meals. A portion would be a whole apple or a banana, about ten grapes or fresh strawberries. Make a treat of exotic fruits such as pawpaw, lychees or a generous slice of pineapple. The 'sweeter' fruits such as mangoes, bananas and figs have a little more sugar than apples or oranges, so I would suggest that you just have one of these a day.

Tinned or frozen fruits can be fine, as long as they are stored in their natural juice rather than sugary syrups.

Besides plain fruit, think about using fruit in recipes: fruit salads, compotes and puddings such as crumbles made with a wholemeal crumble topping. You could also make a fruit shake, with a single fruit or a combination of two or more, liquidized on their own or with yoghurt. (See the recipe on page 72 for some ideas.) Since they can be high in fruit sugar (fructose) I would suggest that you have just one of these drinks a day.

Aim to have at least two helpings of vegetables every day. This could be a lunchtime salad or even a sandwich packed with salad vegetables, a bowl of vegetable soup, a selection of vegetables or side salad with your evening meal.

Again, they don't always have to be fresh vegetables. Tinned vegetables such as artichoke hearts can add a special touch and extra fibre to pizzas or simple snacks. Frozen spinach or peas make excellent soup. Don't forget that 'fresh' vegetables could have been sitting on a dock side or in transit for days before you eat them, whereas frozen and tinned vegetables are subject to strict laws governing the time that elapses between picking and processing.

Remember that potatoes should be considered as part of your high-fibre carbohydrate intake.

- **HAVE A PORTION OF LEAN PROTEIN AT YOUR LUNCH AND EVENING MEALS**

Protein is needed to build healthy body tissues. Choose a lean protein, not highly fatty meat or processed foods such as cheap sausages. Fish is a good choice two or three times a week. Instead of cooking in fat, try marinating protein foods in wine, with herbs and spices. Vegetarians can get their protein from eggs, beans, lentils and other sources.

- **YOU NEED A SMALL BUT REGULAR INTAKE OF DAIRY PRODUCTS**

Dairy products are an extremely valuable source of calcium, which is an important mineral for all women (discussed in What your body needs). Dairy products don't adversely affect blood sugar levels, unless they are also full of added sugar, for example ice cream or milk chocolate.

'Live' yoghurts containing acidophilus and bifidus cultures provide not only calcium but also beneficial bacteria. I recommend that most women should eat a small pot every day (see page 34).

Vegans may substitute soya milk, yoghurt and cheese for the dairy versions. These are sometimes enriched with calcium, which is good, but they may contain added sugar (sucrose), so try to choose unsweetened ones.

- **DRINK PLENTY OF WATER DURING THE DAY**

You should try to have at least two litres (about four pints, or eight to ten large tumblers) of water a day. This will help to excrete excess sugar from your body and also help the fibre in your diet to perform its blood sugar regulatory duties. This amount of water also enables your kidneys and other organs (including your skin) to stay healthy.

- **AVOID FATTY FOODS**

Diabetic women are more prone to developing heart disease because their blood vessels contain more sugar than those of non-diabetic women, causing the blood cells to become more 'sticky' and therefore more likely to pick up circulating fats and cause obstructions. Try to keep your intake of all fats to a minimum, particularly the saturated (mainly animal-based) fats. Choose lean cuts of meat, cut the skin off poultry, use cream and butter sparingly and choose vegetable oils such as olive oil for cooking.

- ### RESTRICT YOUR INTAKE OF SUGARY, LOW-FIBRE FOODS

Sugar comes in many forms, but all have the same effect, even the less refined sugars such as molasses sugar. Honey, chocolate, toffee and other sweets, sugar-coated breakfast cereals, cakes, biscuits and pastries such as Danish pastries, mousses, trifles, sweet sauces and custard are all very high in a type of sugar that is very rapidly absorbed into the blood stream. This causes your blood sugar level to rise very high, especially if they are eaten on an empty stomach. As a general rule this is not advisable, as it makes it very difficult to keep your blood sugar level within the normal range. It was thought at one time that all diabetics had to avoid anything sweet; this is not always the case. Sugary foods can be enjoyed on occasions, but it is important to incorporate them within your meals, and in small amounts.

For example, instead of having a chocolate bar in the afternoon, you should wait until your evening meal and have a small amount of chocolate after the main course. The fibre in the meal enables the sugar from the chocolate to be absorbed more slowly, therefore avoiding high blood sugar levels.

Note If you need to take insulin to help control your diabetes, you should carry some of these rapidly absorbed sugars around with you, just in case your sugar level drops too low, bringing on a hypoglycaemic attack (See page 162).

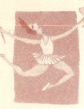

Choose a dry wine rather than something sweet. Almost all red wines are dry, and are excellent with a huge variety of foods. White wines are sometimes labelled (on the shelf or the bottle) on a scale of 1 to 9, 1 being the driest and 9 the sweetest. Try to stay within the 1 to 3 range. Resist Sauternes and all the sweet dessert wines and port. Many of the German wines are also rather sweet.

• THE QUESTION OF ALCOHOL

If you like wine or other alcoholic drinks, you should be able to enjoy them in moderation. What you must do is:

• Check with your doctor, just in case special care needs to be taken.

• Always accompany your alcohol with some food. Choosing wine with a meal is fine, but drinking on an empty stomach should be avoided.

Alcohol can cause your blood sugar level to go too low, by inhibiting the breakdown of sugar from your liver. This may at first sound like a good idea, since diabetics generally need to keep their blood sugar level low. However, alcohol-induced blood sugar drops are not healthy. This is especially important for insulin-dependent diabetics, as it can cause you to suffer a 'hypo' (see page 162). The symptoms of a hypo are very similar to those experienced by anyone who has had too much alcohol to drink, so if you are diabetic you can run into serious problems if you drink alone or the people around you fail to realize that you're suffering from a hypo and not just drunk.

My advice is the same to all women, not just diabetics: cut out futile and dangerous drinking. Above all, diabetics should not drink on an empty stomach. Instead enjoy alcohol with a meal.

• WHICH SORT OF ALCOHOL SHOULD YOU DRINK?

You can more or less choose whatever you like, as long as you just have a small amount of it. Enjoy planning which wine to have with your meal and savour the taste.

If you drink beers or lagers, choose the ordinary varieties, preferably with less than 5% alcohol. Low-sugar beers (such as some Pilsner lagers) – in which more of the sugar has been fermented to form alcohol – tend to be high in alcohol. Diabetic or alcohol-free beers and wines frequently taste disgusting!

You might think that it would be best to mix spirits with a soft mixer such as lemonade. However, since these contain significant amounts of sugar I would suggest that you choose a low-calorie mixer if you don't mind the taste of the artificial sweetener.

PREGNANCY AND DIABETES

If you're a healthy diabetic there is no reason why you should not have a very happy and healthy pregnancy. If you are planning to become pregnant it is a good idea to get your diabetes well controlled beforehand, as it helps prevent any unnecessary complications!

Ask your doctor or nurse to help ensure that all is well before and during your pregnancy. The huge hormonal changes may make you feel a little 'out of sync', but don't suffer in silence, ask for advice. You may find that you need to change the timing of your carbo-hydrate intake, or take extra bedtime or early morning snacks. I suggest you read the chapter on pregnancy for further information on enjoying a healthy pregnancy.

Remember that once you're pregnant the baby will take and use some of your sugar. It is therefore even more important to eat regularly and keep an eye on your sugar and medication levels.

Try to be well prepared, remembering to keep your kitchen stocked with good ingredients and something sweet in your handbag. You may have previously been able to get away with skipping the odd meal, which of course you shouldn't, but with a baby growing inside you you must not take any risks.

• GESTATIONAL DIABETES

Some women develop diabetes when they are pregnant. This most frequently happens after the 26th week and sometimes disappears once the baby is born. However it is likely to reappear, either in another pregnancy or when you're older. There is nothing to worry about as it is easily controlled by your diet. Follow the healthy eating guidelines in this chapter, making sure that you eat regular, small, nutritious and well-balanced meals.

You need to watch that you're not drinking lots of sugary drinks, which can be a temptation when you're not drinking alcohol. Stick to natural, unsweetened juices and squashes, herbal teas and the best health drink of all, pure water.

When diagnosed as having gestational diabetes, women need to take extra care that they don't put on too much weight, as this makes it harder for the body to control the sugar levels. This should not be a problem, as long as your meals are low in fats and sugars and high in fibre.

TROUBLESHOOTING

• IF YOU ARE OVERWEIGHT
Firstly try to reduce your calorie intake and increase your calorie expenditure by taking exercise (see page 165). Losing excess weight will improve your body's ability to control your blood sugar level. Check with your doctor and dietitian before you change your exercise or eating habits, as they will be able to advise you about any changes in medication and any specific food issues. I would also recommend that you read the chapter on weight loss.

• WHEN YOU'RE FEELING UNWELL
If you are feeling ill, the body's natural response is to produce more glucose. Hence blood sugar levels tend to rise. It is therefore vital if you're an insulin-dependent diabetic that your insulin is taken, regardless of whether or not you eat anything. If you don't fancy eating anything solid, you should have a regular intake of easier-to-manage carbohydrates, such as glasses of milk, fruit juice, soup, ice cream or yoghurt.

You should also drink plenty of water, as you will remember that the body's natural way of getting rid of excess sugar and other unwanted substances is by producing urine. When you have a raised temperature your body will also lose a lot of water through sweating, making it doubly important to take in enough water. Carry a small bottle of water around with you during the day and keep a bottle by your bed, so that you can take sips when you fancy. A general rule is to try to have a tumbler of water every hour.

• SOME OF THE MANY RECIPES THAT DIABETICS CAN ENJOY

Pea, mint and lettuce soup

Garlic bean soup

Carrot and orange soup

Spinach borscht

Minestrone

Caramelized artichoke and tomato toasts

Smoked mackerel pâté

Guacamole

Hummus

Radicchio and grape salad

Pear and walnut salad with watercress

Tomato and tarragon vinaigrette

Artichoke and avocado salad

Tabbouleh

Grilled vegetable salad

Christmas salad

Chicken with melon, grapes and asparagus

Grilled peppers with garlic cheese croûtons

Tomatoes stuffed with olives, garlic and parsley

Gado gado

Vegetarian chilli

Baked pasta with ratatouille sauce

Smoked mackerel and spinach fishcakes

Smoked fish casserole

Garlic and herb chicken

Honey and mustard quail

Tropical dried fruit salad

Fruit compote

Mixed berries in Grand Marnier

Vanilla poached peaches

Cinnamon apples and plums

Chilled gingered rhubarb

Apricot filo tart

Prune and bitter chocolate tart

Flapjacks

Barabrith

Banana cake

9 Eating disorders

The aim of this book is to inspire you to make food work for you, but I am only too well aware that the issue of control over food and your body treads a very fine line between constructive and destructive control. Many women spend hours every day preoccupied with food, wondering how they can use it to help them achieve their ideal body and life.

Women are forever being bombarded (in advertising, the press, films and television) with images of 'the perfect body'. On top of these signals the food manufacturing industries spend a lot of money promoting foods that they claim can help you achieve that wonderful body. Food, health and the shape of your body are big business. On the surface this may not seem a bad thing, but the constant exposure to these images and ideas puts women under enormous pressure.

One of the most frightening aspects of our society is that so many women are on diets to help them lose weight that abnormal eating habits have become a part of everyday life. In my practice I see many women who, although they don't consider themselves to be anorexic or bulimic, have a very unsettled relationship with food. They may complain of chronic constipation, lack of energy or a food intolerance. Approximately 65% of women who see me with these problems have been or are going through a phase of a negative attitude towards their body and the effect food has on it. Once they feel they can trust me, many women admit their fears and insecurities over their body and relationship with food, and acknowledge that they have an eating problem.

• **WHAT ARE EATING DISORDERS?**
The main difference between anorexia and bulimia is that anorexics largely starve themselves, whereas bulimics overeat and then purge their bodies by making

themselves vomit or by using laxatives. However, in practice this clear-cut definition does not really exist. There is a broad spectrum of eating disorders, from the severe anorexic who refuses to eat anything at all and whose body weight is so low that she needs medical and nutritional therapy to stay alive, to the more common situation in which a woman suffers occasional anorexic or bulimic tendencies. She may eat fairly normally for most of the time and then starve herself or binge and purge for other periods. These episodes of anorexia or bulimia frequently go unnoticed by other people, as they can be carried out in secrecy, and not all anorexic women are desperately thin.

Most anorexics go through periods of binge eating and purging and bulimics may starve themselves for days at a time. The treatments of the two disorders are quite similar, encompassing psychological support to help you understand and get over the underlying issues and nutritional support to help correct the physical symptoms. The ultimate goal is to help you to cope with eating normally.

While nutritional advice alone cannot cure eating disorders, it can help in several ways: by helping you build a better relationship with food, by improving your health and emotional status, and by getting you into the right frame of mind to seek and cope with psychological help, if you need it.

This chapter aims to enable those of you who are worried that you may be heading down the eating disorder pathway to understand why food is becoming such a negative issue in your life and how you can become more positive about eating. If you have lost a lot of weight or you worry that you may be out of control of your eating habits, I do suggest you see your doctor as he or she will be able to put you in contact with a professional who can help you on a one-to-one basis. If you are already seeing a professional therapist I hope this chapter will help clarify some of the issues.

• WHY DO WOMEN DEVELOP EATING DISORDERS?

When Wallis Simpson, the Duchess of Windsor, said, 'A woman can be neither too rich nor too thin,' she summarized the unrealistic expectations of women with a tendency to eating problems.

Today, it is not only women in the public eye, but at every level of society, who are under phenomenal pressure, both in the home and in the workplace. Our lives are full of obligations, to our work, to our relationships. If we are not achieving high standards in all of them, one of the first things a lot of women do is turn to their body and start criticizing it. Women are meant to look the part; if they don't, they are seen as letting themselves go. The same does not seem to apply to men, which is why nine out of ten eating disorders are suffered by women.

Eating disorders are not something that only wealthy women – with nothing better to do – suffer from. Some people think that if the women who receive most publicity because of their eating disorders had less time and money and had to struggle to make ends meet, they wouldn't be able to enjoy the 'self-indulgence' of being anorexic or bulimic. While I would agree that distractions and changes in priorities can help some women get over an eating disorder, anorexia and bulimia exist throughout society. Lack of parental care and support may well be a predisposing factor in the development of eating disorders and this does not exist only in wealthy families.

Some experts believe that there is a type of personality that makes a woman more likely to develop an eating disorder. For example, a woman who is a high achiever and expects herself and others to achieve perfection in all areas of life. I don't think this is always the case, as very relaxed women can also develop eating disorders.

The eating disorders anorexia and bulimia are the result of insecurities, which are manifested in the need for control. This control is often directed towards food, even though the underlying problem may be unconnected with it. For any woman who has insecurities in her life, including the shape of her body being 'less than perfect', food is one of the easiest things to control on a day-to-day basis.

• WHAT HAPPENS WHEN FOOD BECOMES AN UNHEALTHY OBSESSION?

Life is not always full of happy experiences. When things are not going well, food can be either a source of comfort, or a source of control and conflict. Some women use food to punish themselves for something that, with or without justification, they feel guilty about. We all know that our bodies need food, therefore one way of punishing ourselves is to not eat it. Some women are so deeply emotionally upset that they decide to refrain from eating, to derive a degree of control, pleasure or comfort, however perverse, from resisting food. Many women are forever trying to reach the weight at which they feel as if they will gain all the jewels in life: 'Just a few pounds lighter.'

One thing common to all eating disorders is the love-hate relationship with food. Anorexic and bulimic women may be the finest cooks and really love preparing food for their friends, partner or children, but they cannot cope with eating it and leaving it inside their bodies to 'turn into fat'. They may spend all day reading recipes and preparing food. The ritual of thinking about, preparing and cooking the dish symbolizes a degree of care and affection that deep inside they wish they could show themselves or be given by others. Some women derive a feeling of 'strength' from resisting such delicious food: 'Wow, what a woman I am, if I can sit and watch others eating and not give in.' They will make excuses for not eating: 'I ate with the children' or 'I had a large lunch'.

• THE AGE RANGE

It is not just teenagers who suffer from eating disorders. Women may develop anorexia or bulimia in their late forties or early fifties. The emotional and sociological reasons that precipitate this are quite different from those in a teenager's life.

While some women enjoy the middle years as their 'prime' time, others see it as the dreaded stage when their life loses a lot. As the years go by, relationships change. When your children are no longer dependent on you, you can in theory devote a little more time to yourself. Unfortunately, some husbands may leave their wives to be with a younger woman, or because they, too, worry about growing old and unfulfilled. The emotional upset can lead to an eating disorder.

At this time of life the body starts changing, with weight creeping around the middle, noticeable wrinkles, and possibly menopausal symptoms such as hot flushes, mood swings and osteoporosis, which arise from hormonal, vitamin, mineral and other nutrient imbalances. Many women turn to creams, nutritional supplements and medication to try to prevent or reverse the signs of ageing, as well as fill some emotional and lifestyle gaps.

Women may become very depressed because they see only limited options available to them, as they cannot turn the clock back. Losing weight can become more difficult as you get older, which may be because you have tried 'starvation' diets in the past. Extremely restricted diets can cause your body to drop its metabolic rate to such a low level that, despite a low calorie intake, the body won't lose any more weight. Emotionally it may also be harder to be motivated to stick to diets.

The emotional upset about not being the shape you want or about changing relationships can cause some women to become anorexic or bulimic.

WHAT IS ANOREXIA?

The overriding characteristic of the majority of anorexic women is the desire to become thin. No matter how much weight they lose, they always want to be thinner.

They have an intense fear of being or becoming fat. They think they look fatter than they are and have a very distorted body image. This may not be all over the body; they might focus on one part of the anatomy and describe it as fat, even when it is clearly not. Many women hide their body under layers of baggy jumpers and loose clothing. They frequently exercise to excess and may resort to using diuretics and laxatives to help them lose weight.

• PHYSICAL SYMPTOMS OF ANOREXIA

The most obvious symptom of anorexia is not wanting to eat. What may start off as a harmless diet turns into an unreserved drive to lose more and more weight. Anorexics never reach their ideal weight because the goal posts are always moving. Lack of food leads to extreme fatigue, irritability, loss of hair, poor skin, nails and teeth, a permanent state of feeling cold, and depression. Anorexics frequently suffer from hormonal imbalances and their periods cease. If they resort to using laxatives and diuretics their body's metabolic balance may become so disturbed that, in extreme cases, their heart struggles to function properly. Long-term starvation and/or laxative or diuretic abuse can ultimately be fatal, therefore anorexia must always be treated seriously.

• SEVERE ANOREXIA

Severe anorexics need to go into hospital if their body weight is very low or their hormone and body fluid levels are unbalanced. They require expert medical treatment to enable the body and mind to recover enough to reach the stage where they can accept psychological help. The mind can only cope with therapy if the acute nutritional deficiencies and other medical problems are being tackled; this is where the dietitian should be involved with the doctors. Once the body is out of the acute stage it is very important that the patient receives a combination of psychological and nutritional support.

BULIMIA

Bulimics, like anorexics, have a distorted vision of their body and desire to control it. The main difference is the fact that they eat. The quantities they eat varies, and not all women are bulimic every day. Bulimics generally binge on large amounts of foods in secret, often eating starchy foods such as pasta and bread, or sweet foods such as chocolate and ice cream.

The oral satisfaction is often linked to a 'serotonin rush', which results from taking in a large volume of certain foods that cause a substance called serotonin to be produced in the brain and bloodstream. The serotonin rush, along with the fact that it is done in secret, can give a real 'buzz'. Sometimes bulimic women can binge in public, but the majority prefer eating secretly. They may experience satisfaction in getting away with eating all of the food they want without society seeing and judging them. Other women eat in secret out of shame.

Whether it is secret or public bingeing, a massive guilt attack follows. 'How can I possibly keep all this food inside my stomach when I know in my mind that it will lead to me becoming fat?' They must then purge themselves, either by making themselves sick or by using laxatives.

• BULIMICS WHO DON'T BINGE

At this point I feel it is important to document the other type of bulimic, who seems to be more common in working women. She eats a normal-sized meal, at work or in the evening, and then realizes that she can get rid of the calories by purging herself. She doesn't binge, but eats normally, so that no alarm bells are raised with friends or colleagues, which would tend to happen in the anorexic state or the classic binge-purge scenario. This is also worrying because the sufferer, who doesn't follow the traditional pattern of anorexia or bulimia, sees what she does as acceptable behaviour.

• PHYSICAL MANIFESTATIONS OF BULIMIA

Bulimic activity results in rotting teeth (from the acid contents of the stomach), burst small blood vessels in the eyes and metabolic imbalances caused by losing large amounts of body fluids, through vomiting, diarrhoea or the use of diuretics. If the level of laxative abuse is high, incontinence and severe bowel problems may develop.

SELF HELP

In my practice I find it useful to work through the following exercises with many of the women with a disturbed body image and attitude towards food. They provide ways of helping you to understand how your body works with food and ultimately turn eating into a more positive experience.

• UNDERSTAND THE NUTRIENTS YOUR BODY NEEDS

It is helpful to understand the way that the body works and its requirements in terms of giving you good skin, teeth, eyes and hair, as well as all the less visible functions such as blood, muscles, bones and nervous system, a healthy metabolism and enough energy to function properly and to be able to carry out normal daily activities such as walking. Read the section in Part One of this book on What your body needs in terms of nutrients, vitamins and minerals.

The body puts on excess fat only when it takes in calories it doesn't need. Once you have understood that food has far more uses than simply the negative one of 'making you fat', it is important to try to get your body to a stage where it is a little stronger, without feeling that your weight will carry on going up and up. You will put on a few pounds when you are eating a little more food, but it is important to discuss with your dietitian ways in which you can eat foods that won't send your weight escalating up. There shouldn't be any need to take the manufactured supplemented drinks. They not only don't help you get used to eating fresh food, but they also don't taste very nice. In fact, since they are rich in sugar and fat, these concentrated drinks are normally very unappealing to anorexics. I think it is much better to work at having a little something that tastes nice and makes you feel normal.

• CALCULATE YOUR IDEAL BODY WEIGHT
Use the body mass index table on page 46. Even though it is unlikely that a chart will entirely reassure you that your weight is either too low or just right, I think it is a good idea to see how your weight differs from the ideal range. Remember that it is extremely unhealthy to be very underweight, i.e. with a body mass index less than 17, but if you manage to keep your weight at 18 or above, and feel healthy and happy there, there shouldn't be any reason for you to worry.

• UNDERSTAND THAT THE BODY'S FLUID LEVELS
CHANGE EVERY DAY, SEVERAL TIMES A DAY
Hopping on the scales every few hours or even every day makes you overaware of the natural changes. Try to get out of the habit of excessive weighing; once a week should be the maximum. This is not easy when you have been used to obsessive weighing, so throw the scales out, give them to a friend or put them in a place where you can't see them. When you feel tempted to weigh yourself, distraction therapies such as going for a walk can be helpful.

• MAKE A LIST OF PASTIMES THAT MAKE YOU
FEEL GOOD
Write down your favourite pieces of music or books that you associate with happy times. You shouldn't see exercise as your only pastime, as women with eating disorders frequently exercise to punish the body rather than to make it feel healthier. Gentle exercise can help you to feel good about your body, but punishing two-hour episodes are not what you need. Also, list the friends and relatives who offer you the support you

need. Keep your lists in a prominent place so you can take immediate action when you're feeling vulnerable.

• **MAKE A FOOD LIST**
Divide foods into four groups:
• A foods are those that you feel safe eating.
• B foods are those that you like and can eat a small amount of occasionally, but you consider them to be rather high in calories.
• C foods are those that you like the taste of or idea of eating, but won't eat them because you think they are too high in calories or will upset you.
• D foods are those that you don't like; these are genuine dislikes rather than any psychological fear of eating.

I find that A foods are usually fruits and vegetables, apart from avocados, bananas and pineapples, along with yoghurt, black coffee, canned diet drinks, and occasionally pasta, rice, potatoes and white bread. Some women find the carbohydrate foods such as bread a little scary; they can manage a little but won't eat much, unless they are in a binge mood. Bread or other carbohydrate foods would therefore be placed in the B list. Other B foods might include cottage or low-fat cheese, fish, meat or chicken and breakfast cereals. Many women with eating disorders find the easiest list to compile is the C foods. These are usually fatty and sugary foods such as crisps, pastries, cakes, biscuits, butter, oil, cheese, sauces and full-calorie canned drinks. Some women would place alcohol in the C foods, but a lot of anorexic women drink heavily as it numbs a lot of the emotional upset.

Try to find recipes that make your A foods into something a little more appetizing and substantial. Use herbs and spices to add new flavours with no calories. Bland food doesn't excite anyone. It is good to learn to treat yourself with delicious-tasting food. While the ultimate goal is to get you to be able to include foods from your C group as well as B foods in your eating pattern, start with making your cooking more appetizing.

Once you have done this and also understood from reading Part One the nutrients your body needs to become and stay healthy, try to incorporate some of the C foods in your eating pattern. Do this a little at a time and try to enjoy the experience.

• TRY TO REAWAKEN THE TASTE, TEMPERATURE AND TEXTURE SENSATIONS IN YOUR MOUTH

As you will see from reading page 6 on the appetite mechanism, a lot of the satisfaction we gain from our meals comes from acknowledging food within the mouth. Many anorexics, and to an even greater extent bulimics, don't taste or feel food in the mouth. They see food as the enemy and something that has to be swallowed quickly. Unfortunately what happens with bulimics is that they miss out on many of the potential satiety signals that normally come from chewing and concentrating on the food. They eat a large amount of the same type of food and by the time the stomach acknowledges the food there is so much of it that they feel uncomfortable. Uncomfortable feelings make them feel more guilty and therefore tempted to purge.

It is much better to have small amounts of varied food, which your body can acknowledge in ways other than an uncomfortably full stomach. The ultimate goal of this exercise is to stop the guilt/panic attacks that accompany eating, not to make you take in calories. I give similar advice to people who want to lose weight. Concentrating on and respecting everything that goes into your mouth is very important in being positive about food.

• TRY TO RESIST HAVING YOUR BINGE FOODS IN THE HOUSE

While in the long run you will have to cope with situations where these foods arise, you first need to learn how to eat normally without bingeing. Keeping such foods in the cupboard will make it easier and therefore more tempting to binge. If you have a large list of binge foods (the classic ones are bread, breakfast cereal, ice

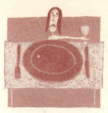

Instead of alcohol, look out for unusual fruit and herb drinks: cordials, syrups, juices, still or sparkling blends. Try elderflower, ginger or lime cordial or a few drops of orange blossom water mixed with sparkling water. My fruit shake (see page 72) is extremely versatile, so experiment with combinations of fruits. Serve your drink in a nice glass and make an occasion of it.

cream, chocolate and biscuits) you may need to find alternatives, foods that nutritionally give your body what it needs, but that don't set you off on a binge. For example, if breakfast cereals are your main binge food, make yourself a varied breakfast of wholemeal bread, fruit, yoghurt and fruit juice to re-educate your eating patterns and avoid the food that sets you on a binge-purge cycle.

- **TRY TO DRINK NO MORE THAN TWO LITRES (FOUR PINTS) OF WATER A DAY**
Some women fill themselves up with water to numb the hunger pangs. Take small sips throughout the day.

- **LIMIT YOUR TEA AND COFFEE INTAKES**
Tea and coffee bind vitamins and minerals in your gut and prevent your body from using them effectively. Being diuretic, they also make your body excrete nutrients in the urine. While you are trying to get your body and mind back into shape you should try to cut them out completely. This will make you feel a lot more energized and healthy. You may have a couple of days of withdrawal symptoms such as headaches, but these should pass. See page 62 for alternative drinks.

- **WATCH YOUR ALCOHOL INTAKE**
While alcohol can be beneficial in some situations, it can confuse your mind and make you feel unsure of what you've eaten so you then feel you need to purge yourself. I think it is best to avoid it when you're feeling vulnerable about your eating habits.

The only circumstance where I think it could be appropriate is when you're trying to get your appetite back. After a long time of ignoring your hunger pangs it can be difficult to recognize them. Alcohol can serve as an aperitif and stimulate your hunger. I would suggest you discuss this with your dietitian before you use alcohol in this way.

- **STOP USING LAXATIVES AND DIURETICS**

They don't help you to reduce your body weight; the temporary loss you see on the scales is because they have made your body excrete abnormal amounts of fluids. This is potentially very damaging to your health. If you feel constipated, read the chapter on constipation. If you feel fluid retention is your problem, read the chapter on periods or seek your dietitian's advice.

- **TRY TO BUILD A STRUCTURE INTO YOUR EATING PATTERN**

Eating three small meals a day, at roughly the same time every day, will give you a sense of being positively in control. Bulimics and anorexics frequently go for long periods of time without eating and then give in to snacking or bingeing urges. It is much better to try to establish a regular eating pattern. Some women find they can cope better with five small meals a day rather than three slightly larger meals. This could be particularly helpful if you suffer from low blood sugar levels. Whatever pattern of eating you decide works for you, I suggest you keep to it so that some normality can start filtering into your life.

Don't rely on your hunger pangs to tell you when to eat; a structured eating plan is much more likely to make you feel positive about eating. Try to make eating as relaxing an experience as possible, in a pleasant environment and with a sympathetic friend. If possible, eat with someone else; eating alone is not a good idea.

- **BREAK YOUR DAY INTO UNITS**

Get into the habit of breaking your day into three units, for example, morning, afternoon and evening. At the end of each unit, look at whether you have reached your eating goals, for instance having breakfast or not bingeing, and give yourself some positive feedback, maybe even write it down. If you have a day with three good units you should reward yourself, with something other than food. For example, see a good friend, buy some clothes.

If you have a bad unit, put the lid on it and start afresh with the next unit, don't think the whole day should be written off. This will give you the maximum opportunity to give yourself a lot of positive feedback and not allow you to get swept into a negative 'punishment' cycle.

• TREAT YOURSELF TO THE OCCASIONAL MASSAGE OR FACIAL
The more positive attention you give yourself, the more likely you are to accept your body for what it is and not struggle for an unachievable image.

• NUTRITIONAL SUPPLEMENTS
The role of nutritional supplements in the treatment of eating disorders is very complex. I worry that women may see taking supplements as a substitute for eating normally. Although they can be useful for correcting vitamin or mineral deficiencies and helping you feel stronger while you are trying to get into the habit of eating normally, vitamins and minerals need to be carefully balanced in the body. While food does this naturally, supplements need to be matched to specific needs, which is best done by a doctor or dietitian.

One mineral that has been advocated in the treatment of anorexia is zinc. Zinc deficiency may result from poor eating habits, stress or taking the contraceptive pill. The deficiency leads to poor appetite and depression. Therefore it is possible that a zinc deficiency can aggravate the symptoms experienced with anorexia and bulimia. I recommend that you discuss the issue of zinc and other nutrient supplements with your doctor or dietitian.

PSYCHOLOGICAL HELP

I hope this chapter can help women who have a disturbed relationship with food and their body to feel a lot healthier and happier about eating. But there will be those of you who recognize that you could use psychological help. It takes a lot of courage for a woman to approach someone who they believe is going to start challenging them about their thoughts. Yet we don't have any problem seeking advice about physical matters, so why should we deny our mind the care it deserves?

The psychological therapy you need depends very much on the root of your problem. Many doctors recommend a combination of seeing a psychiatrist who can prescribe medication to deal with depression, frequently experienced by anorexics, and counselling, conducted by a clinical psychologist. However, not all women with eating disorders are depressed and therefore they don't require medication. It is also important to find a dietitian who is experienced in dealing with eating disorders, as a bad or inexperienced dietitian may damage your recovery as much as a bad psychological therapist. Personal recommendation, from more than one person, is the best way to find a good therapist.

Sadly, some psychiatrists and psychologists dismiss the idea that food is connected with the underlying psychological problem and don't seek nutritional input within the support team. A few even believe that anorexics and bulimics have a very clear, wide knowledge of the nutritional breakdown of foods and therefore have no need for more help in that area. While I would agree that many anorexic and bulimic women know a lot about the calorie and fat contents of food, they do not know how the food affects their body and how they can use food positively to help them get over the eating disorder. The right information can help you feel empowered and in control of food and your eating habits in a healthy way. You will be amazed at how good it feels to release yourself from the eating disorder 'jail'.

10 Fatigue

There is an increasing awareness of the role of nutrition in fatigue, whether this is chronic fatigue, as in the post-viral fatigue syndrome (also known as myalargic encephalomyelitis or ME), glandular fever, or just normal tiredness. Perhaps as a result of an unsympathetic reaction from a conventional health practitioner, many women are attracted to try alternative approaches such as eliminating certain foods from their diet: yeasts (the anti-candida diet), gluten or milk. The danger of self-help remedies or falling into the hands of unqualified 'experts' is that a potentially serious problem could be missed.

If you've been feeling very tired for quite a while and cannot seem to pick yourself up even when you're eating well, you should arrange to see your doctor so that he or she can investigate this further. It may be that you are suffering from a virus such as the Epstein Barr virus, which can cause glandular fever, episodes of severe fatigue, depression and swollen glands. A blood test can confirm the diagnosis. Other causes of chronic and acute fatigue include poor nutrition, anaemia, food intolerances, excess caffeine and alcohol, and lack of oxygen to the muscles.

• LACK OF THE CORRECT NUTRIENTS

Every vitamin and mineral has a vital part to play in energy production or hormone metabolism. Therefore virtually all vitamin and mineral deficiencies can manifest themselves as chronic or acute fatigue. If you eat a well-balanced diet and are otherwise healthy it is very unlikely that you will suffer from nutrient deficiency-related fatigue. I have seen it in women who have a disturbed relationship with food and may have episodes of anorexia or bulimia, and in women who are on extremely restricted diets because of food preferences or allergies. It is not uncommon in women who decide to become vegetarian or vegan; they need to be extra careful about balancing their intake of the different food groups, so that their bodies can absorb and metabolize the nutrients efficiently.

If you think that you may have a vitamin or mineral deficiency you should ask your doctor to arrange blood tests to find out what your body is lacking. Don't just put yourself on a supplement.

• ANAEMIA

Anaemia is one of the most common causes of extreme tiredness in women. It can easily happen in women who have long or heavy periods, unbalanced eating habits, such as young women who eat just fruits and vegetables to stay slim, or individuals training in a lot of sports. There are various types of anaemia, but among women the most common type is iron-deficiency anaemia. In mild cases it can be easily corrected with rest and a diet rich in iron, vitamin C and other nutrients. In more severe cases your doctor or dietitian may advise you to take an iron supplement. See the separate chapter on anaemia.

• FOOD INTOLERANCES

Some people can experience relief from fatigue by avoiding certain foods to which they are sensitive. However, exclusion diets must be executed within a healthy, well-balanced eating plan. It is easy to become malnourished and even more tired as a result of cutting foods out of your diet. Time and time again I see women who have been told that their extreme fatigue is down to a food allergy. They are sent away with a list of things to avoid, but without alternatives to eat and drink. You cannot simply remove something from the diet, without recognizing the body's natural requirements. For example, if you cut out sugar and all yeast products, you need to find other foods that will give the equivalent amount of energy and nutrients.

Beginning an exclusion diet takes effort and careful organization, and this is not very easy when you're feeling chronically or acutely tired. I frequently find that tiredness is simply due to insufficient energy, so instead of following an exclusion diet, try boosting your immune system and general nutritional and energy status by following a healthy diet with plenty of fresh fruit and vegetables. If you then feel you want to explore the food intolerance issue, see the chapter on allergies.

• TOO MUCH CAFFEINE

Caffeine overdose is one of the most common causes of chronic and acute fatigue. I can understand why women drink caffeine-containing drinks such as coffee, tea and colas; they can give a stimulating 'kick start' in the morning or in the middle of the afternoon, when your energy level is falling. Unfortunately, caffeine has two major detrimental effects on energy levels. Although caffeine stimulates your energy, the energy boost is short lived. It upsets the hormone levels in your body, which results in your energy level crashing. When your energy crashes it is very tempting to have another caffeine fix to get you high again, but this is a negative cycle, which cannot help you in the long run. The more you have, the more you need to get the desired effect. Before you know it, you're drinking three or four cups rather than one. Disturbing your natural energy systems means that your body is never able to find a healthy balance. Secondly, caffeine inhibits the efficient absorption of vitamins and minerals from the gut, and also makes your body excrete more vitamins and minerals; your body loses out, in both respects.

I have seen many women feeling completely different after they cut all caffeine out of their daily eating pattern. Some women find they can enjoy a small amount of caffeine, without detrimental effect, if the rest of the diet is healthy. I have suggested some alternative drinks on page 62. I would suggest that you try to limit yourself to a maximum of two or three cups of good tea or coffee a day. Don't drink strong black coffee on its own, as it can give you an exaggerated energy response. It is much better to have it with a wholegrain biscuit or a piece of high-fibre cake.

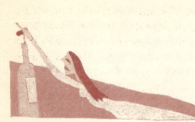

You need an easy-to-open tipple such as screw-top Lambrusco or a good beer or cider. There is such a wide range of beers, and they are far lower in alcohol than wine. Look out for the pale, cloudy wheat beers from Belgium and Germany, Belgium's delicious fruit beers, or England's unusual ciders.

Note If you take caffeine out of your diet, you may find that you suffer from headaches and low energy levels for a couple of days. This happens because your body has become reliant on the caffeine to feel normal. Don't worry – you will soon start to feel truly healthy.

• ALCOHOL

A little alcohol can be fine, but excessive drinking causes your body to become nutritionally unbalanced, because alcohol acts as a diuretic drug, which causes the body to excrete vitamins and minerals. Alcohol suppresses your energy levels in another way if drunk on an empty stomach. Alcohol affects the ability of the liver to release energy, which is stored in the liver as glycogen. This can be used to your advantage; having a little tipple before your meal can help to conquer lack of appetite, which is common in chronic fatigue. But you must follow the alcohol with a meal.

Some women find it much better to stay away from alcoholic drinks when they're tired or suffering from chronic fatigue. If this is the case then you could try the more natural non-alcoholic drinks such as sparkling elderflower water, ginger beer or fruity mineral waters.

• LACK OF OXYGEN IN THE BLOOD

The most common cause of lack of oxygen in the blood is smoking. When you fill your lungs with smoke, you diminish the volume of oxygen you can obtain from each breath. Smoking can therefore cause you to suffer from lack of energy simply because the muscles, brain and other organs are not getting the oxygen they need to function properly. Being a smoker also minimizes the potential benefits you'll receive from eating better, so do try to give it up or at least cut down. Talk to your doctor if you need advice on how to give up. You may like to consider acupuncture, nicotine patches or hypnotherapy.

A lot of women don't breathe efficiently, even if they don't smoke. Learning to breathe using the whole of your lungs – diaphragmatic breathing – can really help you to feel more energized, as you can push more oxygen around your body.

FOOD GUIDELINES

The nutritional guidelines for coping with and curing fatigue focus on three core issues: correcting deficiencies, building a strong immune system and cutting out substances that compromise your immunity and energy levels, especially caffeine, alcohol and nicotine (see above).

• CORRECT ANY VITAMIN OR MINERAL DEFICIENCIES

Your doctor will be able to test your blood to discover whether you lack any of the essential nutrients. You should be able to correct a mild deficiency by eating a healthy well-balanced diet and boosting your intake of the relevant nutrients. If you have a serious deficiency your doctor or dietitian may advise a supplement to get you back to fitness.

• HELP YOUR BODY TO BUILD A STRONG IMMUNE SYSTEM

A strong immune system will help you to fight any secondary infections such as cystitis and colds, which can plague you when your system is down. Glandular fever and chronic fatigue syndrome can stay with you for months, especially if you don't look after yourself. Eating well is a fundamental part of making sure you recover as quickly as possible. Have plenty of fresh vegetables and fruits, lean proteins, wholegrain foods, dairy products and water.

• RESIST THE CRAVING FOR VERY SWEET FOODS

One of the commonest mistakes when low in energy is to eat something very sweet for a 'boost'. Unfortunately, if you take in a sugary snack which contains a lot of rapidly absorbed sugar such as glucose or sucrose, the pancreas responds to the rapid rise in sugar level by producing far too much insulin (a hormone which breaks down sugar). This then leads to a rapid drop in sugar level, which makes you feel even worse.

The best foods to eat are those which are rich in a high-fibre carbohydrate, such as fresh fruit, a whole-wheat biscuit or cake or a slice of wholegrain bread with a pure fruit topping. These foods contain some sugar to give you energy, but the presence of fibre means that the rise in your sugar and energy level is slow and well controlled.

NUTRITIONAL SUPPLEMENTS

There are several nutrient deficiencies that manifest themselves as chronic or acute fatigue. The most common is iron deficiency, and I suggest you read the chapter on anaemia before you take any supplement. Two other minerals, magnesium and zinc, have also been linked with fatigue. When your body is deficient in magnesium and zinc your immune system can become low, making you vulnerable to infections. Although a supplement may be appropriate on some occasions, there are other times, for example when you have a viral cold, that the body purposely lowers its blood zinc levels, as high zinc levels can make you more prone to bacterial infections. People who take a supplement without looking at all the variables may make the situation worse. It's much better to eat a well-balanced diet that includes some of the foods rich in magnesium and zinc, such as green leafy vegetables, shellfish and nuts, as this won't upset the natural balance of the body.

• RECIPES TO FIGHT FATIGUE

Carrot and orange soup

French onion soup

Clam chowder

Spinach borscht

Salmon and lemon lasagne

Spicy fish kebabs

Sausage and bean casserole

Somerset steak and cider pie

Chicken liver pâté

Chicken with melon, grapes and
  asparagus

Christmas salad

Warm goats' cheese salad

Tomatoes stuffed with olives,
  garlic and parsley

Broccoli with roasted tomatoes

Tomato, pesto and olive omelette

Spinach and watercress roulade

Oysters with cream and Parmesan

Smoked mackerel and spinach
  fishcakes

Oranges in caramel

Mixed fruit with butterscotch
  sauce

Poached pears with ginger

Raspberry and blackberry fool

Lemon syllabub

Flapjacks

Barabrith

Date and walnut cake

Banana cake

Fig and orange cake

Fig and ginger parkin

11 Headaches and migraine

Everyone suffers from headaches at some time in their life. Sadly, some people have much of their lives ruined by headaches or, even worse, by migraines. Headaches and migraines are quite different but there are many similarities in their nutritional management.

A headache can be a dull or sharp pain, which can sometimes extend into the neck. Headaches can last for any length of time and if severe can cause sickness and extreme fatigue. Migraines can cause severe pain in the head and neck, nausea, vomiting, lack of balance and complete incapacity. Other migraine sufferers merely have disturbed vision, such as black spots or lines, without any particular pain.

Migraines are more commonly suffered by women than men, but the good news is that more than half of all female sufferers will cease to be troubled by migraines after their menopause. The headaches may recur frequently, as often as several times a week, or only once every few years; they may last from a few hours to several days. Those who suffer migraines frequently live in dread of the symptoms and are understandably always on the lookout for new theories and new preventative measures.

• WHAT EXACTLY CAUSES A MIGRAINE HEADACHE?

A neurologist will tell you that the causes of a migraine are extremely complex. In simple terms, they are associated with the expansion of sensitive blood vessels in the head. If these blood vessels constrict for a period of 15 minutes to an hour and then rapidly expand, it causes pain.

The constriction, or narrowing, of blood vessels that starts off the whole cycle is triggered by a release of serotonin, a hormone-like substance produced in the blood. Serotonin can be released by eating certain foods and drinks, by undue stress or even oversleeping. As your kidneys process the serotonin and its level drops, the sensitive blood vessels dilate rapidly, pressing on surrounding nerves and causing inflammation and a pulsating pain, usually on one side of the head. The pain can last for days as the swelling takes time to go down, even when the blood vessels have returned to normal.

As many as one in five women who suffer migraines know when an attack is coming on because they experience a change in eyesight, known as an 'aura', sometimes described as zig zag patterns or flashes of light.

FOOD AND MIGRAINE HEADACHES

The role that food plays in the cause of migraine and headaches is controversial, but research shows that there is some connection. Books often tell you to avoid the most common 'trigger' foods: chocolate, hard cheeses, caffeine, red wine and citrus fruits, particularly oranges. However, the association is not clear cut and there is no reason why you should not eat any or all of these foods if you feel that they do not affect you adversely. Unfortunately, some people find that even if they avoid these foods they still get migraines and headaches.

• LOW BLOOD SUGAR LEVEL

Before looking at the foods that can cause or aggravate a migraine it is important to realize that one of the most common triggers is a low blood sugar level. In the majority of cases this is not true hypoglycaemia (see page 224), which can be diagnosed only by detailed tests carried out by your doctor, it is just a sugar level that you as an individual are not happy with.

The good news is that this can easily be prevented by sensible snacking. Correcting or preventing a low blood sugar level is not just a question of eating something sugary as quickly as possible. This can cause the sugar level to rise too quickly, to which the body reacts by producing more insulin, the hormone that breaks down sugar, causing the sugar level to fall again: this is known as the 'yo yo' effect. When you feel low in sugar the answer is to eat something that is both high in fibre and sweet. This could be fruit – fresh, poached or as a fruit compote – a slice of wholemeal bread with a topping of banana, pure fruit spread or honey roast ham, or a wholegrain biscuit such as a flapjack. Keep such snacks readily available, at work and at home.

• **'HOT TRIGGER' FOODS**

It is unfortunate that many classic migraine triggers – caffeine, strong red wine, aged cheese, chocolate – are part of what most people regard as a good dinner: a delicious main course that requires a rich, full-bodied red wine, a wonderful cheeseboard, an irresistible chocolate dessert and a strong black coffee served with dark chocolate mints. A familiar scenario, perhaps, and before you know it, the damage has been done. You fall into bed tired and overfed and wake up a couple of hours later feeling awful, your head heavy, eyes cloudy, neck stiff and stomach nauseous. If you have headaches rather than true migraines you can help prevent the headache from taking a hold by taking your pain-killer tablets and drinking a couple of glasses of cool water before you tumble into bed. Migraine sufferers should seek specific medication advice from their doctor.

Before it happens again, why not work out your own personal 'damage limitation' plan? Try eating only one of the 'banned' foods: if it doesn't affect you adversely you can reintroduce it to your diet.

• **OTHER FOODS TO AVOID**

There are other foods that have also proved to be trigger foods in some people, so it is sensible to watch out for them if you are feeling vulnerable. These include processed meats such as salami and other sausages, mangetout, and the flavour enhancer monosodium glutamate (MSG). MSG is found in a lot of ready-made meals, bottled sauces, crisps and often in Chinese restaurant food. Sticking to fresh foods will mean that you avoid MSG, so just get into the habit of asking

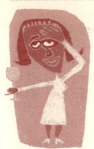

If you find that red wine triggers a migraine, experiment with full-bodied whites; perhaps a Chardonnay or a mature Sémillon. The Hunter Valley in Australia produces 'big and beefy' Chardonnay, which will match meat and other traditional 'red wine' foods. Full-bodied white wines usually have a rich, deep golden colour.

Some sufferers find that white wine triggers their headaches; instead, try a light red such as a Beaujolais or a rosé. France produces good rosés in the Provence and Loire regions, for example the Loire's Cabernet d'Anjou. Serve slightly chilled, at cellar temperature (13°C/55°F).

restaurants to leave MSG out of your dish when you are ordering; it is not necessary, and the best restaurants do not use it.

Remember that not all of the foods outlined below will affect you. Try to keep as many different foods as possible in your diet.

• VASOACTIVE AMINES

Vasoactive amines are commonly found in fermented products, such as pickled fish, hard cheeses, sour cream and wine; they also occur in dried sausages, dry-cured ham (prosciutto), chicken livers, mangetout (and pea pods and broad bean pods) and chocolate. They are capable of changing the size of the blood vessels that carry the blood from your body up into your head. The vessels contract and then expand and the pain cycle starts.

Don't worry unduly if one or all of these foods seem to affect you: once you know what they are it will be easy to avoid them, and you can concentrate on all the things you can eat.

As far as wine is concerned, the Sangiovese grape, which produces Chianti in Italy, seems to have some of the highest levels of vasoactive amines.

• NITRITES

Nitrites are substances that are added to meat products in order to give them a pink or red colour and to preserve them. Unfortunately they can trigger off migraines in particularly sensitive people. Nitrites are found in many sausages – chipolatas, chorizo, hot dogs, salami – and cooked meats such as mortadella and corned beef. If you find that these trigger a migraine, you should stick to unadulterated meats or processed meats that are not coloured red. Try cold cuts of beef, chicken or turkey, or lean ham such as Bradenham, York or Suffolk; the latter has a particularly rich, sweet flavour. For tasty sandwiches, snacks and first courses, don't forget fish such as fresh poached salmon or trout, or homemade fish mousses and pâtés.

• CAFFEINE

Many people find that the more caffeine they drink, the greater the chance of developing a headache or migraine. Coffee is the obvious culprit here, although caffeine is also present in tea, particularly the Indian Assam teas that produce the strong 'cuppa' so beloved of the British. Coffee buffs say that good-quality coffee, made from arabica beans, contains half to one-third the caffeine of cheaper coffee, made from robusta beans; there is also less caffeine in espresso coffee, where the water is forced more quickly through the grains than it is in filter machines.

Caffeine intake in general should be no more than three cups of tea or coffee a day; this should be significantly reduced if coffee affects you adversely. If it's breakfast coffee you like, keep it to the weekend rather than every day.

If you decide to cut caffeine out of your diet entirely, you may suffer from a withdrawal headache. This may develop after about 18 hours without your caffeine fix and is simply 'cold turkey'; your body being deprived of its toxins. Stay with the abstention (drinking plenty of plain water will help), and the headaches should disappear after 26 to 36 hours. You might prefer to lower your caffeine dependence, cup by cup, over a few days. Whichever way you do it, it can only be a cleansing experience for your body.

Try other hot drinks to replace coffee in your day. What about flavoured milk drinks or some of the huge variety of herbal teas such as peppermint, camomile and rosehip? Try orange blossom essence in hot water or hot apple juice and other hot fruit (possibly not orange) juices, you may be surprised how much you enjoy the variety. (See page 62 for more ideas.)

• LACTOSE

This is one of the less common trigger ingredients, but nevertheless one that can cause severe headaches in some people. The problem seems to occur when your digestive system is deficient in an enzyme called lactase, which breaks down lactose, found in dairy products such as cream, butter, yoghurt, cheese, ice cream and milk. In many cases, all that needs to be done is to avoid having too many foods that are high in lactose, although anyone who is particularly sensitive to lactose should avoid it altogether and should read the chapter on allergies. You need to be careful that you don't compromise your calcium status by cutting out dairy products; this could expose you to the risk of osteoporosis. Do see a dietitian if you're worried.

• COPPER

Research shows that the metabolism of people who suffer from migraines is slightly different from those who don't suffer, and it seems that foods that are high in copper can cause problems. These foods include shellfish, nuts, chocolate and wheatgerm (found in wholemeal bread and other wholewheat products). However, you would need to eat quite a lot of these 'coppery' foods before a problem occurred, so my advice is to keep to small amounts rather than completely cutting them out of your diet.

Some foods, particularly citrus fruits such as oranges, lemon, grapefruit and limes, cause the body to absorb more copper, and can therefore aggravate your tendency to have a migraine. Again, try to avoid having a lot of them, especially on an empty stomach. For migraine sufferers, this means getting out of the habit of a morning 'kickstart' of fresh orange juice for breakfast. However, you can include an orange as part of a selection of fruit. Prepare a platter of mango, banana, star fruit or crisp apple, perhaps with a coulis of passion fruit and mango, or make up a bowl of fresh fruit salad to have ready in the refrigerator.

• ASPARTAME

This is an artificial sweetener which manufacturers use in some low-calorie drinks; unfortunately it is also found in a lot of regular squashes, tonic waters and other soft drinks, so look on the label. It can cause sensitive people to develop a migraine after consuming these drinks in any quantity. Note if you've had any such drinks before a migraine attack and avoid them in future.

GENERAL ADVICE

• **KEEP DIARY NOTES**
Make a point of writing down what you're eating and what you're doing, to find out what seems to trigger off a migraine. You may have come to some conclusions already, but when things are written down, a pattern may fall into place that wasn't obvious before. The cause and effect don't necessarily occur within a short period of time. Triggers such as eating cheese can cause a migraine within 20 minutes, whereas other triggers such as extreme exercise or a stressful meeting don't cause a migraine for a few hours.

• **HAVE SMALL, WELL-BALANCED MEALS**
'Little and often', with small, satisfying snacks, is the best plan for eating. Don't allow yourself to go hungry as this can trigger a migraine.

• **AVOID CARRYING TOO MUCH BODY WEIGHT**
Try to keep your weight within the ideal range for your height (see page 46). Being overweight can adversely affect your blood pressure and this heightens the potential for migraine headaches.

• **TAKE TIME, EVERY DAY, TO RELAX**
It is vital to reduce both physical and emotional stress and taking time, even it's only 15 minutes a day, will make a great difference to your well-being. Make a serious date with yourself every day to relax and do it! Even if you can't identify that it's stress that provokes your migraines, you should still take the stress/relaxation aspects of your life seriously.

• **SLEEP**

A most important part of our health schedule, irregular sleep patterns can often contribute to migraines. Oddly enough, oversleeping at weekends can induce migraines as much as undersleeping due to stress. So try to get the same, regular amount of sleep each night.

• **ACT QUICKLY**

As soon as you feel the onset of headache symptoms, act quickly. Once the headache takes a strong hold it becomes more difficult to treat. Ask your doctor's advice about which medication is appropriate for you and take it on time, until the pain lessens. Ride out the pain in a dark, quiet room.

Some women apply cold cloths or soft ice packs on the back of the neck or temples, while others find warmth more helpful. As the pain is caused by the constriction of blood to the head, it helps to relax the muscles at the back of the neck, which are doing the constricting. Standing under a very warm shower has great benefits in easing these tense muscles, as is placing first hot, then warm towels on the nape of the neck.

• **RECIPES THAT CAN BE ENJOYED BY HEADACHE AND MIGRAINE SUFFERERS**

Garlic bean soup
Pea, mint and lettuce soup
Parsnip and apple soup
Sorrel soup
Spinach borscht

Fish terrine
Caramelized artichoke and tomato toasts
Radicchio and grape salad
Baked pasta with ratatouille sauce
Gado gado
Yam biryani
Salmon and asparagus risotto
Garlic and herb chicken
Chicken stroganoff with tarragon
Honey and mustard quail

Minted meatballs with yoghurt sauce

Mixed fruits with butterscotch sauce
Blackberry and raspberry fool
Vanilla poached peaches
Poached pears with ginger
Apple and fig crumble
Fruit compote

Fruit and malt loaf
Date and walnut cake
Banana cake
Barabrith
Fig and ginger parkin
Fruit cake
Flapjacks

12 High blood cholesterol and high blood pressure

High blood cholesterol and high blood pressure are both risk factors in the development of heart disease, one of the major killers in Western society. Nutrition plays an important part in the prevention and treatment of both.

HIGH BLOOD CHOLESTEROL

Many women have problems with their blood fat levels. Some women, especially those with extremely low body weights or an eating disorder such as anorexia nervosa, can suffer from too little fat in their blood, but for the majority, blood fat problems mean too many fats. Hyperlipidaemia is the technical name, which means the presence of abnormally high levels of lipids (cholesterol and triglycerides) within the blood. Blood fat levels are measured as part of routine blood tests and usually quote four values (see the table on the next page).

Many women come to see me confused about what cholesterol and triglycerides are and how they can reduce them, and asking about the difference between 'good' and 'bad' cholesterol. There is so much written about cholesterol and other blood fats in newspapers and magazines, but unfortunately all it seems to do is confuse and depress. Articles tell you what you shouldn't do, yet don't make any positive suggestions as to what you can eat. This chapter aims to redress the balance.

• WHY IS HYPERLIPIDAEMIA A PROBLEM?
Hyperlipidaemia is a silent risk factor condition, in other words it generally doesn't give rise to noticeable symptoms. Occasionally women notice fatty deposits

under the skin, or opticians pick up changes within the eye structure that leads them to suggest a blood fat test, but the majority of women discover that they have hyperlipidaemia when they are having a blood test, either as part of a general screening exercise or when investigating other conditions and symptoms. Since high blood fat levels have been implicated in heart disease, it is in every woman's interest to make sure that blood fat levels are as close to the ideal as possible.

Although nutrition plays a key role in trying to maintain satisfactory blood fat levels, your body produces 75% of your blood fats regardless of what you eat. Therefore the food you eat can only reduce your blood fat levels by 25%, it cannot achieve miracles. However, this 25% reduction can significantly reduce your risk of heart disease and other conditions such as pancreatic cancer, so it is an important issue to address.

REFERENCE AND SUGGESTED 'HEALTHY' RANGES FOR PLASMA LIPIDS IN ADULTS UNDER 60 YEARS

	Reference range mmol/1	Suggested range mmol/1
Total cholesterol	3.5–7.8	<5.2
Low density lipoprotein (LDL) cholesterol	2.3–6.1	<4.0
High density lipoprotein (HDL) cholesterol	0.8–1.7	>1.15
Triglycerides	0.7–1.8	0.7–1.7

mmol/1 = millimoles per litre

Taken from Manual of Dietetic Practice, second edition, 1994.

Edited for The British Dietetic Association by Briony Thomas.

Blackwell Scientific Publications

• UNDERSTANDING YOUR BLOOD FAT READINGS

The figures in the table are given to help you interpret a doctor's test of your blood fats (plasma lipids). The reference is calculated from the mean range of an apparently healthy population. However, sex and age differences need to be considered:

• Triglycerides are higher in men than women. HDL levels are higher in women than men.
• Lipids may increase with age, consequently a cholesterol value in the reference range of 7.0 mmol/1 would be much more noteworthy in a person of 25 years than one of 55 years.

FIRST YOU NEED TO UNDERSTAND THE DIFFERENCE BETWEEN THE VARIOUS BLOOD FATS

• CHOLESTEROL

Cholesterol is a fatty, wax-like substance produced by stress, biochemical and hormonal reactions and food, primarily in your liver, but also in your intestines and other cells within the body. Cholesterol is not all bad news. It plays an essential part in the production of sex hormones such as oestrogen and progesterone, is involved in the synthesis of vitamin D and is also needed in the production of your myelin sheath, the fatty protective substance that surrounds your nerves.

Cholesterol, as with other blood fats, creates a problem only when you have too much of it in your body. Too much cholesterol can promote the production of a fatty plaque that can clog up your arteries. If this happens, the blood flow is interrupted, which in a main heart vessel can cause a heart attack or, in the blood vessel leading to your brain, a stroke. Blocked arteries also cause circulation problems: numbness and pain in your hands and feet.

Nutritionally we need to keep the risk of a fatty plaque blockage as low as possible. In order to do this, you need to understand a little more about the 'good' and 'bad' types of cholesterol.

Within your body the appropriate amount of cholesterol needs to be broken down into a form that can be used by the body and delivered to the cells that need it. Your liver repackages cholesterol, along with a few extra substances, as low density lipoprotein (LDL). As LDL flows through the blood, it latches on to specific receptor sites on the cells that need the cholesterol. When the cells have had enough cholesterol, they stop producing the receptor sites. When this happens, the unused LDL stays in the blood and can start to irritate the blood vessel lining, which then causes a fatty plaque to form.

At this stage, other factors are involved, for example smoking and the presence of other substances such as sugar. Nicotine from cigarettes and abnormally high sugar levels, present in uncontrolled diabetics, irritate the cells in the lining of the blood vessels and make them more susceptible to developing a plaque. But fundamentally the plaque would not be able to form if there wasn't LDL around. If you have too much LDL in your blood, this is referred to as having 'bad' cholesterol.

The 'good' type of cholesterol is high density lipoprotein (HDL). The production of HDL in the liver is stimulated by certain foods. HDL carries the excess amounts of LDL cholesterol back to your intestine, where it is excreted. You generally don't need to worry if HDL levels are raised, as this doesn't cause any health problems.

To reduce the incidence of heart disease and strokes you need to make sure your LDL level is low and your HDL level is high, in order to excrete as much LDL as possible.

• TRIGLYCERIDES

Triglycerides, another type of blood fat, are produced by the body in response to alcohol, hormones and sugar. They are associated with heart disease and pancreatic cancer, therefore you need to try to keep your triglyceride level low.

HOW DO YOU KNOW IF YOU HAVE A BLOOD FAT PROBLEM?

Blood fat levels are measured as part of a standard blood test, so if you are having a blood test for any reason you can ask your doctor for the readings. The only way to find out if your blood fat levels are within the ideal ranges is to have a sample of your blood tested, either by your doctor or by using a self-testing kit, available at many pharmacies. Since the food you eat can raise your blood fat levels, the majority of doctors recommend that you take a 'fasting' sample: you must not eat anything for eight to ten hours before the test. The results will indicate whether you need to alter your eating habits.

Before you implement nutritional measures to change your blood fat profile, there are other influences to consider:

• The female hormone oestrogen alters your metabolism of cholesterol and helps to keep your LDL levels low. This is why women, up until the menopause, have a lower incidence of heart disease than men. After the menopause, when the body's oestrogen levels drop, the protective effect is lost. This explains why our risk of heart disease and strokes increases at this point.

• The contraceptive pill lowers HDL and increases LDL levels, which is one of the reasons why doctors regularly check women taking the pill.

• Hormone replacement therapy (HRT) can lower LDL and increase HDL levels. This is obviously advantageous, but the evidence exists only for women who take a pure oestrogen-based hormone replacement and this is usually prescribed only to women who have had their womb removed. When progesterone is used in the HRT, we are not sure about its effect on the risk of heart disease. See the chapter on the menopause for more information on HRT.

HOW TO BUILD UP A PERFECT BLOOD PROFILE

All women can take steps to improve their blood scenario. A common mistake is to think that in order to reduce the blood cholesterol level you just need to stop taking in foods that contain cholesterol, such as eggs, shellfish and offal (liver, kidney, brain etc.). These foods (dietary cholesterol) do not have a significant impact on the blood cholesterol and LDL levels, because the cholesterol in them is broken down quite efficiently by the body. Obviously, if you have a lot of these foods and very few of the good, cholesterol-lowering foods such as oily fish, garlic and fibre (see below), your blood cholesterol level may be a little high. However, this is not normally the situation in women I see, which is why they get upset about the fact that they seem to be doing the right thing and yet their cholesterol level remains high.

The major influence on the level of LDL in the blood is the intake of saturated fats. These include animal fats such as butter, cheese and cream, and are also found in hard margarines and some vegetable oils. Coconut and palm oil, for example, are highly saturated fats, as is the hydrogenated vegetable oil or fat in hard margarine and used in many manufactured foods, both sweet and savoury. These make the body produce more LDL, therefore in order to keep your LDL level low, you need to make sure that your saturated fat intake is not too high.

The level of LDL in the blood is a result of the balance between the amounts taken in, produced and excreted by the body. In our society, where we are generally ruled by what we cannot eat, many women seem to make the right moves in terms of reducing their intake of saturated fats, but they fail to consider how they can change the balance between intake and excretion, by making the body excrete more. This is how positive nutrition comes into the picture.

You need to make sure that your body has as much HDL as possible, in order to carry the LDL to the intestine to be excreted. You can also encourage the body to excrete LDL by taking in more of other beneficial foods. In addition, you can ensure that your diet contains plenty of the nutrients that prevent LDL from forming deposits in your blood vessels.

• **INCREASE YOUR INTAKE OF HDL-PRODUCING FOODS**
Some foods can stimulate your body to produce HDL. Garlic contains a substance that has this effect, as do oily fish such as herrings, mackerel, sardines, tuna and salmon. The oily fish contain beneficial types of fat called omega-3 fatty acid and omega-6 fatty acid, which help your body to carry more LDL to the intestine to be excreted.

As well as this beneficial function, both garlic and oily fish contain other substances that help reduce your likelihood of developing a blood clot. A blood clot is a collection of blood cells, rather than fat, but this can also block a blood vessel, so the more we can do to prevent this, the better.

I recommend that you aim to have at least two or three meals based on oily fish and/or garlic every week. There are plenty of ideas for soups, dips, kedgeree and risotto in this book, or try freshly grilled sardines or herrings, tuna steaks or salmon.

The fresh garlic, which is in the shops for just a couple of months each year, contains the most anti-clotting substances, but during the rest of the year the older garlic is fine. Scientists haven't decided whether it is significantly better to eat raw or cooked garlic, so I think you should eat it as you like. There is, however, hardly any benefit from using garlic salt.

If you find the smell of garlic a little anti-social, try chewing fresh parsley or coffee beans after you've eaten it, to reduce the potency of the smell.

There are garlic and fish oil supplements on the market, for people who don't want to eat foods containing the real ingredients. I am not convinced by their efficacy; nothing could be more effective than the real food.

• **INCREASE YOUR INTAKE OF FIBRE**
Fibre helps your body in two ways. Firstly, fibre produces substances that enable the body to excrete more LDL. Secondly, the presence of fibre in your meals acts as a buffer: less fat is brought into contact with your blood vessels, which means less fat is absorbed and

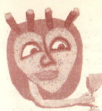

Choose young red wines, as they contain the most tannin and anthocyanin. Wines based on the Cabernet Sauvignon grape, whether from the Médoc region of France or virtually anywhere in the world, are particularly good. So are wines based on some of the most popular Italian grapes, such as Sangiovese, the grape behind Chianti, and Nebbiolo, which makes Barolo, Barbaresco and other northern Italian wines.

more LDL is kept bound within the gut and excreted. Eating vegetables (including dried beans and lentils), fruits and wholegrain cereals, bread, pasta and rice every day really helps to bring your blood fat profile within the ideal range.

Oats have been singled out for praise because they are rich in a particular type of fibre that has proved especially useful in reducing cholesterol levels. Try to include oats in your meals at least once or twice a week, as oatcakes, flapjacks, porridge or in fruit crumbles.

Remember that when you increase your fibre intake you also need to drink more water, in order for the fibre to swell and work effectively.

• INCREASE YOUR INTAKE OF ANTIOXIDANTS

There is little harm in fat circulating around the body; problems occur when it starts to form deposits in the blood vessels. In order for fat to deposit, it needs to oxidize. Nutritionally we can stop this by eating plenty of foods containing antioxidants, nutrients that prevent fat from oxidizing and depositing.

The most powerful antioxidants found in food are vitamins A, C and E. Foods rich in these antioxidants are discussed in the section on What your body needs in Part One; many of them are fresh fruits and vegetables. Ideally you should have five portions of fresh fruits and/or vegetables every day. By a portion I mean a piece of fruit such as a whole orange or a kiwi fruit, or a large helping of salad or lightly cooked vegetables, or a bowl of vegetable soup. Rather than worrying about the scientific size of the portion, I suggest you eat three pieces of antioxidant-rich fresh fruits and include a good helping of vegetables or salad at your two main meals.

Two other powerful antioxidants, called anthocyanin and tannin, are found in young red wine. It is recommended that, unless you have a contraindication to alcohol such as liver or kidney problems, you drink a glass of red wine every day. However, red wine does not contain anything magical, just antioxidants in a different form. If you don't want to drink, you can easily derive just as many antioxidants from other foods.

- **AVOID EXPOSURE TO OTHER RISK FACTORS**
- Stress can cause your liver to produce more fat, in particular LDL cholesterol. Since stress is in itself a risk factor in heart disease and cancer, you should take steps to reduce the stress levels in your life. I heard a lovely phrase recently: 'It's time to be a human being rather than a human doing!'
- Excess body weight can lead to high blood pressure, which is another risk factor linked with high blood fat levels and heart disease. The ideal is a Body Mass Index between 20 and 25 (see page 46). Body weight above this can lead to high blood pressure, but it is equally important not to 'yo-yo' with your weight. Rapid weight loss is as detrimental to your health as rapid weight gain. If you are overweight you should aim to lose around 1–1.5 kg/2–3 lb a week by following a healthy eating plan (see the chapter on weight loss).
- Caffeine and smoking both irritate the blood vessel linings, making them more likely to develop fatty plaques. Try to keep your caffeine intake down and stop smoking.

GENERAL GUIDELINES

- **WATCH YOUR FAT INTAKE**
Keep your saturated fat intake low. Limit the amount of butter, cheese and cream you eat, and choose lean cuts of meat when possible, cut the skin off chicken and eat more fish. The good news here is that game is particularly low in saturated fat. In particular, avoid hard margarines, as they are high in a type of saturated fat known as trans-fatty acids, which can lead to 'free radical' damage within the cells of the body. (See page 296 for further information.)

Look for the vegetable oils with a high proportion of unsaturated fats: polyunsaturates and monounsaturates.

Monounsaturated fats have the positive benefit of stimulating the body to produce HDL, and fortunately one of the most delicious and varied oils, olive oil, is high in monounsaturates. Other useful oils include peanut, corn, safflower, sunflower, soya, rapeseed, hazelnut and walnut. Avocados are high in monounsaturates, and are delicious spread on bread instead of butter, topped with tomatoes for a satisfying snack.

• EXERCISE

Aerobic exercise helps to reduce blood fat levels. It can also reduce your risk of developing heart disease and particular types of cancer. It is therefore a very good idea to try to include at least 20 minutes of aerobic exercise at least three times a week: try running, jogging, swimming, cycling, power walking or brisk walking.

• BOOST GUT BACTERIA

Two bacteria commonly found in the gut, acidophilus and bifidus, have been linked to a decreased risk of heart disease. It is thought that they produce substances that encourage the body to excrete more LDL and possibly raise HDL levels. Research is still in its early days, but it can do no harm to eat a small pot of 'live' yoghurt containing these bacteria (often labelled 'bio') every day.

• EAT SMALL MEALS

Try to eat small meals often, rather than one large meal each day. Leaving your gut without any food for hours and hours and then putting a large meal into it is not healthy. This habit not only puts a strain on your digestion, but it is also thought to raise your LDL levels.

ARE SUPPLEMENTS HELPFUL?

There has been so much interest surrounding antioxidants, in connection with reducing the incidence of heart disease and cancer, that many women wonder whether they should be taking a supplement as well as eating a balanced diet. Many studies seem to suggest that we need to take an antioxidant tablet, but the evidence is not conclusive. One of the most common supplements taken by women is the antioxidant vitamin C. Since it is a water-soluble vitamin, the body does not store large amounts of it. I encourage women to have five portions of fresh fruits or vegetables every day, so that the body will easily meet the daily recommended intake of 60 mg of vitamin C. Contrary to popular belief, consuming more than 1000 mg a day does not have clearly proven benefits. If you try to eat plenty of fresh fruit and vegetables and keep the cooking time to a minimum you should get sufficient vitamin C not only to prevent LDL from depositing in your blood vessels, but also to benefit from its anti-cancer properties.

As long as you are eating a well-balanced diet consisting of at least five portions of fresh fruits or vegetables every day, I believe you should not need a supplement.

HOW TO CORRECT RAISED BLOOD FATS

Before you embark on any sort of eating plan, you need to establish which form of hyperlipidaemia you have. Although a lot of the nutritional principles apply to both cholesterol and triglycerides, there are differences in emphasis. Remember that any nutritional action has only got the chance of reducing your blood fats by 25%, so it is often the subtle, finely-tuned changes that make a real difference.

People are often told that they have a raised cholesterol level, without any further information. You really need to know which of your cholesterol levels is raised: LDL or HDL? Remember that it doesn't matter if you have high HDL, in fact it is beneficial. If you don't have access to the exact analysis I suggest you assume that your LDL is raised, as this is the harmful cholesterol.

There are three potential problem scenarios:

If you find that since you have reduced one of the most concentrated sources of calories, i.e. fats, your body weight drops, I suggest you increase the amount of carbohydrates such as pasta, rice, potatoes and bread. These will give you a healthy energy supply.

• RAISED CHOLESTEROL LEVEL (WITH A NORMAL TRIGLYCERIDE LEVEL)

If you are told that you have a raised cholesterol level it is likely that your doctor means you have too much LDL in your blood and not enough HDL.

Make sure that your body weight is within the ideal range (see page 46). If it is above this I suggest you reduce it: a reduction in body weight commonly brings your LDL level down. A healthy-eating weight-reducing diet is a good basis to start from, but place particular emphasis on fat. You must make sure that as well as reducing your total fat intake, you keep to unsaturated vegetable oils and avoid saturated, LDL cholesterol-forming fats such as butter and hard margarines.

If you are of ideal body weight you should:
• Reduce the total amount of fat in your diet, by avoiding fatty foods and using the minimum amount in cooking.
• Make sure that any fat you use is of the most beneficial, HDL-producing kind.
• Make sure that you are not over-indulging in the cholesterol-rich foods, such as eggs, seafood and offal. Enjoy them as a treat, don't eat them every day.
• Increase your fibre intake.
• Increase your intake of antioxidants, garlic and water.
• Avoid the other risk factors: smoking, stress and caffeine.

• RAISED TRIGLYCERIDE LEVEL (WITH A NORMAL CHOLESTEROL LEVEL)

Women with raised triglyceride levels are at far greater risk of developing heart disease than men with the equivalent triglyceride level. However, this situation is a little less common and requires different advice to the other two scenarios. Triglycerides are produced in your body, but rather than being a by-product of saturated fats they are created in response to sugary foods and alcohol.

If your weight is above the ideal (see page 46), I suggest you go on a healthy weight-reducing diet and your blood triglyceride levels should decrease.

If your weight is normal I suggest you:
• Reduce your intake of sugary foods.
• Increase your intake of oily fish.
• Reduce alcohol intake, as alcohol can cause your liver to produce and store excessive amounts of triglycerides.
• Increase your intake of antioxidants, garlic and water.
• Try not to use too much of the hard margarines, as they contain trans-fatty acids, which can cause damage within the body's cells.
• Avoid the other risk factors: smoking, stress and caffeine.

• RAISED CHOLESTEROL AND TRIGLYCERIDE LEVELS

Reduce your weight if you are over the upper end of the ideal range (see page 46).

If your weight is acceptable you should:
• Increase your fibre and antioxidant intakes.
• Reduce your total fat intake.
• Any fat you use should be an HDL-producing fat such as olive or sunflower oil. If you need to use a hard fat, use a small amount of butter rather than a hard margarine. Although butter produces cholesterol, I think it is much better to have the natural product.
• Think of the cholesterol-containing foods, such as seafood and eggs, as a treat and not part of your everyday eating plan.
• Keep your sugar and alcohol intakes moderately low. Try to resist very rich cakes and lots of biscuits. If you fancy something sweet, have fresh fruits.
• Eat plenty of starchy foods: pasta, rice, potatoes and bread. Since you have reduced three of the most concentrated sources of calories in the diet – fat, sugar and alcohol – you may find that your weight drops. Keep up your energy levels with pasta and other starches.
• Increase your intake of oily fish and water.

Always remember that food should never be something you feel deprived over. Cholesterol is a risk factor, not a disease. If you fancy having a seafood supper or a platter of cheese, then have it. Don't let it become an everyday habit at the expense of other more ideal foods, but see it as a treat and treasure it.

HIGH BLOOD PRESSURE

Blood pressure is the force exerted by the blood on the inner walls of the blood vessels, and is related to the elasticity and diameter of the vessels and the force of the heart beat. A blood pressure measurement is expressed as one number over another, e.g. 120/80. The upper (systolic) value reflects the force with which the heart pumps blood around the body and the bottom (diastolic) value is the pressure in the blood vessels when they are relaxed. Normal blood pressure readings for women are in the region of 120/80. The bottom (diastolic) pressure is the important one in terms of establishing whether you have hyper-tension, which is the medical term for high blood pressure. A diastolic pressure of 90 to 105 is considered mildly hypertensive; 105 to 120 is moderately hypertensive; and above 120 is severely hypertensive. Blood pressure rises gradually as you get older, but when someone has high blood pressure it means that the pressure in the relaxed blood vessels is higher than ideal. Hypertension may be caused by several factors, including kidney and heart problems, but in the majority of cases there is no known cause. Your doctor will be able to deal with kidney and heart problems, but simple hypertension can be managed quite successfully by modifications to nutrition and lifestyle.

Excess weight, stress and high blood fat levels all aggravate hypertension, so it is important to reduce them as much as possible. If hypertension is ignored it can lead to an increased risk of heart disease, strokes or kidney problems. Some women need medication to help control their blood pressure, but most doctors will explore all of the non-drug remedies – weight, blood fat and stress reduction – before they give you any drugs. All drugs have side effects and they are also expensive and invasive. It is much better to tackle the problem through nutrition and general lifestyle.

GENERAL GUIDELINES TO CORRECT HYPERTENSION

Keeping your body in good shape means that your blood vessels are more likely to remain elastic and unclogged.

Try to take regular aerobic exercise. Exercise helps keep the heart and other muscles strong and efficient. If you laze around all the time the heart may become less efficient and may struggle when you then exert pressure on it. It is much better to do some regular exercise that exerts a controlled pressure on your heart. Check with your doctor before you embark on any exercise programme, but good aerobic exercises include brisk walking, swimming and running.

Try to reduce stress. Stress causes your body to release hormones such as adrenaline (the 'fight or flight' hormone), which increases the blood pressure within the body in anticipation of sudden movement. High blood pressure often improves if you reduce the amount of stress in your life. Take the time to relax, through hobbies, stress management classes, and by listening to music you love.

If you smoke, try to give up. Smoking causes your blood vessel linings to become more sensitive to developing fatty plaque deposits.

NUTRITIONAL GUIDELINES

If you have hypertension you should make an effort to eat a well-balanced diet, as discussed in What your body needs, in Part One. A healthy diet will provide your body with all the foods it needs to help reduce your blood pressure. In addition it is important to consider the following:

• **TRY TO KEEP YOUR WEIGHT WITHIN THE IDEAL RANGE**
Refer to the chart on page 46; if your weight is on the high side, you may well find that losing weight will

lower your blood pressure. It may even cease to become a problem. Excess weight around the waist and chest is particularly dangerous, as this places undue strain on your blood vessels and heart. Obviously there are disadvantages of carrying too much weight anywhere, but because the important blood vessels leading to and from the heart are located in the chest and tummy regions, excess fat can reduce the diameter of the blood vessels and cause a rise in blood pressure. If you are overweight you should reduce your weight slowly and sensibly, by following the advice in the chapter on weight loss. It is very important not to 'crash diet', as this can place stress on your heart.

• WATCH YOUR CHOLESTEROL LEVEL

Cholesterol, as discussed earlier in this chapter, can deposit in the blood vessels and cause the pressure within them to rise. If you have a high cholesterol level, try to do as much as you can to keep it down. Remember that stress can cause your body to produce more cholesterol.

• LIMIT YOUR INTAKE OF SALT

For many women, watching the amount of salty foods they eat can help reduce blood pressure. Salt, or sodium chloride, is found naturally in small amounts in many foods. It is used in greater quantities in manufactured foods, both as a preservative and as a flavour enhancer. It is virtually impossible to avoid all foods with salt or sodium in them, but far easier to reach a sensible, palatable compromise, by taking small steps to reduce your sodium intake without detracting from the enjoyment of eating.

• Try to get out of the habit of adding unnecessary salt in cooking. Taste food before you add salt. It is one of the greatest insults to a cook who has spent hours creating the balance of flavours to add salt before you taste the food. Try to wean yourself off salt and experiment with subtler flavours, using herbs and spices.

• Resist very salty foods. Your taste buds are the best

judge, but the following are very high in salt: smoked salmon, dried fish, tinned and cured anchovies, pickled herrings, smoked bacon, dill and other vegetable pickles, sauerkraut, salt dried beef and ham such as bresaola, prosciutto (e.g. Parma ham) and the Spanish jamon serrano, plus many other salt preserved meats. Instead of the salty preserved foods, choose the fresh alternative, for example, fresh salmon or trout, lean beef, fresh vegetables.

• BOOST YOUR POTASSIUM INTAKE

Sodium and potassium are elements that exist in balance within your body. Generally, if the sodium level is high, the potassium level is low. Therefore boosting your potassium intake is one of the most effective ways of lowering or maintaining an acceptable level of sodium within your blood. Potassium is found in abundance in most fruits, vegetables and wholegrain products. The following are especially rich fruit sources: apricots, bananas, cantaloupe melons, figs, grapes, peaches and plums, being even higher in the dried versions such as raisins and prunes. Among vegetables, good sources are: tomatoes, squash, broad beans, potatoes, beetroot, spinach and avocados.

A generally healthy eating pattern provides plenty of potassium. You should not take any form of potassium supplement unless this has been prescribed by your doctor. They are potentially very dangerous.

• INCLUDE SOME DAIRY PRODUCTS IN YOUR DAILY DIET

Milk and dairy products such as yoghurt, fromage frais and cheese are the major source of calcium in the Western diet. Calcium has been found to be helpful in correcting high blood pressure, so you should try to include some milk and dairy products in your diet. If you're watching your weight or your saturated fat intake, remember that semi-skimmed milk and low-fat yoghurt contain plenty of calcium. If you don't like dairy products, other food sources of calcium include white bread, spinach, ready-to-eat apricots and sesame seeds, although the calcium in these is more difficult for the body to absorb. You may need to take a calcium supplement, but discuss this with your doctor.

• OTHER BENEFICIAL FOODS

There are several other nutrients that can help to reduce blood pressure, both in their own right and by helping to prevent blood fats from depositing in your blood vessels. These include fish oils (omega-3 and omega-6 fatty acids, found in fish such as salmon, mackerel and herring), garlic and antioxidants (found primarily in fresh fruits and vegetables, but also in young red wines such as Beaujolais).

• RECIPES TO REDUCE HIGH BLOOD CHOLESTEROL

Garlic bean soup

Minestrone soup

French onion soup

Baked garlic bruschetta

Hummus

Guacamole

Smoked mackerel pâté

Caramelized artichoke and tomato toasts

Chicken with melon, grapes and asparagus

Warm duck breast salad with apricots

Artichoke and avocado salad

Grilled vegetable salad

Grilled peppers with garlic cheese croûtons

Tomatoes stuffed with olives, garlic and parsley

Broccoli with roasted tomatoes

Grapefruit, smoked salmon and avocado salad

Pasta bows with courgettes

Baked pasta with ratatouille sauce

Salmon and celery kedgeree

Salmon and asparagus risotto

Salmon and lemon lasagne

Smoked fish casserole

Smoked mackerel and spinach fishcakes

Honey and mustard quail

Garlic and herb chicken

Coconut chicken

Raspberry and blackberry fool

Vanilla poached peaches

Apple and fig crumble

Mixed berries in Grand Marnier

Fruit compote

Tropical dried fruit salad

Flapjacks

Barabrith

Staffordshire oatcakes

Oatcakes

13 Hypoglycaemia

Hypoglycaemia is the medical term for a low blood sugar level. When the level of sugar in your blood drops below a level at which your body is comfortable, which varies under different circumstances, you are likely to feel very unwell. The most common symptoms are weakness, shaking, mood swings, insomnia, migraine and headaches, pallor, irritability, nausea and fatigue.

Many women find that they feel low in sugar just before they start their period, when they are under stress or when they have exercised vigorously. Our sex hormones, oestrogen and progesterone, as well as our stress hormones, such as adrenaline, appear to be crucial players in dictating whether we feel low enough to suffer from hypoglycaemic symptoms. True hypoglycaemia can be diagnosed by a blood test. It takes two forms: fasting hypoglycaemia, which occurs when you haven't eaten for six or more hours, and reactive hypoglycaemia, which occurs any time from half an hour to four hours after a meal. You should also be aware that some medication can precipitate hypoglycaemic symptoms. For example, many women taking Metronidazole, used to treat thrush and other infections, suffer from symptoms such as shakiness, but this usually disappears when the medication is stopped.

Treatments for hypoglycaemia range from those supervised by your doctor and dietitian to simple nutritional and lifestyle adjustments. The majority of women who experience symptoms of hypoglycaemia find that the symptoms can easily be rectified by adopting good eating habits.

• WHY DO SOME WOMEN SUFFER FROM HYPOGLYCAEMIA?

Hypoglycaemia, whether it is fasting or reactive, suggests that your blood sugar regulatory system is not functioning effectively. Usually, when you eat a meal containing sugar, either in a simple form such as a sugary food or in a more complex form, a natural carbohydrate such as bread or potato, the body secretes a hormone called insulin. The insulin enables your body to use the sugar as fuel or store it for later use. If your body secretes too little insulin the blood sugar level remains too high and this means you are a diabetic. Hypoglycaemia is the opposite condition and is thought on many occasions to be caused by too much insulin being produced. The effect of insulin on too little food is to lower the blood sugar levels, producing the shaking, pallor and other symptoms similar to those experienced by a diabetic who has injected insulin and then not eaten.

A low blood sugar level after not eating for six or more hours is less common and more serious than reactive hypoglycaemia. Fasting hypoglycaemia may be a symptom of your body not managing your insulin and sugar levels if you're diabetic, a tumour of the pancreas (the organ that secretes insulin), liver damage, starvation (as with anorexic women), or cancer. Hypoglycaemia may also be a symptom of an underactive or overactive thyroid gland. If you suffer from any of the symptoms, it is important that you seek the advice of your doctor, who will be able to check for these conditions.

• TESTING FOR HYPOGLYCAEMIA

It is relatively easy to test for fasting hypoglycaemia. The most common test used is the Glucose Tolerance Test (GTT). This entails taking a very sugary drink and testing the blood sugar levels at regular intervals, to see how your body reacts. If your blood sugar level behaves in an abnormal fashion, your doctor may diagnose either fasting hypoglycaemia, or a sensitivity to sugar. Other tests will probably be arranged to determine the cause. If no serious conditions are found you should follow the advice in this chapter.

A sensitivity to sugar causes your body to overreact to sugary food by producing too much insulin, making your blood sugar level drop too low. A third possibility is that the test shows no evidence of an abnormality, in which case the symptoms can be put down to periodic hypoglycaemia (see page 231).

GUIDELINES FOR PREVENTING AND MANAGING HYPOGLYCAEMIA

The nutritional principles are aimed at keeping your blood sugar level as steady as possible. The foods you eat and the pattern of eating should prevent your sugar level from rising and falling rapidly. In women who don't have an abnormal GTT it is very often the rapid rises and falls in sugar level that make them feel unwell, rather than the sugar level itself.

• EAT A WELL-BALANCED DIET
Focus your eating plan on fresh vegetables, fruit and wholegrain cereal foods, with lean proteins, small amounts of fat and plenty of water. See What your body needs and Healthy eating for life in Part One.

• EAT SMALL MEALS, OFTEN
You can help stabilize your blood sugar levels by making sure that you have small, regular meals. Try not to leave more than three or four hours between your snacks or meals. This eating pattern prevents your blood sugar from dropping too low and helps you refrain from overeating at meal times. Overeating could overload your body with large quantities of sugar-containing foods. It is much better to space meals out and give your body a chance to digest food well, rather than go for long periods of not eating and then overeating.

The majority of women I see find that they feel a lot better if they have five or six small snacks, rather than three large meals. This need not cause weight gain as long as the total amount you consume throughout the day is not greater than you would consume in three normal meals. Separating your main meals into two or more courses can provide a healthy eating pattern that shouldn't increase your weight. For instance save your dessert until three hours later. If you find that you crave sugary foods, or more food in general, just before your period is due, I suggest you read the chapter on periods, as this will help you to conquer your cravings.

Regular meals not only help to keep your blood sugar level steady, they also help protect your stomach from too much acid and ensure that there is a regular flow of food through the bowel.

• KEEP SNACKS HANDY

Make sure that you have a supply of snacks readily available so that you can have something appropriate to eat every few hours. Choose foods that are high in neither fat nor sugar. Fresh or dried fruits, cake or biscuits made with wholewheat flour or oats are good to keep in your handbag or at work.

• AVOID SUGARY FOODS ON AN EMPTY STOMACH

If you eat a sugary food on an empty stomach, the level of sugar in your blood rises quickly. The rapid rise in sugar level causes your body to secrete too much insulin, which then causes your sugar level to fall quickly. I recommend that you avoid these foods as much as possible, and if you feel that you can't live without them or you really enjoy them as a occasional treat, have them after a meal containing a lot of fibre, i.e. a meal with lots of vegetables, wholegrains or pulses. The fibre will have a cushioning effect and help to slow down the rise in sugar. Some women seem to be able to control hypoglycaemic symptoms in this way.

- **AVOID DRINKING ALCOHOL ON AN EMPTY STOMACH**

Alcohol has much the same effect on your blood sugar as sugary foods, ultimately resulting in falling blood sugar levels and distressing low-sugar symptoms. The extent to which you have to avoid alcohol varies according to the severity of your symptoms. Some women manage to enjoy a little alcohol with food. Other women find that they can drink 'drier' alcoholic drinks such as Champagne. If you wish to drink alcohol make sure you have it with a meal that contains some fibre, which will help to cushion the adverse sugar effects.

- **AVOID CAFFEINE-CONTAINING DRINKS**

Caffeine, present in coffee, tea, cola-based drinks and hot chocolate, stimulates your pancreas to secrete more insulin. This aggravates sugar sensitivities and low-sugar symptoms. Some women can tolerate small amounts of caffeine provided it is not drunk on an empty stomach. However, I recommend that you try to cut out all caffeine, for at least two or three weeks, and prepare to be amazed at how much better you feel. See page 62 for alternative drinks.

- **TRY TO KEEP YOUR BODY WEIGHT STABLE AND WITHIN THE IDEAL RANGE**

It is important to make sure that your body weight is acceptable (see the table on page 46) and doesn't fall or rise rapidly. 'Crash' dieting frequently causes hypoglycaemic episodes; if you need to lose weight, see the chapter on weight loss. If you are underweight your ability to control your blood sugar level may be compromised.

- **TRY TO GIVE UP SMOKING**

Be aware that smoking compromises your ability to control your blood sugar levels. Nicotine, present in cigarette smoke, increases the production of insulin and decreases the production of another hormone called glucagon. Glucagon is secreted in the liver in response to low blood sugar levels. Glucagon's role is to stimulate the liver to release glucose which has been stored in the liver as glycogen. If you smoke your body may find it very difficult to regulate its sugar levels, as it is forever reacting to a dose of nicotine.

• **TRY TO KEEP HEALTHY IN BODY AND MIND**
A healthy body and mind is much less likely to suffer from conditions such as hypoglycaemia. Try to set aside time for yourself to relax every day and exercise at least three times a week.

• **DO YOU NEED A CHROMIUM SUPPLEMENT?**
Chromium is a trace element, i.e. a mineral that is found in the body and needed in minute quantities. It is essential for the production of insulin, the hormone that the body produces to control blood sugar levels. Low levels of chromium in the body have been linked with poor blood sugar control.

Some people ask if they should take a chromium supplement. I don't advocate this as we are not sure how much chromium we need and taking a concentrated dose could be inappropriate. I advise women to make sure that they have some of the more concentrated sources of chromium as part of their daily diet. These include: scallops, clams, oysters, cheese, black pepper, brewers' yeast (found in beer and sold in health food shops for sprinkling on cereals and yoghurt), baked beans and wholewheat products.

REACTIONS TO SUGAR

Although there are various types of sugar in food, such as sucrose, glucose, fructose (fruit sugar), molasses and honey, they all have similar effects on blood sugar levels, and should all be treated with caution if you are sensitive to sugar level changes. There is very little difference in the speed at which these different sugars affect you. The effect depends less on the type of sugar and more on the fibre content of the food. This is the reason why a piece of fruit will produce a less dramatic effect than a piece of chocolate.

If you avoid sugary foods you will probably find that your blood sugar levels will not cause any symptoms. Don't feel that you need to read the sides of packets and avoid everything that contains sugar. Just follow your taste buds and resist the things that taste very sweet. If you fancy something sweet-tasting you should choose a dessert that contains some fibre, to cushion the sugar. Cakes and desserts made with fresh or dried fruits should do the trick: think of apple crumble, apricot tart or carrot cake.

• ARTIFICIAL SWEETENERS

There are several types of artificial sweeteners, some used in manufactured products, some sold for use as direct sugar substitutes in drinks or in cooking. Although they taste sweet they do not usually affect blood sugar levels in the same way as normal sugars. Therefore if you have hypoglycaemia they can help give you a sugary taste that won't alter your blood sugar level.

However, as with all food substitutes, I don't advocate that you go out of your way to use them. The taste is inferior to the real thing, and they can give you a false sense of security; the more you get used to the sweet taste the harder it will be to break the sugar-craving cycle. You need to give yourself other types of treats, rather than sweet foods, if you are to re-educate yourself.

High dosages of certain sweeteners such as aspartame and saccharin have been linked to particular cancers, so this is another reason to try to re-educate your sweet tooth and avoid using sweeteners in any quantity. Fructose, often used in diabetic products, may have a laxative effect.

PERIODIC HYPOGLYCAEMIA

If your sensitivity occurs at a particular time of the month, this is probably caused by changes in your hormone levels. As the levels of oestrogen rise about one week after ovulation, blood serotonin levels fall. The fall in serotonin can make you feel hypoglycaemic, although it is highly likely that if you measured your blood sugar level it would not be low. This hypoglycaemia may also account for pre-menstrual symptoms such as mood swings and tiredness.

Stress can also cause periodic hypoglycaemia. The stress hormones, such as adrenaline, can cause the pancreas to secrete more insulin, leading to a drop in your blood sugar level. When you are stressed you should make sure that you are eating regular, small, healthy meals to cushion this increase in insulin. Try to reduce the level of stress in your life, as food can only help to a certain degree.

Other women experience hypoglycaemic symptoms when they exercise vigorously. This is a result of an increase in the amount of sugar your muscles use as fuel, which means that your blood sugar level drops. When you don't have enough sugar in your blood to fuel the muscles and maintain a normal level, you start to feel shaky and cold. You can help prevent this by having a light, high-fibre snack about half an hour before exercising: this could be a banana, a handful of dried apricots, a wholemeal or oat biscuit, a slice of banana cake. It is also very important that you do not drink sugary drinks during exercise as this will cause your blood sugar level to swing uncontrollably. Sips of water are best, just enough to prevent dehydration. If you feel hypoglycaemic after you exercise I suggest you have another high-fibre snack and then rest until you start to feel normal. If you start to feel hypoglycaemic before you exercise, have a snack and rest for 20 minutes before proceeding. If you are worried, seek the advice of a sports dietitian.

- **WHAT TO DO IF YOU FEEL VERY HYPOGLYCAEMIC**
- Eat something that has sugar in it to help bring your sugar level up to normal. However, don't choose something very sugary, such as a full-calorie canned drink or chocolate. A rapid rise in blood sugar will stimulate your body to produce a lot of insulin, which will then cause your sugar level to drop even further. Choose a food that contains some fibre to cushion the sugar.
- Eat a well-balanced meal as soon as possible.
- Rest. Don't do any form of vigorous exercise as this will make you feel worse.
- You may find it helpful to make yourself warm by wrapping yourself up with a rug or having a hot, non-caffeine-containing drink (see page 62).
- If you are diabetic you should read the chapter on diabetes, as the treatment of a diabetic hypoglycaemic attack is a little more complicated than this.
- If you have a medical condition such as Crohn's disease, your doctor or dietitian will be able to give you specific advice.

- **FOODS FOR SNACK ATTACKS**

Dried fruits: succulent prunes, tangy mango, sweet raisins

Oatcakes topped with pure fruit spread or bananas mashed with honey

Staffordshire oatcakes with golden syrup

Date and walnut cake

Banana cake

Carrot cake

Flapjacks

Fruit shake (use sweet fruit, such as banana, mango, pineapple, strawberries, raspberries, or add a little sugar)

14 Indigestion

Indigestion is a symptom of many stomach and intestinal problems, some more serious than others. If you regularly suffer from indigestion you should consult your doctor, in case there is something that needs to be corrected surgically or medically with tablets. Once you have established that you do not have anything more serious than simple indigestion, there is a lot you can do, both nutritionally and in your general lifestyle, to reduce your symptoms.

Simple indigestion usually means that you have an acid stomach, wind and frequently burp a lot. An acid stomach may be felt either in the stomach itself, in which case it is called gastritis, or further up, in the oesophagus, the feeding tube leading into the stomach, where it is technically called oesophagitis. Indigestion may also manifest itself as an acid taste in the mouth.

Oesophagitis is more commonly known as heartburn, because the pain is felt around the area of your heart. Some women think they are having a heart attack, as the pain is sometimes very severe. It is most important that you consult your doctor and do not simply diagnose yourself as having 'just a little indigestion'. Heartburn occurs when, for various reasons, the acid contents of your stomach leak up into the oesophagus. The oesophagus is made up of muscles that like an alkaline environment, the opposite of the acidic environment in the stomach. Therefore if the oesophagus is exposed to acid from the stomach it becomes irritated and you feel pain. The pain may occur either before or after eating, as a reaction to something you have eaten or as a result of not eating. Oesophagitis is sometimes caused by a leaky valve at the top of the stomach, but one of the most common causes is the development of a hiatus hernia, when the oesophagus may become twisted and very sensitive.

• ULCERS

Stressed women are particularly prone to an acid stomach. When stress is constant, acid levels in the stomach tend to be rather high, which may make the stomach more sensitive than usual. In times of extreme stress the combination of a high acid secretion, a sensitive stomach and generally poor eating habits mean that the stomach becomes severely inflamed. This is made worse if the stomach is left empty for long periods, which may happen if you have other things on your mind. If this situation develops one stage further, an ulcer may appear in the stomach, oesophagus or lower down in the intestine. An ulcer is an open wound on the surface of the muscle lining. It occurs as a result of the acid wearing away the protective lining of the organ.

Ulcers can cause a great deal of discomfort and if untreated may burst and cause internal bleeding. However, the advice for avoiding indigestion should also help to prevent ulcers; and if you do get them, treatment is now far more positive than in the past.

Traditional remedies either just decreased acid production or neutralized the acid. Medical treatment of ulcers has improved dramatically since the discovery that the bacterium *Helicobacter pylori* is often found at the site of ulceration. This means that doctors can now prescribe antibiotics to kill the *Helicobacter pylori*, which enables the ulceration site to heal.

AVOIDING INDIGESTION

Once your doctor has confirmed that your problem does not need further treatment, the nutritional and lifestyle guidelines for oesophagitis, gastritis and ulcers are very similar. You may feel that some of the suggestions do not apply to you, but it is helpful to consider them all.

- **TRY NOT TO LEAVE YOUR STOMACH EMPTY FOR LONGER THAN FOUR HOURS**

If you go for long periods without putting anything in your system the body reduces the production of digestive enzymes, as they are not needed. If you then put a large quantity of food in your stomach, especially if you eat it quickly, the stomach does not have enough time to prepare itself and produce the necessary enzymes. The food sits 'heavily' in your stomach without being digested appropriately. Eventually the food will be broken down, but this situation should be avoided.

In addition, if you are ravenously hungry there is a tendency to grab foods that are not the healthiest: they are frequently high in fat and sugar. If you know that you are going to be in a situation where you will not be able to get anything to eat, take something with you: fruit, or one of the cakes or biscuits in this book, which are relatively low in sugar and high in fibre. Make sure you have a good stock of such snacks in your office. If you are at home you can easily cut yourself a slice of wholemeal bread and add a topping of a pure fruit spread or a piece of lean ham or chicken.

Don't worry that you will put on weight if you start eating every few hours. You should need less at main meal times, which gives you room for regular small snacks. Over a 24-hour period your intake does not increase. The pattern of small regular meals enables your stomach to anticipate and react to the foods that you put into it.

- **MAKE SURE THAT YOUR MAIN MEALS ARE HIGH IN FIBRE**

Try to include some wholegrain bread or other cereal fibre, along with fresh vegetables or fruits, at each main meal. These are digested slowly, so the stomach stays full longer.

• AVOID TOO MANY FATTY FOODS, ESPECIALLY ON AN EMPTY STOMACH

Fatty foods may cause the valve at the top of your stomach to become lazy, because when you ingest fat, hormones are released that make the muscles in this valve relax. Concentrate on lean protein foods – lean cuts of meat, chicken and fresh fish – and starches such as pasta, rice, potatoes and breads.

• TRY TO KEEP MAIN MEALS HEALTHY AND WELL-BALANCED

Choosing fresh and varied ingredients will do wonders for your general feeling of well-being. Large amounts of any one food – fatty or sugary food or even fruit and vegetables – may be difficult to digest.

• AVOID FOODS THAT YOU FIND HARD TO DIGEST

This may sound obvious, but some women don't put much thought into what they are eating, especially if under stress. Many women feel uncomfortable when they eat a lot of raw foods, especially cucumber, apple, chocolate and soft bread. Others find citrus fruits such as oranges and grapefruits too acidic. Try to choose plain, starchy food such as a pasta, rice or potato dish, rather than a huge salad. A bowl of warming leek and potato soup would be perfect.

• AVOID HIGHLY SPICED FOODS

Chillies and certain spices, such as dried coriander, may aggravate and inflame the stomach. Instead, enhance your food with mild spices, garlic (which gives a very subtle flavour when baked) and fresh herbs, which often have a positive effect on digestion.

Fresh herbs make it easy to titillate the taste buds without using chillies or other hot spices. Cooking is both science and art: you need the basic science to know how to make an omelette, but the artistic cook can add basil, parsley, chervil or tarragon for very different effects. Even the simplest touches, such as adding a little chopped fresh dill, can turn a tuna fish and tomato

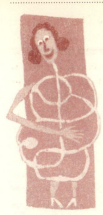

Some women find that a tot of whisky helps to settle the stomach, or a glass of wine that is low in acidity. Most Chardonnays grown in sunny climates are suitable. As an alternative to alcohol, try sparkling elderflower water. If you take time to relax over a glass, the combination of elderflower and bubbles is very settling.

sandwich into something quite delicious and digestible. See page 57 for some ideas as to which herbs go particularly well with certain flavours.

In addition to providing food with a subtle interest that shouldn't irritate the gut, there are many herbs that are thought to help digestion and remedy indigestion, particularly mint, camomile and ginger. Ginger is technically a root, but a slice of fresh ginger in boiling water can really help ease an acid stomach.

• AVOID EXCESSIVE COFFEE AND TEA

Coffee, tea and many other drinks contain caffeine and/or tannin, both of which irritate the stomach and oesophagus linings. Drink plenty of water (frequent small sips rather than gulping down pints at a time) and experiment with herb teas such as camomile and mint (see page 62 for other caffeine-free drinks).

• AVOID EXCESSIVE AMOUNTS OF ALCOHOL

Alcohol can irritate the stomach, especially if you are stressed or you have a very empty stomach. The effect of alcohol is very individual: some women find strong spirits irritating, whereas others find an after-meal 'digestive' of brandy or whisky helpful. I suggest that you primarily avoid drinking on an empty stomach and sip small amounts of your favourite drink with meals.

• AVOID DRINKING LARGE AMOUNTS WHILE YOU EAT

Just have sips to help the food go down and to refresh your palate.

• TRY TO EAT AND DRINK SLOWLY

Take small mouthfuls and sips of food and drink. Try not to gulp large amounts or eat quickly, as you will take in air, which can be very painful inside a sore stomach. Taking food and drink in small amounts also means that you can taste and enjoy it more.

• **SIT DOWN, ENJOY YOUR FOOD AND MAKE AN OCCASION OF EVERY MEAL**

Before you say it takes too long, remember it's a question of prioritizing your time. Many of my patients notice a big difference in their efficiency level when they take the time to sit down and enjoy a small meal, three times a day. If you think about what you're eating you will get more sensory stimulation from it. The brain requires nourishment, it does not perform well when you're hungry.

Business meals are a case in point. It's surely a shame to go to a gorgeous restaurant on business and end up not noticing or remembering what you've eaten! Even if a lunch takes an extra 30 minutes out of your hectic schedule it's nevertheless a great deal more efficient than spending the time going to the pharmacy in search of indigestion pills or spending hours doubled up!

• **ALLOW TIME AFTER EATING**

Try to wait at least 30 minutes after finishing your meal before you rush off to do something else or go to bed. If you rush, your stomach will be sent into spasm and this may lead to heartburn. If you are exercising you should allow a couple of hours after eating; ideally you should exercise before you eat.

• **GIVE UP SMOKING**

Smoking severely aggravates the stomach and oesophagus; you should really try to give up if you have recurrent indigestion or an ulcer.

• **MAKE SURE THAT YOU ARE NOT CARRYING TOO MUCH FAT AROUND YOUR MIDDLE**

Excess body fat around your midriff can cause your stomach and oesophagus to be squeezed, causing acid to be nudged into your oesophagus. Frequently, if you lose this excess fat the indigestion disappears. See the chapter on weight loss for advice.

TREATING INDIGESTION

If you feel an attack of indigestion coming on, there are several things you can do to alleviate the symptoms.

• RESIST THE TEMPTATION TO DRINK MILK

Milk may seem the natural, inoffensive and perfect thing to cool and soothe your stomach, and many women with indigestion or a tendency towards an acid stomach believe they should eat milk puddings and drink endless glasses of cold milk. This is an outdated belief and potentially very damaging, because substances within the milk cause the stomach to produce even more acid, which means the initial cooling effect is followed by extreme indigestion. The only exception I know of is those women who have an ulcer in the jejunum, the feeding tube that leaves the stomach. In these cases milk can help, but this is not a common complaint and, unless you have been given this diagnosis, I suggest you avoid milk.

It is far better to make sure you have regular, small, high-starch snacks, which don't have the same 'knock-back' acid effect.

• TRY DRINKING MINT TEA

Peppermint is a very soothing flavour, so try drinking mint tea. It is best served warm, rather than icy cold or very hot. Drinks of extreme temperatures may cause the muscles to go into spasms, which will aggravate the situation.

• APPLY A LITTLE WARMTH OVER YOUR STOMACH

Warmth can help the stomach muscles to relax and hence become less painful. A hot water bottle can be very helpful. Alternatively you could try having a warm bath, listening to some relaxing classical music; Mozart's mass in C minor is a personal favourite. Several aromatherapy oils are particularly soothing, such as lavender and neroli. Add a few drops of these to your bath or use an aromatherapy burner while you're soaking in the suds.

- ### TRY TO GET SOME REST
Remember to rest with your head slightly raised, so that gravity can keep the acid stomach contents down in the stomach, not in the oesophagus.

- ### INDIGESTION REMEDIES
Don't spend your days chewing indigestion tablets, as they can mask more serious problems. In fact, since they neutralize stomach acid, they may interfere with the absorption of vitamins and minerals from the gut. They are fine as a short-term, infrequent remedy, but don't let them become a habit. If you follow the positive approach outlined in this chapter you should be able to keep them as a last resort, not something you automatically take after every meal.

Aspirin irritates the stomach, so you should avoid aspirin preparations; this is particularly important for ulcer sufferers.

- ### RECIPES TO SETTLE AND SOOTH

Chilled mint and cucumber soup

Parsnip and apple soup

Carrot and orange soup

Garlic bean soup

Sorrel soup

Minestrone soup

Smoked salmon ramekins

Goats' cheese and aubergine crostini

Cheese fluff

Artichoke and avocado salad

Chicken with melon, grapes and
    asparagus

Potatoes with basil

Pasta bows with courgettes

Pasta with wild mushrooms

Salmon and lemon lasagne

Chicken stroganoff with tarragon

Staffordshire oatcakes

Bread and butter pudding

Poached pears with ginger

Blackberry and ricotta pancakes

Banana cake

Lemon cake

Carrot cake

15 The menopause

Sooner or later, all women go through the menopause. In most women the onset is gradual, between the ages of 50 and 55, but in some cases it can be hastened or suddenly brought about by an emotional trauma, shock or surgery. The earlier you start your periods, the later you seem to start the menopause. There is also evidence to suggest that the better nourished you are, the later your periods cease.

The menopause is not something to be dreaded, as gone are the days when 'the change' signalled an inevitable decline in health and quality of life. Since women are now living longer, keeping healthier and taking a greater part in the workplace, many women see this period as one of reappraisal, before they meet new challenges. It is, for many of the women I see, the first time in their lives that they have some space to enjoy what they want to do, rather than caring so much for others. It may be a time of sheer self-indulgence as, if you are lucky, you will have a little more money to buy foods and wines that previously would have been too costly. Many enjoy having the time and resources to cook something just for themselves or two, or go out to eat, rather than having to feed children every day. Sadly, other women have a rougher time because of ill health, hormonal imbalance or lifestyle situations that hinder their ability to stay well and happy. Women come to me depressed about getting older, not being the major person in their child's life, worried that their husband will leave them for a younger woman or just fed-up with feeling 'menopausal' and 'middle aged'.

Whatever your situation, changes in your nutrition and lifestyle can help you to minimize your problems and maximize your health and energy status.

• SYMPTOMS

About 15% of women suffer from symptoms they consider extremely distressing, but a majority may experience some of the following: hot flushes, dry skin, hair loss, mood swings, depression, tiredness, poor concentration, headaches, vaginal dryness and loss of sexual desire. High levels of pollution and substances found in medicines, nutritional supplements and some cosmetics have been found to aggravate some of these problems, so making lifestyle changes such as exercising in fresh air and avoiding drugs, capsules and creams unless you absolutely need them can help to reduce symptoms.

• HORMONE CHANGES AND REPLACEMENT THERAPY (HRT)

The symptoms are caused by hormonal changes in your body. These usually occur gradually, but at some point the hormones reach such low levels that your body enters the menopause and your periods stop. The two important female sex hormones, which regulate the monthly cycle of ovulation and menstruation, are oestrogen and progesterone. As the levels of these hormones drop and the balance between the two fluctuates, during the start of the menopause, some or all of the symptoms may occur.

Although this is a perfectly natural process, there are many reasons why some women choose to replace these hormones within their body, by hormone replacement therapy, usually known as HRT. The replacement hormones must be prescribed by a doctor. They may be taken as tablets, in a patch, an implant placed just under the surface of the skin, or as a cream.

Throughout the reproductive period of a woman's life, oestrogen provides a protection against heart disease and osteoporosis, a disease in which the bones become less dense and more brittle. As women enter the menopause, oestrogen's protective effect is lost and therefore the risk of developing these conditions increases. This increased risk and/or the distress caused by menopausal symptoms makes many women consider whether they should stop their body from entering the menopause. HRT can positively change many women's lives, but you shouldn't feel pressurized to defy nature, and you should be aware of the risks.

HRT is associated with an increased risk of developing problems with the uterus (womb) and endometrium (the membrane that lines the womb), including fibroids (benign tumours). It has also been linked with an increased risk of breast cancer in women who are at high risk, and it can activate so-called dormant cancer cells. Women who still have their womb must take a combination of progesterone with the oestrogen to reduce the risks of endometrial cancer, but women who have had their womb removed usually take a pure oestrogen type of HRT.

The issue of the different types of HRT, and their benefits and risks, is something to discuss with your doctor. Some women are unable for medical reasons to take HRT, others feel that they don't want to take a drug. For both types of women there is an alternative.

NATURAL HORMONE REPLACEMENT

There is much debate about whether natural, plant-based substances are viable alternatives to the traditional HRT drugs currently on the market. I think it is well worth considering natural foods; in some cases they really seem to help balance the hormones and give relief from awkward symptoms such as hot flushes and vaginal dryness.

• FRUIT AND VEGETABLE SOURCES
In the United States, some interesting research has been carried out by a Dr Lees of Portland, Oregon. He claims that it is the non-production of progesterone in menopausal women that causes many of the painful symptoms associated with imbalance of hormones. He believes that we should use nutrition to try to boost the progesterone level in our blood. Beans, pulses, root vegetables and fruits are good sources of progesterone

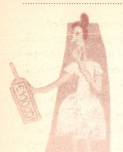

This is the time to splash out and spoil yourself: drink the wines you've been storing or buy some really good vintage wine and vintage or luxury cuvée Champagne. Your taste buds tend to decline as you get older, so you really ought to drink the best you can afford now, before it's too late! Grand Cru burgundies are rich and subtle, very expensive but well worth trying. Make friends with your wine merchant: he or she will value your custom and once they know your tastes will look out for wines they think you'll like.

precursors (substances that stimulate the body to produce progesterone). Research on the Mexican yam (what we in Britain call sweet potato) has shown that it is particularly high in progesterone precursors, as is the herb sarsaparilla, once used to flavour a refreshing drink in the hot climate of America's deep south.

It has yet to be proved conclusively how effectively these precursor sources can balance the hormones. However, I think it is worth including beans, pulses, fruit, root vegetables and tubers such as sweet potatoes in a balanced diet, since it is quite possible that they could help minimize the symptoms.

• HERBS

Certain herbs can be useful in relieving menopausal symptoms, but studies don't really explain why. Several of my patients find Chinese medicine very helpful. Chinese medicine has long recommended dong quai, schizandra and white peony as hormone balancers at this time of life. There is also some evidence that the vitamin E found in evening primrose oil and starflower oil can help reduce hot flushes. However, the body has the ability to adjust to these substances, making the beneficial effects wear off after a while, which can be disconcerting if you have come to regard the capsules as part of your daily life. Sometimes a short break of a month or so gives the body a chance to respond once more when the dose is resumed.

NUTRITION FOR MIDDLE AGE

A well-balanced, healthy diet, including plenty of vitamin C and vitamin D, calcium and magnesium, will help to keep your body tissues healthy, maintain a good bone mass and reduce the incidence of menopausal symptoms. Women who have a healthy diet, high in fresh and preferably organically grown vegetables and fruits, with a smaller proportion of dairy products and meat, seem to pass through the menopause more easily than those whose healthy eating habits have lapsed.

It is important to see replenishing your gut with good ingredients as a first priority. Read the information in Part One on What your body needs and Healthy eating for life. I see a lot of women who have not managed to eat and live healthily during their late thirties and early forties. This may be through lack of time or inspiration, or because they have been totally turned off eating by articles telling them what not to eat. Many women feel they need to eat manufactured foods with 'healthy eating' labels, reduced-fat and low-sugar products, rather than unadulterated, simple, fresh foods. They often feel ten years younger once they start eating proper, healthy food and remove excessive amounts of over-refined 'new' food. Finding foods that suit your body and are also tasty, 'real' foods can be a very empowering experience. Some of you might like to follow the weekend cleansing programme (see page 68) for a good 'kickstart' to a healthy eating plan.

- **CLEAR OUT THE SUPPLEMENTS!**

I suggest that you stop taking any vitamin, mineral or other nutritional supplements unless you have been advised to take them by your doctor or dietitian. Some of them are full of tablet 'filler' rather than nutrients, others are ineffective if taken with another supplement, and in the worst cases, or when taken in excess, they can be harmful, causing bowel problems, fatigue or even liver damage. I understand why women take them, in desperation for a healthy body, but supplements should be treated with caution. Once your body is cleared and replenished with proper foods, you will feel so much better.

DEALING WITH MENOPAUSAL PROBLEMS

The two most common complaints of women going through the menopause are weight gain and fluid retention. They may also suffer from stomach and bowel problems, headaches and difficulty in sleeping.

• WEIGHT GAIN

Many women find that when they start taking HRT, the weight piles on. This is partly because oestrogen can change your appetite and body fat levels, but an increase in weight, especially fat, ultimately comes from an excess of 'unused' calories.

Some women, even those not on HRT, get very upset as they find they are unable to eat the same foods as they did when they were younger without putting on weight. They don't seem to be eating larger quantities, there just seems to be a change in their body's metabolism and/or energy expenditure. Other women find that their appetite changes, both in terms of degree and preference of foods; many women develop cravings for sweet foods.

It is very frustrating that the body seems to change its ability to metabolize food, but I suggest that you read the chapter on weight loss just to make sure that you are doing everything possible. I very rarely see women who can't lose any weight once they follow the advice outlined in that chapter. Problems may arise when there is a lack of exercise, a hormonal imbalance or an emotional problem that means that they look for something more from food than just the nutrients; in some cases it is called 'comfort eating', although I am not suggesting that all women who are unable to lose weight are comfort eaters. See your doctor if you suspect that your hormones are excessively unbalanced. It might be a question of changing to a different form of HRT, or starting HRT if you don't already use it. Although HRT can cause weight gain, in some cases it can make you feel so much better, both physically and emotionally, that you can lose some weight.

I would encourage those of you who have a body mass index of over 25 (see chart on page 46) to do as much as you can to bring it down, because the more weight you carry into later years the greater your risk of heart disease, joint problems and some cancers.

Warning It is not advisable for you to go below a body mass index of 19 or 20. Women with a very low body mass index are at increased risk of developing osteoporosis. It is essential not to allow your body to become malnourished by going on a crash diet. If you do this while you are going through the menopause you will run into even more problems.

• **FOOD CRAVINGS**

Some women find that the menopause can bring about changes in food preference. I have seen many women, especially those taking HRT, who develop a very sweet tooth. As with the cravings associated with periods, these are primarily caused by fluctuations in the levels of various hormones in the blood, which can account for mood changes, depression and tiredness, or may just make the body feel 'low in sugar'. However, the worst thing you can do is to eat a 'quick fix' sugary food, as this will set up a vicious circle of energy and mood swings. It is much better to choose a high-fibre carbohydrate food, such as a wholemeal biscuit or a piece of fruit, or a food rich in protein, such as a lean ham or chicken sandwich made with wholemeal bread. The chapter on periods gives further advice on conquering cravings.

• **FLUID RETENTION**

Some women suffer from quite severe fluid retention, especially if they are taking HRT. If you are worried about this I suggest you see your doctor, who can check that there is no underlying problem. The chapter on periods gives more information on dealing with fluid retention. To sum up, I suggest you:
• drink two to three litres (four to five pints) of water a day
• reduce your intake of caffeine-containing drinks (coffee, tea, cola-based and chocolate drinks)
• eat plenty of fresh fruits and vegetables
• keep your salt intake down. Resist salty foods and use plenty of fresh herbs and spices such as coriander, mustards, garlic or chillies to enhance flavours
• exercise regularly to maintain a good circulation and fluid balance within your body.

● DIURETICS

Any long-term use of diuretics should always be under
the supervision of your doctor, as he or she will be able
to check how your body is responding. Taking diuretics
regularly without supervision is dangerous nutritionally
because they cause your body to excrete several important minerals. If you lose a lot of these nutrients you
could develop a deficiency that may make you feel tired
and run down or cause muscle cramps.

Instead of taking diuretics, make sure that your
diet contains plenty of fresh fruits, vegetables and
wholegrain products; these foods will help reduce the
problem. Even if you need to take diuretics for medical
reasons, following a healthy diet may mean you can
lower the dosage.

● ABDOMINAL AND BOWEL PROBLEMS

The digestive system consists of a collection of muscles
and glands, which are very sensitive to blood oestrogen
levels. Therefore as you enter the menopause your gut
may change its ability to absorb and metabolize nutrients.
Symptoms that suggest that your bowel is malabsorbing
include constipation, stomach and bowel bloating, and
stomach cramps. Some women find that the menopause is the time at which they develop food allergies
and intolerances. If you suspect you have a food sensitivity, read the chapter on allergies. Constipation may
be helped by HRT, but you would not be prescribed it
for this reason; the chapter on constipation should help.
Remember that stress adversely affects the gut so try to
keep this to a minimum.

● SLEEPING PROBLEMS

Some women have difficulty sleeping when they're
going through the menopause. Sometimes, even though
you seem to sleep through the night, you don't feel
refreshed in the morning. Try the following:
● Stop drinking any beverage with caffeine in it after 3
o'clock in the afternoon. This includes coffee, tea, cola-
based drinks and chocolate. You may not believe that

the caffeine in your afternoon tea can affect the body for that long, but when I cut it out I found that I woke up the next day feeling a lot fresher.

• Try to avoid foods that cause your blood sugar to yo-yo, especially in the evening. Rapid changes in the levels of sugar and related hormones such as serotonin in your blood may cause disturbed sleep. Instead of foods high in refined sugars, such as cakes, chocolate and biscuits, choose higher-fibre carbohydrate foods such as pasta (preferably wholewheat) with a vegetable accompaniment, or a large bowl of soup with wholemeal bread. These foods will bring about a slow, steady release of comfort and resting hormones.

• Try having a glass of cold milk or a mug of warm milk before you go to bed. This can be very soothing (and also gives you an opportunity to boost your calcium intake). If you don't like milk, try a herbal tea such as camomile.

• Make sure that you're neither too full nor too hungry before you settle down. A full stomach can cause indigestion; hunger can lead to stomach rumblings.

• If you suspect that you may be a little stressed, take measures to reduce this before you go to bed. You may like to try sprinkling drops of relaxing aromatherapy oils such as lavender on your pillow, or buy one of the little aromatherapy or herbal sleep pillows.

• Avoid taking any vitamin and mineral supplements late at night as they can affect sleep patterns.

• HEADACHES

The hormonal changes that occur during the menopause can cause you to suffer from headaches or even migraines. The chapter on headaches and migraine suggests a number of ways you may be able to use nutrition to prevent and treat them.

DISEASE PREVENTION

As you go through the menopause and your oestrogen levels fall, you lose their protective effect against heart disease, osteoporosis and breast cancer, unless you are taking HRT, which replaces your natural oestrogen. If you have a family history of heart disease or breast cancer, I suggest you read the chapters on high blood cholesterol and cancer, to see how you can minimize your risks. Osteoporosis is discussed below.

You should examine your body at least every month to check that there are no lumps, which might be a sign of a medical problem. Keep in regular contact with your doctor. Having said this, many women go through the menopause without any serious medical or emotional problems.

• EXERCISE

Regular exercise throughout life helps to build up a strong muscular frame and strong bone mass. Most importantly it helps to reduce the rate of bone loss after menopause, which is when bone mass starts to diminish at a greatly increased rate. Every woman should exercise for at least 20 minutes on at least three occasions every week. This is not only important in helping to preserve your bone mass and prevent osteoporosis, but it also reduces your risk of developing heart disease and some cancers.

The exercises that achieve the best results are known as load-bearing exercise, in other words they involve resting your weight on your limbs, for example, running, hockey, tennis, brisk or 'power' walking. In the gym, using a step machine, treadmill or rowing machine are all good.

• GIVING UP SMOKING

Smoking harms your body in many ways. This is particularly relevant during middle age, as smoking damages your skin, making you more likely to develop wrinkles, increases your risk of heart disease and some cancers, and contributes to bone loss (and possible osteoporosis) through malabsorption of calcium.

OSTEOPOROSIS

One of the most common causes for concern among women entering the menopause is avoiding osteoporosis. In recent years there has been a great deal of press coverage on the subject, so women are aware of the issue and may be very worried about it. Although osteoporosis is one of the greatest causes of disability in women over the age of 50, the good news is that it is a condition that in most cases can be prevented and treated. Women today live longer than ever before and more women are now having health checks which help to highlight possible problems.

There are many different forms of osteoporosis, including infantile osteoporosis and those associated with anorexia nervosa, but here I shall address the form that is a result of growing older and experiencing hormonal changes and a deteriorating bone mass. Whatever the cause, the key feature is the same: low bone mass, which enhances bone fragility and increases the risk of fracture.

The best time to build up good bone mass is during childhood and the teen years. Thereafter, it's never too late to focus on doing as much as possible to prevent bone loss after the maximum level has been achieved. There is an increased risk of developing osteoporosis if you are too thin. I frequently tell my young, thin, female patients that while it may seem a good idea to be thin at the moment, they will run into problems if they don't take great care to eat a varied and balanced diet.

NUTRITIONAL PREVENTION OF OSTEOPOROSIS

There is clearly a correlation between nutrition and osteoporosis. The most readily understood association is that calcium builds strong bones. There is somewhat conflicting evidence as to whether lack of calcium leads to osteoporosis, but all research tends to agree that women benefit from a diet that meets their calcium requirement from childhood onwards. Young children need approximately 525 mg of calcium a day, adult women about 800 mg. The adult requirement can be found in 660 ml (just over 1 pint) of semi-skimmed milk, about 100 g (3 1/2 oz) of Cheddar cheese, or 400 g (14 oz, a large pot) of natural yoghurt. So you see that you can easily obtain sufficient calcium if you incorporate some milk and other dairy products in your daily diet.

If you don't like dairy products, calcium is found in several other food sources, including spinach, broccoli, sesame seeds (which are used to make tahini paste, an ingredient of hummus), dried fruits, especially apricots, and calcium-enriched soya products, such as tofu. However, the body does not absorb this calcium as easily as that from dairy sources, and you may need to take a supplement to meet the shortfall; seek professional advice. (There is no benefit to be gained from taking excess calcium, and several medical conditions, such as kidney problems, may be aggravated by excess calcium.)

Once you are going through the menopause it is particularly important that your calcium intake remains at 800 mg a day (or 1000 mg if you are taking a supplement). The reason for the difference is that calcium is much better absorbed from dairy products and other foods, packaged by Mother Nature, than from a supplement.

As well as ensuring that your intake of calcium is adequate to maintain good bones there are several other nutritional factors to consider. Smoking, excess caffeine and excess fibre should be avoided, whereas vitamins D and E and the minerals magnesium, zinc and copper are needed in small amounts. Vitamin C is vital as part of any healthy eating pattern, so don't forget to include lots of fresh fruit and vegetables in meals and snacks.

• VITAMIN D

Vitamin D is needed together with calcium to create and maintain strong bones. Although osteoporosis is not a vitamin D disorder, you need to make sure that your vitamin D status is good. Vitamin D is produced in the skin when it is exposed to sunlight, so if you are an active woman who regularly goes outside you shouldn't have any problems with your vitamin D status. However, as you get older your skin becomes less efficient at metabolizing vitamin D, so it is a good idea to include some vitamin D rich foods in your eating plan, just to be sure. The best sources are the oily fish, such as sardines and salmon, and vegetable oils.

• VITAMIN K

This is needed to help form strong bones. Vitamin K is mainly produced by bacteria in the bowel – little is derived from food – and if you have a normal healthy gut your vitamin K status should be good. However, since such a lot of women I see seem to have an imbalance in their gut flora, as a result of antibiotics or a highly refined, low-fibre, high-fat, high-sugar diet, with very little rest, it is often a good idea to take a small pot of 'live' yoghurt with acidophilus and bifidus cultures every day. These will help restore the balance of healthy bacteria in your gut.

If you have any gut problems, such as irritable bowel syndrome, Crohn's disease or rheumatoid arthritis, you should see your doctor or dietitian to discuss ways of ensuring that your vitamin K level is satisfactory.

• MAGNESIUM, ZINC AND COPPER

All of these minerals are needed to make and preserve healthy bones. However, I do not believe that we need to take them as a supplement, as the possible effects of excessive amounts have not been documented and, in any case, nature provides all these nutrients in abundance in a varied and well-balanced diet. Rich sources of zinc include shellfish and fish, lean beef, oxtail and liver, eggs, wholewheat bread and pasta, cheese and nuts. Nuts and wholewheat products are good suppliers of magnesium.

• AVOID EXCESS CAFFEINE

In addition to keeping the body supplied with vitamins and minerals we should make sure that it can use them effectively. Caffeine inhibits the absorption of calcium and other nutrients, so try to limit your daily caffeine intake to three cups of tea, coffee or other caffeine-containing drinks.

• AVOID EXCESS FIBRE

High-fibre foods are part of any healthy, well-balanced eating plan, but the key word is balance. Fibre-rich foods contain substances that can inhibit the absorption of calcium and other nutrients from the gut, so if you are concerned about your calcium intake, don't fill yourself up with too much fibre.

IF YOU HAVE OSTEOPOROSIS

The only way to diagnose osteoporosis is by a bone density scan. Once it has been diagnosed, it becomes even more important to take steps to prevent further bone loss; in some cases you may even be able to reverse the process. Nutritionally you can maximize your current and future bone status by following the above guidelines on the prevention of osteoporosis.

Emotionally it is a difficult condition to deal with, as you don't really see any signs of improvement, other than changes in the bone density scans. But since these are carried out infrequently, for other health reasons, you may become despondent and worried that you're doing everything possible. It's not as if you feel unwell when you have osteoporosis, unless of course you have a fracture. You just need to trust that you're doing everything you can. Living and eating well can be empowering; think positively as osteoporosis can be managed extremely effectively if you look after yourself.

• WEIGHT AND OSTEOPOROSIS

It is a good idea to keep your weight within the ideal range (see page 46). If you are overweight this can place inappropriate pressure on your joints and may even cause fractures. Losing weight can help to reduce the risk of fractures, but it must done in a healthy way, as explained in the chapter on weight loss. Crash diets (unbalanced diets where your food intake is severely restricted) will increase bone loss and therefore aggravate osteoporosis.

If you are underweight you should make sure that you are eating a well-balanced diet. There is a big difference between being slim and healthy and being thin and malnourished. A healthy, varied and balanced diet is absolutely crucial in managing osteoporosis.

• RECIPES TO CUSHION THE CHANGE

Chilled mint and cucumber soup
Clam chowder
French onion soup

Goats' cheese and aubergine crostini
Hummus
Smoked mackerel pâté
Brie and porcini tart
Spinach and goats' cheese soufflé
Cheese fluff
Spinach and watercress roulade
Warm goats' cheese salad
Smoked haddock and spinach pasta
Smoked cheese and olive pasta
Yam biryani

Oysters with cream and Parmesan
Salmon and lemon lasagne
Salmon and asparagus risotto
Chicken stroganoff with tarragon
Garlic and herb chicken
Minted meatballs with yoghurt sauce

Oranges in caramel
Blackberry and raspberry fool
Bread and butter pudding
Fresh figs filled with almond cream
Blackberries and ricotta pancakes
Lemon syllabub
Brown bread ice cream
Coconut ice cream

16 Periods

Although some women seem to sail through their monthly cycles without any problems, others suffer with painful periods or find the physical and emotional symptoms and stress a great encumbrance. The symptoms include weight gain, fluid retention, food cravings, bloating, constipation, diarrhoea, breast and abdominal tenderness, headache, fatigue, energy crashes, irritability and depression. Of course these symptoms can be felt at any time of the month, but they are most common during the week before the period and can last into the first few days.

Women who suffer in this way are said to suffer from pre-menstrual tension (PMT) or pre-menstrual syndrome (PMS). Nutrition can help to prevent and minimize the degree of PMT, and help you cope with the symptoms.

Every woman's menstrual cycle differs, both in length and symptoms experienced. The usual oestrogen and progesterone hormone cycle rotates around a 28-day pattern, with five to seven days of menstrual bleeding, a state we refer to as a 'period'. The healthier and better nourished you are, the earlier you start your periods, the more regular they will be and the longer you will have them. Sadly the women who are victims of 'thin is fashionable' pressure may experience great problems with their periods. Not only are they irregular, they are frequently painful and heavy. In the extreme, women who allow their body weight to drop too low may lose their periods altogether. Many women temporarily lose their periods if they lose weight quickly. This may also happen if you experience a stressful situation in your life, such as the break-up of a relationship, but in these cases they usually reappear after a couple of months. Also women who come off the contraceptive pill sometimes miss a period or experience a few months of irregular periods.

However appealing the loss of periods seems, seek

medical opinion if your periods disappear, as it is very important to assess and if necessary reverse the situation. Unless you are pregnant, the lack of periods signifies hormonal imbalance, which may lead to osteoporosis and other debilitating conditions.

• PMT

The physiological symptoms are mainly down to fluctuations in the levels of oestrogen and progesterone (the sex hormones) in the body. The severity ranges from a little pre-menstrual fluid gain and stomach cramps to severe pain and suicidal thoughts. If you suffer from severe PMT, I would recommend that you see your doctor to find out whether there is any physiological cause and treatment. Don't just suffer in silence.

Women most commonly suffer from PMT symptoms in the week leading up to their period. Often, once the period starts, the symptoms decrease, perhaps with the exception of period pain. The abdominal period pains or 'stomach cramps' may be linked to one or more of the other symptoms, so try the suggestions for the problems that sound closest to your own.

Many pre-menstrual symptoms can be alleviated by following a healthy eating plan (see Part One), along with a positive state of mind and low level of stress throughout the month, but especially during the week before the period starts. Some studies have even shown that a healthy vegetarian diet, i.e. one that is high in vegetables, fruits, pulses and seeds, causes the body to excrete more oestrogens and progesterones than a meat-based diet. Since it has been suggested that a woman with lower levels of oestrogens and progesterones is much less likely to suffer from PMT, you should try to boost these foods and cut back on meat, at least for the week before your period.

• EXERCISE

Exercise causes your body to produce endorphins, chemicals that make you feel exhilarated and happy. It also helps the body maintain good fluid circulation and tissue drainage, which can alleviate fluid retention.

• THE POWER OF THE MIND

Food can be a great healer and preventer of PMT symptoms, but it can only help if you're not overstressed or agitated by your periods. I see quite a few women who suffer more than they need to from PMT. As soon as they acknowledge the fact that their menstrual cycle is an important physiological process and adapt their life around it, their symptoms decrease. I'm not saying that all PMT is all in the mind but stress definitely aggravates it. If you are going to make food work for your body, you need to begin with a positive state of mind and relieve your life of as much stress as possible.

WEIGHT GAIN

This is the most common PMT symptom. It can lead to a number of physical problems, such as pain due to pressure exerted on organs surrounding the womb, bowel problems, breast tenderness and pain in the joints. You may put on as much as 3 to 3.5 kg (6 to 8 pounds) during the week leading up to your period, with symptoms such as puffy eyes and distended tummy. Fitting into clothes becomes a nightmare. Before you make any changes to your diet you need to establish whether the excess weight is fluid, fat or gas.

The most common cause for the weight gain is an increase in fluid retention, but food cravings and eating habits can also put weight on. Do you have an increased appetite and eat more during the week before your period, which causes an increase in fat? If you only feel bloated around the middle, this is likely to be excess gas. Some women suffer from all three problems.

Basil is one of my
favourite herbs.
Try a fresh basil leaf
in a tomato sand-
wich with some
freshly ground black
pepper, or some
chopped basil leaves
in a potato salad.

FLUID RETENTION

Fluid retention can make your whole body feel puffy, the worst-affected areas being the waist, feet, face and hands. It can be the result of poor protein and vitamin and mineral intakes, but this is extremely unlikely in generally healthy and well-nourished women. Kidney and heart problems can cause fluid retention, but this is unlikely to be the case if you just suffer from temporary fluid retention around the time of your period and generally feel well.

For the majority of women, PMT fluid retention occurs because there is a temporary rise in the body's sodium level, which causes the body to retain excess fluid to dilute the sodium concentration in the tissues.

- CUT DOWN ON SALT

Putting less sodium into your body is the obvious way to reduce the sodium level, and most of the sodium we eat is in the form of sodium chloride, or salt. A decrease in the level of salt you eat reduces the amount of fluid you gain.Cutting down on the amount of salt you put on your food and avoiding salty foods such as crisps, chips, olives, anchovies, pickled vegetables, smoked and salt-cured fish and meats, such as ham and bacon, helps your body to correct this balance. Look to other ways of enhancing flavours.

- Instead of salt experiment with herbs and spices (see page 56 for ideas).
- Wine is a wonderful flavour enhancer. When it is boiled the alcohol evaporates, leaving behind the aromatic 'essence' of the wine.
- Mustard really brings out the flavours of cheese.

You will gradually adjust to a less salty diet and learn to appreciate the more subtle flavours that were hidden by the overriding tang of salt.

Warning If you live in an excessively hot climate where you sweat a lot, or you're going to a hot country during the time leading up to your period, make sure that you don't cut back on your salt intake too much, as this could interfere with your fluid balance. Seek the advice of your doctor.

• INCREASE YOUR WATER INTAKE

I frequently see women who restrict their fluid intake, because they think it will solve the problem of fluid retention. In fact the opposite is true. Increasing the volume of water you drink helps your body dilute the salt level in your tissues and enables it to excrete more salt and fluid. You should aim to drink at least two to three litres (four to five pints) of water a day, especially in the week before your period. Some women find that still water lies in the stomach more easily than sparkling, as it doesn't contain gas.

• REDUCE YOUR TEA AND COFFEE INTAKE

A mistake women often make is to think that coffee and tea count as part of a healthy pre-menstrual fluid intake. Most women know that caffeine is found in coffee, but many don't realize that it is also found in traditional Indian and China tea, chocolate, cola-based drinks and even some medications such as over-the-counter painkillers. Although caffeine is a diuretic, the water it makes you lose from some parts of your body actually impedes the excretion of excess salt and fluid from your tissues.

Caffeine also aggravates the majority of hormone-based problems such as breast tenderness, headaches and the general feeling of muzziness.

Herb teas are a good alternative when you want a caffeine-free hot drink. There is a huge variety available, some specially blended to give you early morning zest, others, such as camomile, for evening soothing.

• BOOST YOUR POTASSIUM INTAKE

Potassium and sodium are two minerals found in cells throughout the body. The levels of the two minerals are constantly fluctuating as they find the balance that is right for the work your body needs them to do.

Boosting your intake of potassium-rich foods is an effective way of bringing down the body's sodium level. Remember, however, that you need to consider potassium, sodium and water together, and reduce your salt intake and increase your fluid intake at the same time as eating plenty of foods high in potassium, such as bananas, tomatoes, green leafy vegetables, wholegrains, and fresh fruit juices.

Warning Do not think about taking a potassium supplement for fluid retention, unless your doctor has prescribed it.

• DIURETICS

There are a number of diuretic preparations for sale without prescription. While these can be useful for occasional PMS fluid retention episodes, for instance if you need to fit into a dress in the evening, they should never be used on a regular long-term basis as they can affect the balance of fluids, vitamins and minerals in your body.

FOOD CRAVINGS AND VORACIOUS APPETITE

Women can suffer the most horrendous cravings around the time of their period. I see women who would drive for miles or get up in the middle of the night to buy bars of chocolate or loaves of bread! The most common food cravings are for chocolate, white bread, pasta and generally sweet foods. Physiologically this is caused by changes in the balance of hormones within the body. Some people believe that women who crave chocolate are desperately trying to get a 'fix' of phenylethylamine, a substance found in chocolate that has a similar hormonal effect to dopamine, making you feel comforted and happy. Unfortunately the sugary, starchy and phenylethylamine-containing foods can set up addictive and negative cycles: the more you have, the more you need to satisfy yourself. You need to tackle this nutritionally.

Some women find that rather than sugar cravings, they forage for salty foods. A similar 'the more you have the more you want' cycle can easily be set up, which of course makes fluid retention worse. An additional side effect of eating salty foods is weight gain, mainly because salt and fat together provide a very moreish combination, as many food manufacturers are well aware.

- **TRY TO RESIST THE FIRST BITE OF VERY SUGARY FOOD OR CHOCOLATE**

Once you take in a small amount of these rapidly absorbed sugars your blood sugar rises. This gives you a temporary 'fix', but unfortunately the body then secretes a lot of insulin, the hormone that breaks the sugar down. The surge in insulin then causes your sugar level to crash, giving you a sugar low. This vicious circle cannot be conquered, unless you avoid starting it.

- **USE HIGH-FIBRE FOODS WITH SOME SUGAR AS SNACKS**

When you have a sugar craving, you should eat a food that has a little sugar (preferably natural fruit sugar) to satisfy your craving, but also contains fibre. The fibre releases the sugar slowly into your system and therefore helps avoid any sugar peaks and crashes. Good snacks for when you have a sugar craving include a piece of fresh fruit, a bowl of fruit compote or poached fruit, a flapjack, wholemeal or fruit scone, or a slice of cake made with wholewheat flour and/or dried fruit such as figs, dates or raisins.

- **TRY TO CONQUER YOUR INCREASED APPETITE**

Remember that the satisfaction you derive from your meals comes from a variety of sources; read the appetite mechanism on page 6. If you make sure that your meals give you as much satisfaction as possible, you will be less likely to experience hunger pangs. Also remember that a large part of appetite is psychological, so do something to distract yourself from eating.

CHROMIUM AND
MAGNESIUM
Some women feel
that these help
reduce sugar and
chocolate cravings,
but the results are
not conclusive.
If you would like to
see whether you
respond favourably
to an increased
intake of chromium
and magnesium you
should concentrate
on boosting the
following foods:
brewers' yeast (which
can be sprinkled on
cereal), wholewheat
bread, seeds and
nuts, green leafy
vegetables (magne-
sium is a component
of chlorophyll the
green pigment in the
vegetables), shellfish
(especially winkles,
shrimps, prawns),
cheese, calves' liver,
soya beans and black
pepper.

Having discussed conquering your cravings, I think it is important to acknowledge that we have many cycles within our lives: physical, emotional and ordinary life events. While you should do as much as you can to minimize and cope with the weight gain, you shouldn't let it get you down too much. If your weight goes up a little just before your period and then comes down again afterwards, this shouldn't be a big issue. Negative feelings will increase your stress levels which will then aggravate your PMT.

BLOATING

Bloating is a condition that makes you feel gassy around the middle and generally 'windy'. This may just make you feel uncomfortable and anti-social, but in severe cases it can cause a lot of pain. The bowel and womb are very close to each other and any distension in the bowel may press on the womb.

• HORMONAL CHANGES

The muscles in the intestine are extremely sensitive to oestrogen and progesterone. This means that at different times of the month your gut may be slightly better or slightly worse at digesting your food. In a premenstrual period this can lead to the over-production of gas and the bloated feeling.

• APPETITE CHANGES

Because your appetite frequently changes just before your period, your food intake changes. This in turn brings about changes in the gut flora, and for a period of time your gut may contain bacteria that produce more gas than its usual bacteria. The solution here is to try to put as many good bacteria as possible into the gut, so that the bad, gas-producing bacteria don't have the opportunity to grow. I would therefore suggest that you take some 'live' yoghurt, containing acidophilus and bifidus cultures, every day.

'I have friends who
begin with pasta, and
friends who begin
with rice, but when-
ever I fall in love I
begin with potatoes...
I have made a lot of
mistakes falling in
love, and regretted
most of them, but
never the potatoes
that went with them.'
Nora Ephron

Some foods contain substances that produce more gas than others. The most common culprits are cabbage, cauliflower, broccoli and pulses such as baked beans, lentils and chickpeas, so reduce your consumption. Choose other vegetables such as spinach, carrots, mangetout, broad and French beans.

Irregular and hurried eating habits can also increase bloating. If you leave your gut empty for a long time the secretion of digestive enzymes slows down slightly. If you then eat a lot it can over-load the gut which can cause more gas. Also, you tend to gulp more air when you eat quickly. So eat small, regular meals, slowly.

CONSTIPATION

Many women find that in the week or so before their period they become constipated to some extent. This is caused by changes in the body's hormone levels. At this time of month it is particularly important to try to keep your bowels moving regularly, because constipation will add to the general feeling of bloatedness and discomfort. Forcing yourself to 'go' may press on your swollen womb and other inflamed tissues. If you find you are becoming constipated, make a point of eating high-fibre foods and drinking plenty of water, as discussed in the chapter on constipation.

DIARRHOEA

Women often find that they have a touch of diarrhoea once they start bleeding. As with other symptoms, this is the result of hormonal changes that cause your bowel to be upset. It is quite normal and shouldn't be a cause for great concern, unless the symptoms persist. If you have diarrhoea for more than one day you should see your doctor for advice, as you may need to take something to help bind your stool and stop your body from losing too many nutrients. There are a number of steps you can take to alleviate the situation.

• Drink at least two and a half to three litres (four and a half to five pints) of water every day, to make up for the water you lose in your stools.

• Keep your fibre intake low on the days when you have diarrhoea. Choose white breads, such as French bread, ciabatta and focaccias, white pasta and white rice, rather than the wholegrain versions.

• Avoid large amounts of vegetables and fruits. Citrus fruits in particular can aggravate diarrhoea, but other fruits may be better; try pears, apples, mangoes, papayas, bananas, grapes, strawberries.

You may also like to experiment to see whether the temperature and structure of the vegetable or fruit influences your tendency to diarrhoea. Some women find that they can tolerate them cooked better than raw. Try vegetable soups, chargrilled or puréed vegetables, baked apples or poached pears, instead of salads and raw fruit.

• Bananas, pasta, rice and potatoes can be rather good bowel 'binders', so try basing meals around these foods.

• Choose lean protein and starchy dishes rather than fatty foods. Fatty foods are difficult to digest. This may lead to too much fat in the lower bowel, which causes irritation and diarrhoea. The technical name for this is steatorrhoea (fatty stool) which makes your stools very smelly. Replenish your body with easily absorbed low-fat foods such as white rice and pasta, potato dishes, fish and shellfish, lean meat and poultry.

• Resist spicy foods, as these can aggravate diarrhoea. Instead, look to fresh herbs to enhance the flavours of your dishes (see page 57).

• Avoid caffeine-containing drinks (see page 260), as these may irritate the bowel. Camomile or mint tea are particularly effective at relieving diarrhoea.

IRRITABLE BOWEL SYNDROME

Irritable bowel syndrome (IBS) is a condition with many different symptoms, ranging from indigestion, diarrhoea, constipation, bloating and pain, to blood in the stools. Women who suffer from IBS may have a particularly bad time just before their period. The bowel is located near the womb, so any swelling can cause the womb to press on the bowel or pull on surrounding ligaments. In addition, hormonal changes alter the tone and function of the bowel muscle, which can make pain, diarrhoea and/or constipation worse.

BREAST TENDERNESS AND PERIOD PAIN

Tender breasts may be caused either by excessive fluid in the tissues, or inflamed breast tissue. I suggest you first read the advice earlier in this chapter on how to reduce fluid retention. Many of my patients with tender breasts find the condition much improved if caffeine is reduced or avoided completely for the week before the period (see page 260).

You might consider boosting your intake of oily fish or taking evening primrose oil. The special fatty acids found in these oils may help reduce the inflammation that results in breast tenderness and womb/period pain.

• You should ask your doctor or dietitian about the dosage of evening primrose oil you require. Some of the proprietary preparations do not contain significant amounts of the healing oils and are a waste of money.

• These oils can help reduce inflammation only if you have a diet that is low in saturated fats. If you are following the healthy eating guidelines set out in Part one you will already have reduced your saturated fat intake. If you need to use fat for cooking, choose a vegetable oil such as olive or sunflower oil.

VITAMINS AND MINERALS

Many claims have been made that certain vitamins and minerals can alleviate PMT symptoms. Some recent studies have concentrated on the role of vitamin B6. These studies are inconclusive and may encourage women to take unnecessary vitamins, potentially causing toxicity. Instead of taking supplements, I recommend that you eat foods rich in the B vitamins. The B vitamins, luckily, tend to be found together, in similar foods, so you do not need to become obsessed with them individually. Good food sources include yeast extract, fortified breakfast cereals, whole grains such as oats and wheat, found in wholewheat bread and pasta, meat, milk, yoghurt, cheese, eggs and dark green leafy vegetables.

• RECIPES TO RELIEVE PMT

Leek and potato soup
Carrot and orange soup
Pea, mint and lettuce soup
Parsnip and apple soup

Goats' cheese and aubergine crostini
Radicchio and grape salad
Pear and walnut salad with
    watercress
Christmas salad
Warm goats' cheese salad
Tomato and tarragon vinaigrette
Grilled vegetable salad
Warm duck breast salad with
    apricots
Gruyère potatoes
Potatoes with basil
Tomatoes stuffed with olives, garlic
    and parsley
Tomato, pesto and olive omelette
Spinach and watercress roulade

Baked pasta with ratatouille sauce
Pasta bows with courgettes
Smoked cheese and olive pasta
Salmon and asparagus risotto
Salmon and celery kedgeree
Monkfish and mussel paella
Chicken stroganoff with tarragon
Garlic and herb chicken
Winter vegetable and oxtail pie

Fruit compote
Tropical dried fruit salad
Blackberry and raspberry fool
Bread and butter pudding
Poached pears with ginger
Cinnamon apples and plums
Carrot cake
Date and walnut cake
Fig and ginger parkin

17 Pregnancy

Nutrition directly and indirectly affects your ability to get pregnant, the progress of your pregnancy and your chances of giving birth to a strong healthy baby. However, as with all nutritional issues, it is vital that you are relaxed about eating; don't let it become an obsession. Before you become pregnant, stress will not help either your own or your partner's libido. Don't turn meal times into a battleground, forcing yourselves to eat piles of alien food in the hope of conceiving; it doesn't work this way. Equally, when you become pregnant, don't let choosing food and eating become a stressful activity. I see women who are so worried about what to eat and what to avoid that they lose some of the enjoyment of being pregnant and may even suffer from high blood pressure and other serious conditions. Food is important in conception and pregnancy, but so is relaxation and peace of mind.

CONCEPTION

Any changes in diet and lifestyle aimed at increasing the likelihood of conception should ideally be made at least three months before the intended time; however this doesn't always work out! There are several key issues to address when planning to get pregnant:
• body weight
• alcohol intake
• vitamin and mineral intake

• BODY WEIGHT

Your weight takes on an increased significance when you are planning to become pregnant. Society as a whole encourages women to have body weights below the ideal range. The ideal range is best expressed as a body mass index (BMI) of 20 to 25 (see the table on pages 46–47). When the amount of body fat is low, your periods may become irregular or even stop altogether. This is because body fat helps maintain regular hormone cycles. As a result women with a very low BMI, especially anorexic and bulimic women, may have problems both in conceiving and in carrying a healthy baby to term. This does not mean that you should worry that you may not be able to get pregnant if you are naturally thin and your periods are normal. However, it can only help to build up reserves, because, almost from the moment you conceive, the growing baby has first call on your nutrients.

Overweight women may also find it difficult to conceive, as excess body fat may interfere with ovulation. Doctors are concerned that overweight women are likely to experience complications such as high blood pressure and pregnancy onset diabetes (see page 173), both of which are more common if you are overweight before you get pregnant. Many overweight women also worry that when they become pregnant they will start piling on even more weight. This is very often the case, so do try to lose some if you are overweight and planning to get pregnant. Even a small weight loss can greatly increase your ability to conceive and have a healthy pregnancy. It is important for you to lose the excess weight healthily; follow the advice in the chapter on weight loss, aiming for a body mass index of around 20–25. Don't go on a crash diet or take diet pills as these can stop your periods and adversely affect your health.

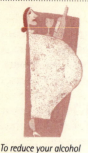

To reduce your alcohol intake, you could mix white wine with sparkling mineral water and make a spritzer. Or try the light, grapey sparkling wine Asti Spumante, which has only around 8% alcohol by volume. Wines from southern Europe tend to be higher in alcohol than those from further north. German wines, and some English wines, often have an alcohol level of 9–10% by volume, compared with 12% in many wines from France, Italy and Spain. There is a complicated system for recognizing the good from the poor German wines, but the general rule is the longer the name, the better the wine! The phrase to look for is Qualitätswein mit Prädikat (QmP), which means that the wine was made without any added sugar. I can recommend the Riesling wines produced in the Rheingau region.

• **ALCOHOL**

A little drop of alcohol will not affect your chances of becoming pregnant, assuming that your diet is well rounded in all other aspects. However, excessive amounts of alcohol have the opposite effect, adversely affecting your libido and sexual performance, so I recommend that women who are trying to get pregnant should have no more than five glasses of wine, single spirits or half pints of beer a week. If you are trying to lose weight it will be a little easier if you cut out excessive drinking.

• **VITAMINS AND MINERALS**

If you have never paid much attention to healthy eating before, take this opportunity to turn over a new leaf and think of not only yourself but also your baby. Read the advice in Part One on What your body needs and Healthy eating for life. A good, well-balanced diet contains plenty of fresh vegetables and fruit, lean proteins, high-fibre carbohydrates and some dairy products. Women's protein and fat intakes are as important as vitamin and mineral intakes, as low intakes of either protein or fat may lead to impaired fertility. Try to eat a varied diet, including fresh, unprocessed foods, preferably organic. This should provide all the nutrients you need, with adequate vitamins and minerals, to maximize your chance of a healthy pregnancy. Certain nutrients – folic acid, iron, zinc and manganese – are particularly important.

• **FOLIC ACID**

There has been a great deal of research into the link between folic acid (a B vitamin) and neural tube defects such as spina bifida. Mothers who are deficient in folic acid are at increased risk of having a baby with such problems. Anyone planning to become pregnant should ensure that their diet is rich in folic acid. Some women like to take a supplement to ensure that their intake is adequate, but I think it is much better to firstly try to achieve the required folic acid intake by boosting the amount of folic acid-rich foods in your diet. The required dosage of folic acid can be met if you have two to three good portions of the following foods in your daily diet: asparagus, raw or freshly boiled beetroot, curly kale, spinach, okra, Brussels sprouts, spring greens, Savoy cabbage, fresh peas and green beans, broccoli. Folic acid can also be obtained from yeast extract, wholemeal bread and fortified breakfast cereals. Blackeyed beans and chickpeas may be high in folic acid, but much of the nutrient is lost in the canning process. Folic acid is unfortunately one of the vitamins which is easily lost during storage and cooking (this is covered in more detail on page 23). If you doubt your intake is adequate, consult your dietitian.

• IRON

Iron-deficiency anaemia can adversely affect your ability to conceive. If you suspect that you may have iron-deficiency anaemia I suggest you read the chapter on anaemia for advice. As you will see, there is much you can do nutritionally to treat this condition. There are also various types of iron supplement available, but it is very important that you ask your doctor, pharmacist or dietitian to recommend one that is appropriate for pregnant women.

• ZINC AND MANGANESE

Deficiencies in these two minerals can lead to low libido, sterility or birth defects. Zinc deficiency is quite common in women who have been taking the contra-ceptive pill for any length of time. So if you have just come off the pill I suggest you try to include plenty of zinc in your daily healthy eating plan to improve your zinc status and your chance of becoming pregnant. I do not recommend a supplement; instead you should try to eat plenty of foods rich in these nutrients such as shellfish and fish, lean red meats, eggs, cheese, milk and yoghurt, wheatgerm and wholegrain cereal foods and nuts.

WHEN YOU ARE PREGNANT

The first thing to realize is that although you are supporting two people, the old adage 'eating for two' does not literally mean consuming twice as much, for a number of reasons:

• during pregnancy your body absorbs more of the nutrients from the gut, and therefore uses more of the calories you have taken in
• you excrete less of these nutrients
• a foetus is not as big as an adult!

However, when you are pregnant your need for certain nutrients does increase, and even doubles in the case of vitamin C and calcium, so you do need to take extra care that your diet is nutritionally balanced. You should be able to meet your needs with a regular healthy diet which is:

• rich in high-fibre carbohydrates
• rich in fresh fruits and vegetables
• moderate in lean proteins and dairy products
• low in fats and refined sugars

• FIBRE

When you are pregnant it is particularly important that your diet is high in fibre – and, of course, plenty of water to help the fibre do its work in keeping your digestive system working healthily. Pregnant women often suffer from constipation, at the time they need it least: straining to go to the loo can be very uncomfortable, and is likely to lead to post-natal piles (haemorrhoids). To avoid problems, increase your intake of high-fibre foods, including fresh fruit and vegetables, wholemeal bread and cereals, brown rice, wholewheat pasta, pulses (red kidney beans, baked beans, lentils, chickpeas).

- ### ENERGY

In theory pregnant women need to increase their intake of energy-rich foods. However, this should be covered by your increased intake of fibre-rich foods suggested above. Many women expend a lot less energy when they're pregnant, especially in the late stages. I generally advise that you should follow your appetite and eat what you fancy, maintaining a healthy balance overall.

Don't be scared by the stories you hear of women completely changing their body shapes, from a 'thin' to a 'fat' person, when they have children. Women may put on weight during and after pregnancy, but it is neither hormonal nor inevitable. It is simply down to the fact that they eat more. If you stick to a healthy eating pattern and avoid high-fat and high-sugar low-fibre snacks you should not put on too much weight.

- ### PROTEIN

There is no need to increase your protein intake, as long as it follows general healthy eating principles and includes some fish, chicken, lean meat, dairy products, eggs, grains, nuts, pulses and seeds (sunflower, sesame, pumpkin).

VITAMINS AND MINERALS

- ### IRON

If you are not anaemic or don't have a history of iron-deficiency anaemia you should try to maintain a good iron intake. If you are anaemic I suggest you read the separate chapter on anaemia and seek the advice of your doctor.

Examples of well-absorbed iron include lean red meat, game and kidneys; liver, although the richest source of well-absorbed dietary iron, should be avoided during pregnancy because of its high vitamin A content (see below). Since you won't be eating meat every day, you can also find a lot of iron in eggs, baked beans and other pulses, green leafy vegetables such as spinach, broccoli and sorrel, dried apricots and prunes, and wholegrain cereals, wholemeal bread and wholewheat pasta. Iron from non-meat foods is not quite as easily absorbed by the body, so you need to eat more of them to gain the equivalent amount of iron. For iron to be absorbed efficiently you also need plenty of folic acid and vitamin C in your diet.

• VITAMIN A

The vitamin A from animal sources, if taken in excess, can build up in the liver and cause serious damage. In the tiny liver of the baby growing inside you, it does not take much to tip the delicate balance. For this reason, doctors generally recommend that pregnant women should avoid foods that are rich in vitamin A. These include liver and liver pâté, and cod liver oil. You should also be aware that some supplements are high in this form of vitamin A. However, the form of vitamin A derived from green, orange and yellow vegetables and fruit (known as carotene) has positive health benefits, and is plentiful in sweet potatoes, carrots, red and yellow peppers, broccoli, watercress, kale, apricots.

• VITAMIN C

In order to help your body absorb and effectively use iron and other nutrients in your food, you should eat plenty of vitamin C. Good sources include the citrus fruits – oranges, tangerines, grapefruit, fresh lemon juice – kiwi fruits, blackcurrants, strawberries, rosehips, tomatoes, peppers and green leafy vegetables. Aim to have five portions of fresh fruit or vegetables every day.

• SUPPLEMENTS

Although many women believe that they need to take vitamin and mineral supplements when pregnant, supplements are in the majority of cases unnecessary; most of us can easily get all the vitamins and minerals we need from a varied diet that includes plenty of fresh food. In some cases supplements may even be harmful, and pregnant women in particular should take supplements only on medical advice. They may be necessary when you have a specific problem such as extreme sickness, and folic acid may be a useful supplement, but avoid taking it as part of a very general vitamin and mineral package. It is all too easy to take an excess of certain nutrients, especially the fat-soluble vitamins A and D, and toxicity may occur. Remember that it's not just your own life you're putting at risk, but also your baby's.

COFFEE AND TEA

The caffeine found in tea, coffee and many soft drinks such as cola interferes with your body's absorption of iron and other nutrients, which your baby needs. It is also diuretic, therefore you lose other important nutrients in your urine. All these drinks can fill you up so you are less inclined to eat the healthy foods you really need, and they are addictive, an addiction that can be passed into the baby in your womb. Finally, coffee and tea are likely to aggravate nausea. Do you need any more reasons to limit your intake of tea and coffee to no more than two cups a day during pregnancy?

FOOD POISONING RISKS

Pregnant women should be very careful not to expose themselves to any risk of food poisoning. Food poisoning is always very unpleasant and potentially dangerous, but when you're pregnant and a little more vulnerable it may be very serious and can in the cases of toxoplasmosis and listeriosis cause deformities in your baby. However, if you follow the guidelines below your risk of contracting these infections is very low.
• Wash your hands carefully after you have touched any animal.
• Make sure that meat and poultry are cooked and hot through before you eat them.

• Wash all vegetables and fruits thoroughly before you eat them. This will get rid of soil and some potential food poisoning organisms, and also reduces the amount of wax and other appearance-enhancing chemicals.

• Always keep cooked and raw foods separately in the refrigerator, so that the bacteria from raw foods do not infect the cooked foods.

• Use separate chopping boards for raw and cooked meat and fish, one for vegetables and fruits. (Or at least clearly mark separate sides of two chopping boards.)

Botulism Although extremely rare, this can be fatal. It may be found in tinned food where the tin is damaged or blown at the ends.

Clostridium perfringens This may be found in rice that has been cooked and left in a warmish environment, and then not properly reheated. If you choose a rice dish in a restaurant, make sure that it is piping hot all the way through.

Listeriosis This is caused by a bacterium called *Listeria monocytogenes*. Listeriosis produces flu-like symptoms of slight fever and fatigue, but in pregnant women can cause miscarriage (spontaneous abortion). Listeria may be found in soft cheeses, especially mould-ripened cheeses such as Brie and Camembert, in pâté and in chilled ready-made meals and salads. Many people think that as long as they avoid unpasteurized soft cheeses they won't contract listeriosis, but this is not the case: listeria is just as likely to be found in pasteurized soft cheese. Avoid all soft cheese, pâtés and prepared salads such as coleslaw and potato salad. Chilled ready-made meals should be reheated thoroughly until piping hot to destroy any bacteria present.

There are so many gorgeous hard cheeses on the market, you certainly won't lack variety.

• From the British Isles there are various styles of Cheddar, Cheshire, Derby and Sage Derby, Single and Double Gloucester, Lancashire, Red Leicester, Wensleydale and many local cheeses made from cows', ewes' and goats' milk.

• French hard cheeses include Beaufort, Cantal (Fourme de Salers), Comté, Saint Nectaire and Tomme de Savoie. Gruyère and Emmental is made in France and in Switzerland. The Netherlands produces Edam and Gouda; look out for the tasty mature versions. Italy's Parmesan is excellent for cooking or nibbling.

Salmonellosis Salmonella thrives in foods that are insufficiently heated to kill the bacteria, particularly eggs, poultry and unpasteurized milk. It causes diarrhoea and vomiting, and possibly fever and headache, 12 to 48 hours after eating the infected food, and in rare cases has proved fatal. The very young and elderly, pregnant women and people recovering from an illness, whose immune systems are not working at full strength, are particularly vulnerable and should be treated by a doctor immediately. To avoid salmonella poisoning, steer clear of foods containing raw and lightly cooked eggs, such as mayonnaise and some sauces and mousses. Egg dishes should be freshly and thoroughly cooked. All poultry and meat should be well cooked. Take extra care at parties, where food is left in warm rooms and the bacteria grow quickly.

Toxoplasmosis This is rare, but can cause birth defects or miscarriage in some women. It can be diagnosed only by a blood test, but sadly the symptoms don't usually appear until two to three weeks after contracting the disease. There are mild flu-like symptoms, such as a slight fever, fatigue and swollen glands, and possibly a rash. It is transmitted mainly through animal faeces, but also via raw meat and the soil on vegetables.

• Keep cat litter and pet mess completely away from food. Wear rubber gloves to clean up any mess.

• Don't feed raw meat to your cats or dogs, as this provides a possible route for infection.

• Avoid eating undercooked or raw red meat, such as steak tartare.

• Wash vegetables and salads carefully, to remove soil.

GINGER TEA
Place a very thin slice of fresh root ginger in a small cup. Add boiling hot water and leave for 3–5 minutes. Remove the ginger and drink in small sips.

TROUBLESHOOTING

• NAUSEA AND VOMITING

It is common to suffer from some morning sickness, especially in the first three months of pregnancy. It can range in severity from just feeling queasy to being unable to keep anything down, and it may not confine itself to the mornings. If you go for more than a day without being able to keep anything down, do seek the advice of your doctor. The following suggestions may help.

Check your iron supplement. If you are taking iron supplements, stopping these sometimes makes the nausea go away. Check with your doctor, and ensure that you are eating plenty of iron-rich foods (see page 28).

Have small meals often. This is much better than going for long periods without eating. Even if the nausea is very bad you should try to have something, as an empty stomach may make you feel even worse. Base your snacks on carbohydrate-rich foods such as bread rolls, plain biscuits, crispbreads, pasta, rice or potatoes. If you can manage to add some protein to these dishes, such as a little ham, cheese or egg, this would be ideal. It is better to have a little bit of something than to stress yourself out about not eating enough. A bowl of soup can be very settling, but resist creamy ones, as these can aggravate nausea. Enjoy vegetable soups hot or chilled, with a swirl of yoghurt.

Avoid fatty foods. These may be hard to digest and can 'sit' heavily in your stomach. The fat also causes the muscle rings around the top of your stomach to temporarily weaken. If you are feeling sick, this can make the situation worse.

Make sure that you are not drinking too much tea or coffee. Caffeine and tannins (found in coffee and tea) both aggravate nausea and vomiting. As alternative hot drinks, ginger (see margin), peppermint and camomile tea are all very soothing. I would also suggest jasmine tea or a few drops of orange blossom water in boiling water. Some patients find rice water settling; unpleasant as it sounds, it can work wonders. Just save the hot water in which you have cooked the rice and take small sips.

Take small sips of fizzy drinks. Avoid caffeine-containing drinks, but the bubbles in other fizzy drinks can reduce the sickness feeling quite substantially.

Stick to foods that don't take a lot of preparation.

Experiment with the temperature of your foods. Cold foods are often more appealing when you're feeling sick. Try a little piece of your favourite cheese with walnut or seeded bread or some smoked salmon with cherry tomatoes and wholewheat bread. Grapes or sliced fruit are quite easy to manage.

Catch up on good days. On days when you are feeling less sick, try to get into the habit of making larger quantities of dishes that you can freeze in small amounts. Then on days when you can't face spending time in the kitchen you can quickly reheat something nutritious.

Keep a stock of biscuits in a tin by your bed. It can help to nibble one before you get up in the morning. Homemade or bought ginger biscuits are particularly good as many people find that ginger helps reduce nausea.

Try to get a little fresh air before eating. If you can fit in the time, it is often very beneficial to go for a stroll before eating. This can help build up a little bit of an appetite and should also reduce the stale feeling of sickness. If you are not feeling well enough for a walk, try to sit outside (weather permitting!).

• WHAT TO DO IF YOU ARE GAINING TOO MUCH WEIGHT
The usual increase in body weight during pregnancy is: 9 kg (20 lb) for women who start their pregnancy within the ideal range; 7.5 kg (16.5 lb) if you are overweight before you become pregnant; 13.5 kg (30 lb) if you are underweight before pregnancy.

However, this is only a rough guide: many women don't gain this much, whereas others gain a little more and still give birth comfortably, to healthy babies. The best way to make sure you are gaining weight at an acceptable level is to keep in touch with your doctor or obstetrician. It is not only the total weight gain that is important but also the pattern and rate of gain. It is advisable to reduce your weight if it is too high as this will help prevent complications such as raised blood pressure (which may lead to the dangerous condition, pre-eclampsia) and pregnancy onset diabetes (see page 173).

Crash diets are never a good idea, and if you are pregnant they may endanger your baby. Read the chapter on weight loss and make sure that you are eating a healthy, well-balanced diet, without any excess fatty or sugary foods.

If you can establish a healthy eating pattern your weight should not increase too much. You will also feel better and will be laying down a good foundation for your baby's health. However, you will not regain full control of your body for several months after the birth. Let nature take its course.

• INDIGESTION

This frequently occurs once the baby grows to the size at which its body starts pressing on your stomach. The hormone changes during pregnancy may also cause the muscles at the top of your stomach to over-relax, which makes it more likely that the acidic contents of your stomach will leak back into your oesophagus causing an unpleasant sensation. It is often worse at night when you are lying down. I suggest that you read the chapter on indigestion.

• TASTE ALTERATIONS

Some women find that they develop a strong aversion to certain flavours when they are pregnant; others find that things simply don't taste the same. This is caused by hormonal fluctuations. Don't worry about it, as it is only a short-term change. Some of the most common changes in taste relate to coffee, English-style tea, alcohol and fatty foods. See page 62 for alternative hot drinks.

Cravings for strange or unlikely foods usually pose no threat to either you or the baby as long as you still manage to consume a well-balanced diet. If you crave something high in refined sugars or fats, something that may put you at risk of food poisoning or something really peculiar such as coal or sand, seek the advice of your doctor or dietitian as soon as possible.

• RECIPES TO ENJOY DURING PREGNANCY

Chilled mint and cucumber soup

Carrot and orange soup

Lentil soup

Pea, mint and lettuce soup

Gado gado

Tomatoes stuffed with olives, garlic
 and parsley

Warm spinach salad with French
 beans and pancetta

Pasta with wild mushrooms

Smoked cheese and olive pasta

Pasta bows with courgettes

Yam biryani

Smoked mackerel and spinach
 fishcakes

Smoked fish casserole

Salmon and asparagus risotto

Chicken stroganoff with tarragon

Sausage and bean casserole

Tropical dried fruit salad

Fruit compote

Mixed fruit with butterscotch sauce

Oranges in caramel

Apple and fig crumble

Chilled gingered rhubarb

Vanilla poached peaches

Cinnamon apples and plums

Prune and bitter chocolate tart

Flapjacks

Date and walnut cake

Fig and orange cake

Fig and ginger parkin

Fruit cake

Banana cake

Carrot cake

Lemon cake

18 Sex

Nutrition affects sex in many ways. Nutritional deficiencies, excess food and body weight can physiologically and/or psychologically cause you to suffer from poor libido. While there are often other factors involved, such as hormone levels, stress and unhappiness, the foods you eat and the way you treat your body can have profound effects on both your libido and your ability to conceive (more about which in the chapter on pregnancy). It is important to use the information in this chapter as support, rather than becoming obsessed with ways of increasing your sexuality. Stress can reduce your enjoyment of sex; sexual arousal may diminish if you are worried about work, money, relationships or the food you eat.

• SEX AND YOUR PSYCHE

The way you feel about your body frequently manifests itself in the bedroom. Some women who have a poor opinion of their own body find it very hard to feel sexy. We, in the 'thin is beautiful' West, have a very fixed idea of how a good body should look. The fashion for being toned and thin causes some women to feel so unhappy with their body that they cannot enjoy a full and satisfying sex life. Others manage to have an extremely active sex life, although they aren't really happy with themselves underneath. They feel loved and appreciated only when they are in bed with someone.

For many women food is the only thing they can really control in life, which is why so many women focus excessively on their body and food. As babies we associate food given to us by our mothers with affection. As we get older we tend to realize that cooking and eating is a way of communicating how we feel about ourselves and others. A lovely way to show you care about someone is to give them food. Women may spend hours cooking for partners and children, which is fine as long as they enjoy it and do not resent time spent in the kitchen. This association can backfire if the person rejects the food; it is seen as a rejection of love, which can be very upsetting. Other women spend hours cooking for someone else, but they do not allow themselves to eat the food; they either don't feel they are worthy of eating it or they get a kick out of resisting, as in the case of many anorexics or women obsessed with their bodies.

A woman who is sexually unhappy may become anorexic or bulimic, take solace in comfort eating or drinking or generally have poor eating habits. All of these affect your ability to enjoy a good sex life. The destructive food and sex cycle needs to be changed to establish a pattern of healthy eating and sex.

• YOUR HORMONES AND LIBIDO

Many women find that their libido varies as their hormone levels fluctuate. Many feel very sexy at the mid-point of their menstrual cycle, others feel most sexy when they're actually having their period. Lack of sexual desire can be a signal that you are entering the menopause, but this does not apply to all women. Some menopausal and post-menopausal women have the highest libido. At last they can have sex without fear of becoming pregnant! While we are not all designed to have a high libido all of the time, any noticeable or prolonged loss of libido should be investigated by your doctor. She or he will be able to check whether there is any physiological cause for this, such as a hormonal imbalance or a nutritional deficiency. You may be advised to take certain hormonal preparations to improve the situation. Bear in mind that other drugs, such as antibiotics, can adversely affect your libido. Whether or not you require professional treatment, I believe it is worth exploring the possibility that food can help you gain or regain a good sex life.

• VITAMINS AND MINERALS: THEIR ROLE IN YOUR SEX LIFE

The first thing to do if you have a poor libido, or simply want to protect your healthy sex drive, is ensure that your diet is well balanced, including lots of fresh vegetables, fruits, wholegrain foods, water and lean protein. Read the information on What your body needs in Part One of this book. Once you have done this, question whether the foods you eat are affecting your sex life.

Poor nutrient levels, in particular the B vitamins, zinc and iron, can affect your libido, the production of sex hormones and reproductive tissues such as those of the vagina and lower abdominal muscles. Iron deficiency anaemia (see separate chapter) can result in lack of energy, depression and chronic fatigue, which can cause a low libido. If you follow a varied diet you should consume enough of these nutrients to ensure that your ability to become a lover and/or parent is not compromised. If you worry about not feeling sexy, make a point of including some of the following foods in your healthy eating plan; they are all rich in these important nutrients. Fresh oysters, prawns, mussels, clams; lean red meats such as beef, venison, liver; nuts such as pecans, hazelnuts, almonds, walnuts, brazils; egg yolks; milk; wholewheat products; vegetables, especially the green leafy varieties, fresh parsley and garlic.

I would not suggest that you take a supplement, unless you don't regularly eat any of the foods listed above. Always seek professional advice before you take a supplement, as there is a great deal of evidence linking vitamin toxicity (caused by excessive vitamin intake) with birth defects. You may not intend to get pregnant while you are trying to improve your libido, but it is possible.

• HOW WEIGHT AFFECTS YOUR SEX DRIVE
The composition of your body can affect your sex life in several ways. Body fat is needed for the metabolism of the sex hormones, including oestrogen and progesterone; if you are too thin, with a body mass index of less than 17 or 18 (see chart on page 46), your libido could suffer. Even women with normal body weight, but very low blood cholesterol levels, may have problems metabolizing sex hormones. If you have a very low

cholesterol level, below 3mmol/l (see page 207), or percentage of body fat, you should consult your doctor or dietitian, who will be able to advise you as to how you can correct it, healthily.

Anorexic women and women who control their body weight or fat level at a low level by restricting their food intake, which includes serious athletes, may develop nutritional deficiencies which can directly affect their sex drive.

If you have an eating disorder such as anorexia or bulimia I suggest you read the chapter on eating disorders, which should help you to come to terms with the situation. If it is a long-term problem, please seek professional advice.

• EXCESS WEIGHT

Some overweight women have a problem feeling sexy. Unless you are extremely overweight, with a body mass index greater than 25 (see page 46), there is usually not a physiological, but more often a psychological reason for this. If you are overweight and feel it is interfering with your sex life, I suggest you read the chapter on weight loss. It is important to see losing weight as an empowering experience, not one of deprivation. If you lose weight slowly and devote time and attention to your body, your libido is much more likely to return. Don't punish your body by going on a crash diet: this won't work and certainly won't make you happier. Many of my patients find having regular massages a good way of receiving some body pampering, which serves as a real incentive to carry on losing weight. Remember the more positive you can become about losing weight and your body the more likely you are to succeed.

• ALCOHOL AND SEX

Many people use alcohol as part of their arousal. They try to get themselves in the mood for sex by having a tipple. While it is well known that too much alcohol adversely affects the performance of the man, few of us understand that this is also the case for women. The odd drink can help you relax and enjoy sex, but excessive intakes don't. Some women turn to the bottle to give them solace if their libido is low. If you cut down your alcohol intake you may well find that your libido increases.

URINARY TRACT INFECTIONS

There are many women who do not enjoy sex as much as they could because of a urinary tract infection, the best known of which is cystitis. Discomfort and pain can set up a vicious circle, as they worry that sex will aggravate the condition. Most women have at some time suffered from painful urination, blood in the urine or swelling around the opening of the urethra, the tube that leads from the bladder to the outside of the body.

The majority of urinary tract infections, including cystitis, are caused by the bacterium *E. coli,* which sticks to the walls of the bladder and urethra and inflames the tissues, which may even bleed. The bacteria either travel up the urethra into the bladder or spread from elsewhere in the body. Women are particularly susceptible to developing infections in the urethra after sexual intercourse, as the friction can cause the tissues around the urethra to become a little bruised. In a few cases infections are caused by an obstruction, such as a stone in your kidney.

• SELF-HELP FOR URINARY TRACT INFECTIONS

As soon as you have any of the above symptoms you should implement the following self-help regime. If after 48 hours your symptoms don't improve you should seek your doctor's advice, as it may be that you need to take antibiotics. Urinary tract infections can develop into kidney infections, which if untreated can damage your kidneys. It is especially important for pregnant women not to ignore a urinary tract infection, as it can lead to high blood pressure or infections within the womb.

Since cranberries have a beneficial role in preventing and curing cystitis, you could either drink cranberry juice (which looks very much like a light red wine if served in a wine glass) or look out for cranberry wine, made in the USA.

Beers have a diuretic effect, which can help flush the offending bacteria out of your system. If you fancy something fruitier, try cider. Good ciders have a balance between bitterness and sweetness and contain 4–5% alcohol; they may be still or sparkling, dry or sweet. English cider is traditionally made in Somerset, Hereford and Worcestershire. There is also a cider-making tradition in Normandy and northern Brittany in France.

These have serious consequences for you and the baby.
• The primary aim is to flush the bacteria out of the bladder, by drinking at least three litres (about five pints) of water every day. Generally, you can never drink too much water, unless you are taking certain drugs that disturb your perception of thirst, so drink as much as you can manage.
• Empty your bladder regularly. Don't ignore the urge to go.
• Avoid tea and coffee, as these can irritate the bladder and urethra.
• Look to the cranberry for help (see below).
A word of warning. Since vitamin A is needed to help maintain a healthy urinary tract, some people think that it may be helpful to take a vitamin A supplement when they have a urinary tract infection. This is not only unnecessary, it may cause other serious problems. Keep to a healthy balanced diet and your body should receive all the nutrients it needs to fight infections.

• THE CRANBERRY

The treatment of urinary tract infections improved dramatically when it was found that the cranberry has the ability to prevent the *E.coli* bacteria from sticking to the bladder and urethra walls. There are several cranberry juices on the market, but the unsweetened ones available from health food shops are the most effective. You can also buy dried cranberries, which are very 'moreish'. The fresh ones are a little bitter and are best used in sauces and stuffings to accompany turkey and other meats. However, since the aim is to flush out the bladder, I think it is best to drink cranberry juice.

• PREVENTION

All women should be able to prevent themselves from getting urinary tract infections if they drink at least two to three litres of water a day, eat a healthy diet and empty their bladder regularly, especially after sexual intercourse. Tight underwear, made of man-made fabrics such as nylon or polyester, should be avoided as it doesn't allow the skin to breathe, but keeps it warm and moist, which is the environment bacteria love. Wear natural fibres such as cotton or silk as these enable air to circulate, keeping you dry and cool. Bubble baths and bath salts can irritate the bottom, especially if you leave the residue to dry on the skin, which can provide the bacteria with a sticky environment to infest. Always thoroughly rinse and completely dry. Never use perfumed moisturizing products on your bottom.

Always pay attention to the hygiene of the lavatories you use. Urinary tract infections can be transmitted via toilet seats, so either use one of the paper covers that many public toilets stock, or just crouch above the toilet seat.

APHRODISIACS

Throughout history, some foods have been thought to be aphrodisiacs. Ask anyone in Britain which foods they consider to be aphrodisiacs and they will probably say oysters, caviar, Champagne, with a more recent suggestion of lentils raising an eyebrow or two. But in other parts of the world different foods are considered to be influential. There is little scientific evidence to support these theories, although chocolate contains substances similar to those produced by the brain when we are in love, so in the right circumstances luxurious chocolates or chocolate desserts can be highly aphrodisiac. Our perception can make certain foods a real 'turn on'. This may be because they are expensive and make you feel pampered, or because their texture or smell has sexual associations for you. I find it very suggestive to crack the top of a crème brûlée and find the creamy centre. Here are some guidelines to help you set the scene for a deeply sexy dinner.

Whatever gets you in the mood! This could be a favourite drink that has happy, sexy associations or the more traditional bottle of 'champers'. Gently removing the cork from a bottle of Champagne can be very suggestive. Size isn't everything, but a magnum would be impressive! I suggest you crack open a bottle, drink half, then put a special Champagne stopper or a metal spoon in the top of the bottle to stop the bubbles from disappearing, leaving the rest for later.

Relax and enjoy. Don't create stress for yourself by cooking something complicated. Choose simple dishes that you have cooked before. There is no bigger turn off than having conversation interrupted by frequent visits to the kitchen. Many sexologists recommend that you eat out to avoid stress in the kitchen, but I disagree. There are many simple and delicious things you can eat at home, and eating in allows the evening to progress at your pace and not at the hands of waiters. If you do eat out, choose a relaxed restaurant where you can feel pampered but not hassled, and eat at a time when you feel at ease. Choose dishes that are easy to eat: unless you are completely confident about twirling spaghetti or pulling shellfish out of their shells, avoid potentially messy food. On the other hand, if you're eating in, using your hands to eat can be very sensual. If you eat something with a strong flavour, such as garlic, make sure that your partner tries it too, otherwise the smell can be a real turn-off.

Plan ahead. Think about the dishes you are going to prepare well in advance and check that you can get all of the ingredients. Getting to the day of the dinner and then finding out that they are not available is very stressful.

Think about visual appeal. Plan menus to look appetizing. Choose ingredients with different temperatures, textures and colours, to stimulate the senses.

Imagine aromas. Aromatherapists believe that cinnamon, orange and ginger oils are very relaxing. You could have these burning in an oil burner, or why not cook an apple and cinnamon pudding or an orange pudding, served with a ginger sabayon sauce?

Don't overeat. Feeling bloated is not sexy.

Try not to drink too much. Too much alcohol, especially on an empty stomach, may lead to an overindulgent eating session, as alcohol increases your appetite. It could also make you sleepy or, even if you do stay awake, adversely affect your sexual performance.

• APHRODISIACS FOR MODERN LOVERS

Oysters: raw or grilled with cream
    and Parmesan
Caviar
Asparagus
Parma ham with cantaloupe melon
Smoked salmon and scrambled eggs

Apple, dolcelatte and walnut strudel
Pear and walnut salad with
    watercress
Spinach and watercress roulade
Spinach and goats' cheese soufflé

Pasta vongole
Salmon and asparagus risotto
Chicken with melon, grapes
    and asparagus
Honey and mustard quail

Exotic fruit salad made with
    mango, passion fruit, kiwi,
    bananas
Mixed berries in Grand Marnier
Vanilla poached peaches
Coconut ice cream

19 Skin

The skin is the largest organ of the body. It consists of millions of cells that rely on a regular supply of oxygen and nutrients. Adverse changes in either the balance of nutrients or your general health quickly show in your skin, as skin cells have a very short life span: remarkably, they are replaced every few days.

Some women seem to be born with fantastic skin, others battle with spots or more serious skin conditions such as eczema, acne or psoriasis, but even if you are born with good skin, you still need to look after it. Women spend millions of pounds every year on skin creams and lotions, designed to prolong youthful appearance and tackle spots and dry skin. While creams play an essential part in a woman's skin health routine, it is not enough just to tackle the surface. You need to look deeper, to find out why your skin is as it is and how nutrition can help to improve it. Poor skin may be caused by a nutrient deficiency, an imbalance of nutrients, hormones or other chemicals, or by emotional problems, which need to be addressed if you are to improve your skin. Naturally, your skin is as responsive to negative life events and feelings as any other organ in the body. Many women go through good and bad skin times, very few of us manage to keep a glowing healthy skin 24 hours a day for life; it takes work. If you want to look good and stay looking good your skin needs a regular supply of nutrients, water and oxygen, along with a beneficial skin care routine.

In the first part of this chapter I aim to help you create and preserve good healthy skin and show how to reduce the appearance of wrinkles. Later, I will tackle the nutritional issues that can help deal with skin problems.

• A PROFILE OF THE SKIN

The skin consists of three layers. The deepest layer is the subcutaneous layer, which contains the main blood vessels, fat, and two types of protein called collagen and elastin. The middle layer, the dermis, protects the subcutaneous layer and contains small blood vessels. The dermis also supplies the upper layer, the epidermis, with new cells when they become damaged. The epidermis provides a home for the hair and nail beds. Therefore without adequate nourishment your hair and nails may suffer as well as your skin. To complete the skin profile, there is an outer layer of dead skin cells, which swell in response to water. These cells are shed and replenished every day.

HOW TO KEEP HEALTHY-LOOKING SKIN

• EAT A WELL-BALANCED DIET

To remain healthy, your skin needs a regular and well-balanced supply of nutrients. You shouldn't need to take any supplements, provided you look after your skin and you are generally healthy. Try to eat at least five portions of fresh vegetables or fruits every day; this should be quite easy if you have three pieces of fruit as desserts or snacks, plus a salad or vegetable dish with two meals.

Bad skin is not generally caused by any one food, unless it is an allergic reaction (see under Skin problems, page 298), but particular foods can aggravate poor skin.

The myth that chocolate, sweets and other fatty and sugary foods cause spots is not entirely unfounded: an eating pattern high in these foods and low in fresh fruits, vegetables and other constituents of a healthy diet means that your skin is unlikely to be getting all the nutrients it needs. Women who would rather eat a bar of chocolate or a bag of crisps than an orange, for example, may lack vitamin C. This can make your immune system less able to fight infections, including those on the skin – spots. In addition, women often eat more chocolate at times when they are feeling down, whether emotionally, hormonally or physically, which also has a negative effect on the skin. If you already have spots, a diet that is high in sugar or fat may make your system even more susceptible to bacterial infections, which may further aggravate spots and other skin conditions.

• DRINK PLENTY OF WATER

In our society, where many of us have central heating and lead active lives, one of the commonest causes of tired-looking skin is dehydration, both on the surface and throughout the body. Aim to rehydrate your body by drinking two to three litres (four to five pints) of water a day.

This should ideally be taken as plain or lightly flavoured, unsweetened water and not as tea, coffee or other caffeine-containing or sugary drinks.

• CUT DOWN ON TEA AND COFFEE

Women who drink a lot of tea, coffee, hot chocolate and cola-type drinks are more likely to have tired-looking skin and to suffer from conditions such as greasy skin and spots. This is because these drinks contain caffeine, which prevents your body from making good use of the vitamins and minerals from your food. Try to drink no more than three cups of coffee, tea or other caffeine-containing drinks a day. See page 62 for some refreshing alternatives.

• KEEP YOUR ALCOHOL INTAKE LOW

Excessive alcohol intakes may lead to skin problems such as split veins. Try not to drink more than the recommended 21 units a week (a unit is the equivalent of a glass of wine, a standard measure of spirits or half a pint of beer, lager or cider of ordinary strength).

Some women have a skin allergy to some alcoholic drinks, which usually manifests itself as hives. Hives are little itchy red spots that appear under the surface of the skin and make it feel hot and sensitive; they are

Oats are rich in biotin, so porridge is a perfect 'skin food'.

sometimes known as nettle rash. The most common allergic reaction is to salicylates, substances that occur naturally in some foods, such as grapes, bananas, beans, strawberries and other berry fruits. If you get a rash after eating some of these foods, beers may affect you in the same way, since they are often high in salicylates. Instead, choose wine, gin, vodka or whisky.

• TRY TO GIVE UP SMOKING

Nicotine does not help you keep a healthy skin. It attacks the blood vessels that feed the skin with nutrients and oxygen, as well as those that drain away the waste products from the skin. Your skin therefore becomes poor at ridding itself of unwanted substances and in severe cases also starts to lack oxygen.

Other substances produced by smoke can age the skin greatly and affect the nail beds and hair follicles, which nestle in the epidermis. If you want to have a youthful, healthy appearance, try to give up smoking.

• SPECIFIC NUTRIENTS FOR GOOD SKIN

Vitamins A and C and the mineral zinc are all strongly linked with good skin. They are considered part of a healthy balanced diet, and there is usually no need to take them in supplement form. Both vitamins should be provided from your regular intake of fresh fruits and vegetables. Foods rich in vitamin A include carrots, spinach, watercress, broccoli, yellow-fleshed sweet potato and melons such as cantaloupe. Good sources of vitamin C are peppers, green leafy vegetables, strawberries, kiwi fruit, oranges and grapefruit.

Zinc is excellent for problem skin. It helps reduce the inflammatory processes within the body and aids healing. The body is more efficient at absorbing the zinc from foods such as beans and other pulses, shellfish and fish, wholegrain foods, nuts and dairy foods, rather than from tablets. If you feel your diet doesn't include some of these foods most days, you may wish to take a daily 15 mg supplement. Do not exceed this dose as high zinc levels make your body more susceptible to bacterial and viral infections.

Another nutrient that seems to be perfect 'skin food' is biotin, a member of the vitamin B complex (although it is also known as vitamin H). It is mainly synthesized by bacteria in your gut, but is also found in some foods. Women who are on long-term antibiotics, which adversely affect the bacteria within the gut, or who suffer from any sort of gut malabsorption condition such as Crohn's disease or severe irritable bowel syndrome, could be rather low in biotin. A deficiency of this vitamin causes dermatitis (inflammation of the skin), loss of hair and, in my experience, brittle nails.

Biotin-rich foods include eggs, peanut butter, wholegrain foods (especially oats) and liver. Note that raw eggs bind biotin in the gut and therefore will not help if you are looking to boost your biotin intake.

Warning Although some doctors prescribe vitamin A based creams for skin complaints such as acne, there is no benefit to be gained from taking additional vitamin A in the form of a supplement. It is potentially dangerous to take a vitamin A supplement without the supervision of your doctor, as it is stored in the liver and an excess can cause severe liver damage. Vitamin A supplements taken while a woman is pregnant may lead to birth defects.

• SUPPLEMENT YOUR DIET WITH ACIDOPHILUS AND BIFIDUS

I suggest you eat a small pot of 'live' yoghurt containing bifidus and acidophilus bacteria every day. These will help to rebalance the bacteria in your gut, and will particularly help those of you who take antibiotics to control skin problems. I see many women who have been taking antibiotics for anything from a few weeks to years. In doing so, their bodies suffer from side effects such as thrush and irritable bowels. The antibiotics kill the bacteria that exist within the healthy gut, which under normal circumstances produce anti-inflammatory substances, anti-cancer substances, vitamin K and energy. A good balance of bacteria needs to be re-established in order to protect the skin against inflammation and the body against other problems. The yoghurt can be eaten on its own, flavoured with chopped or puréed fruit, poured on to fruit or cereal, or swirled into soup or casseroles.

HOW TO AVOID WRINKLES

As described on page 292, the deepest layer of the skin, the subcutaneous layer, contains two types of protein: collagen and elastin. Collagen provides the skin with a strong, firm texture, and elastin makes it resilient. To avoid wrinkles, you need to try to preserve these two components in your skin. Wrinkles start to appear as the collagen and elastin fibres deteriorate. The nutritional principles behind preserving collagen and elastin fibres focus on preventing free radicals from damaging the skin.

• FREE RADICALS

The most destructive ageing element we all have to face is the sun. Avoiding direct sunlight will not only keep your skin looking younger, it will also render you less likely to develop skin cancer (see page 303). However, sunlight is just one of a number of factors that promote the production of free radicals within our bodies. They are also produced by tobacco smoke, air pollution and environmental toxins, and are found naturally in our bodies. Free radicals are highly reactive molecules that stabilize themselves by attaching themselves to other cells. This causes the cells to behave abnormally, which manifests itself as ageing, or as diseases such as cancer, heart disease and duodenal ulcers. Although free radicals are part of the normal digestion process in the body, it is when we take in or produce too many that problems may occur.

Some people have a genetic predisposition to free radical damage: look around and you will see some women who get lines around the eyes and mouth in their twenties, while others remain unwrinkled into their forties. Nevertheless, we can all take steps to limit free radical damage to the skin.

• *Make sure that our diet contains plenty of substances that protect us from their damage.* The most effective nutrients in protecting us against free radical damage are the antioxidants: beta-carotene, vitamins C and E and selenium. A good intake of antioxidants can fight free radicals and reduce damage to the collagen and elastin fibres. For information and good food sources, see page 32.

• *Make sure we don't eat foods that contain or produce excessive free radicals.* One of the foods thought to increase the number of free radicals produced in the body is margarine made with hydrogenated fat or oil. When vegetable oils are heated to a high temperature, as in the hydrogenation process, their molecular structure changes in a way that is harmful to the body's cells. It can be confusing, because there are so many vegetable margarines in the shops that people are tempted to use them in preference to butter, believing that they need to reduce their intake of saturated fats. However, while it is appropriate to do this, you should also be looking to reduce your overall fat intake as part of your healthy eating plan. When you do use fats, try to choose those that are as natural as possible, such as butter and olive oil.

• *Make sure that you thoroughly wash vegetables and fruits before eating.* Chemicals, pesticides and the wax coating used on some produce, together with exhaust fumes from the harvesting equipment or transport, may be present on the skins and have been implicated in the free radical damage scenario. Choose organic suppliers whenever possible.

• **EXERCISE**

Exercise helps keep a good blood flow to the skin. Blood supplies the skin with oxygen and nutrients and helps the body excrete unwanted substances from the skin. Regular cardiovascular exercise (such as swimming, running, brisk walking) will help keep your skin and the rest of body fit and younger looking. Facial exercises help preserve good tissue drainage and muscular structure.

• **TRY TO KEEP A STEADY NORMAL BODY WEIGHT**

Rapid changes in body weight make the skin stretch and sag. If you lose weight gradually your skin has a chance to change gently and you will be less likely to develop wrinkles and sagging. If you want to lose weight healthily, read the chapter on weight loss.

SKIN PROBLEMS

Vitamin and mineral deficiencies frequently manifest themselves as a skin problem, such as scurvy or pellagra, but this degree of nutrient deficiency is rare in developed countries. Skin problems more commonly occur as a result of an imbalanced nutrient intake, an allergy, or a medical condition such as eczema, acne, psoriasis or skin cancer. These conditions are not directly caused by food, but they can all be helped by adjusting your nutritional intake.

• **ALLERGIES**

If you suspect that you have a skin allergy, whether to a particular nutrient or another irritating substance, seek medical advice before you try to treat yourself with food. Once you have established the nature of your allergy, I suggest you read the chapter on allergies to see whether you can reduce your symptoms by adjusting your food intake.

ACNE

Acne vulgaris, the most common form of the skin complaint, is most common in young women, but women continue to suffer throughout their middle and later years, or may start suffering from acne during the menopausal years.

Acne is the result of the overproduction of a substance called sebum, which is produced by the oil glands of hair follicles. When the pores become clogged with sebum, the result is blackheads, pimples and large spots, which usually erupt on the face, chest and back.

- TACKLING ACNE THROUGH NUTRITION
- A well-balanced healthy diet is the first thing to achieve (see pages 292–3). You may like to boost your intake of vitamin A and zinc, as these two nutrients can be particularly helpful in tackling acne. (See pages 294–5)

It used to be thought that fatty and/or sugary foods such as chocolate caused acne, but this is not exactly the case. It is more the fact that a diet high in these foods is likely to be low in other, more beneficial foods.

- *Reduce your stress level.* People are more likely to eat chocolate or other fatty or sugary foods when stressed, low in mood or general health. When you are low, you are more likely to pick up infections, so the acne may get worse.
- *Eat 'live' yoghurt.* Many women I see are taking antibiotics to control acne. Unfortunately the antibiotics kill the bacteria that live in the healthy gut. These bacteria fulfil several important functions, one of which is to produce anti-inflammatory substances that the body would normally use to fight infection and redness. To re-establish a good bacterial balance I suggest you take a small pot of 'live' yoghurt containing acidophilus and bifidus every day.
- *Boost your intake of oily fish.* This may also help reduce the inflammation of the skin (see under psoriasis, below).

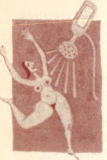

*Wines which comple-
ment oily fish need
to carry a good level
of acidity and weight,
to counteract the
oiliness. White
Burgundy or a very
good Chardonnay
from California or
Australia would be
excellent choices,
as would a good
Riesling.*

• NUTRITIONAL IMPLICATIONS OF THE PILL

Some women's acne is strongly related to their hormone levels. Doctors may prescribe a contraceptive pill to manage acne as it can help correct any slight hormonal imbalance, which can even eliminate acne in some cases. However, women need to be aware of the nutritional implications of the pill, including possible fluid retention, weight gain and zinc deficiency.

PSORIASIS

Psoriasis is a common, chronic skin disorder characterized by red, dry patches, covered with a mass of white scales. There may also be spots and sores that bleed and become infected. Women seem to have particularly bad patches on their elbows, knees, legs and scalp. We do not know the exact cause of psoriasis, but there seems to be a genetic link.

Many of my patients go through good and bad periods. Bad episodes seem to occur when they're stressed, run down or have a bacterial infection elsewhere in the body, such as a bout of thrush, a sore throat or a cold. Psoriasis can also be triggered by drastic changes in body weight. Although there is no cure for psoriasis, nutrition can have a dramatic effect. But the effect takes several weeks to show, so don't expect an overnight cure.

• OILY FISH

One of the most exciting findings in recent years has been the positive effect oily fish can have on psoriasis. Oily fish such as herrings, mackerel, tuna and salmon contain types of fatty acids called omega-3 fatty acid and omega-6 fatty acid. These fatty acids have been shown to alter the body's biochemistry and reduce the inflammatory reaction that is thought to bring on psoriasis. I have seen so many 'miraculous' recoveries that I strongly recommend that you boost your intake of these oily fish. Try to include some every day, perhaps as kipper pâté, a sardine sandwich, chargrilled tuna, or one of the recipes in this book.

At the same time you must reduce your overall fat intake, especially the saturated fats, to enable the omega-3 and omega-6 fatty acids to do their work.

• TRY TO KEEP YOUR BODY ON TOP FORM

It helps to try to make sure that your body does not become 'run down' and therefore more susceptible to bacterial infections. Eat a healthy diet including plenty of fruits and vegetables, get plenty of rest and try to reduce the amount of stress you suffer. Since psoriasis is a condition that involves inflammation, you may find it helpful to take a daily dose of 'live' yoghurt containing acidophilus and bifidus (see pages 295–6).

A bad psoriasis attack may follow rapid weight loss or gain. Try to ensure that your weight changes are gradual; if you wish to lose weight, do so slowly and carefully, following the advice in the chapter on weight loss.

• NON-NUTRITIONAL TREATMENTS FOR PSORIASIS

One of the most effective treatments for psoriasis sufferers is the use of the sun's healing rays. Thousands of psoriasis sufferers travel to special resorts around the Dead Sea to benefit from what appear to be 'healing' salt waters in conjunction with sun. The same sun shines in your own back garden. Discuss the issue of sun creams with your dermatologist. Alternatively, your dermatologist may suggest a special sun lamp, and/or a synthetic form of vitamin D.

Some interesting research suggests that if you have a diet rich in certain vegetables and fruits your body's response to the sun's rays may be enhanced. The compound thought to be responsible for this is psoralen, which is found in limes, lemons, lettuce and parsley. Since these ingredients can be deliciously combined into salads such as tabbouleh, many of my patients like to try this.

ECZEMA

Most, though not all, women who suffer from eczema have a genetic predisposition to other types of hypersensitive reactions to food, dust, pollen and other external irritants. The main symptom is red, itchy skin, and the most common sites are the face, hands and legs, although eczema can affect any area of the body. Constant itching and the need to scratch or rub may cause the skin surface to break, causing bleeding and weeping. On occasions the eczema sites become infected. Sufferers may be kept awake with the itching, which can lead to extreme tiredness, subsequent stress and a susceptible immune system.

• NUTRITIONAL TREATMENT OF ECZEMA

The aim of any treatment is to reduce the inflammation and irritation, thereby breaking the irritation-itching-wound-infection cycle.

In terms of reducing the inflammation of the skin, many women find a diet rich in fish oils to be very beneficial (see under psoriasis, page 300).

Exclusion diets can be a useful tool to identify any food sensitivity that might be aggravating the eczema, but unless they are carried out appropriately they may lead to malnourishment and many physical and emotional problems. If you have severe eczema you require specialized advice; don't try to treat it yourself. However, women with a milder form of eczema may find a marked improvement through boosting certain foods and avoiding others.

Some women find that a milk-free and/or egg-free diet dramatically improves their eczema. In order to try out the theory or learn to manage a milk- or egg-free diet I suggest you read the chapter on allergies.

Women occasionally find that chicken, azo dyes found in red cheese or other coloured foods, and benzoates, often found in processed foods, aggravate eczema. Always remember that there are plenty of good, fresh foods you can eat; don't worry if there are one or two you can't.

• NON-DIETARY TREATMENT OF ECZEMA

Weak topical steroid creams and moisturizers may help reduce the inflammation and dryness. Try to avoid biological washing powders and synthetic bedclothes and undergarments, as these may aggravate the skin. Cotton is the best fibre to choose. Your doctor might also suggest that you take steps to keep the amount of house mites and pet mites to the minimum.

SKIN CANCER

Skin cancer is one of the most prevalent forms of cancer. There are many different types of skin cancer, and the majority, if caught early, can be treated very successfully. However, there is a particularly serious type of skin cancer called melanoma, which causes a great deal of distress and many deaths. All women should keep a regular check on skin blemishes, moles, freckles and other bumps to monitor any changes such as increase in size, weeping, soreness or itchiness. If you have any doubts get your doctor to check it out.

The best way to avoid skin cancer is to avoid unprotected exposure to the sun's rays. You should cover your skin with specially formulated suncreams whenever you go out in the sun, for however short a period.

If you don't feel happy without tanned skin there are many excellent fake tan products available. Applied carefully, you will not be able to tell the difference between them and a sun tan, but they will protect you from unnecessary suffering.

Food neither causes nor cures skin cancer, but it can improve both your ability to fight the cancer and your response to therapies. The nutritional aim in treating any form of cancer is to make your immune system strong. I suggest you read the chapter on cancer for advice on how to do this.

• SKIN FOODS

Clam chowder
Carrot and orange soup
Chilled mint and cucumber soup
Spinach borscht
Pea, mint and lettuce soup
Parsnip and apple soup

Smoked salmon ramekins
Smoked mackerel pâté
Chicken liver pâté
Guacamole
Tabbouleh
Artichoke and avocado salad
Tomato and tarragon vinaigrette
Brie and porcini tart
Apple, dolcelatte and walnut strudel
Radicchio and grape salad
Chicken with melon, grapes and asparagus
Pear and walnut salad with watercress
Spinach and watercress roulade

Gado gado
Pasta vongole
Salmon and lemon lasagne
Smoked mackerel and spinach fishcakes
Salmon and asparagus risotto
Salmon and celery kedgeree
Chicken stroganoff with tarragon
Somerset steak and cider pie
Minted meatballs with yoghurt sauce

Fruit compote
Mixed fruit with butterscotch sauce
Oranges in caramel
Apple and fig crumble (with oat topping)
Cinnamon apples and plums
Blackberry and ricotta pancakes
Flapjacks

20 Weight loss

This is where I get on my soapbox and let rip at the slimming industry and the highly questionable clinics and quacks who claim to offer a quick way to lose weight. One way or another they are conning people, whether their suggestions mean enduring injections, taking pills, spending hours on the loo, or just chomping through disgusting bars and ready meals or swallowing drinks that shouldn't even be used as wallpaper paste.

We were not put on this earth to eat slimming products, still less to abuse our bodies to the point where we deliberately change our metabolism. One of the main reasons people don't lose weight is that they eat meals that contain things alien to their taste buds, feel unsatisfied after they have eaten, and are hence more likely to pick or binge between meals. They don't respect food or their bodies and end up abusing both. It is also the case that once you start dieting, food will be on your mind even more. Before you notice you may become obsessed and unable to break out of the 'diet cage'.

The first thing to do is to try to instil in your mind the idea that you need to start liking and enjoying food. Don't do as some women do and buy food that you don't particularly enjoy in order not to eat too much of it. Once you appreciate what Mother Nature has provided, and start thinking of exciting things you can do with it, you can fill your shelves and refrigerator with good ingredients and throw out all the 'calorie-counted this' and 'reduced-fat that'. No one should spend their lives eating inferior food. Whatever situation you're in there is always something marvellous you can eat.

POSITIVE WEIGHT LOSS

The secret to happy and successful weight loss is to learn to enjoy good, fresh, lean products and use complementary flavours, spices and herbs to enhance your food. Having small delicious meals that are full of new treats means that you can enjoy smaller portions and still feel satiated. This automatically cuts down your calorie intake and makes you less likely to eat unhealthy snacks between meals. The overall aim is to reduce the amount of calories you put into your body and increase the number you expend.

I find that showing women how their body and appetite work is a very successful way to encourage positive weight loss. The principles are explained in the section on the appetite mechanism, on page 6. The messages that are sent to your brain by your eyes, nose, ears (believe it or not!), mouth and stomach all contribute to the feeling of fullness and contentment known as satiety. Understanding satiety allows you to plan meals with minimum calorie intake that leave you contented.

Lose weight the fun way. Treat yourself to new foods and wines and see the whole process as an adventure not a diet.

• DECIDE HOW MUCH YOU WANT TO LOSE

The table on page 46 gives you some idea as to how much you should weigh. The ideal body mass index of 20 to 25 is considered to pose minimum health risks, while weights above and below the ideal are less healthy. Do be realistic, don't aim for a weight you have no hope of achieving. If you used to be a steady weight and then increased, set this as your target weight, as long as it's not too far removed from where you are now. If you have spent many years 'yo-yo' dieting, you will not be able to judge your natural weight, i.e. a weight which you seem to be easily able to hold. In these cases I recommend women take weight loss steadily, without setting a final target weight.

• INCORPORATE INTERMEDIATE GOALS ON THE WAY TO YOUR TARGET WEIGHT

The ideal weight loss is 1–1.5 kg/2–3 lb a week, so set monthly or fortnightly targets. This means that you can take every little step at a time and succeed regularly. You will not lose the same amount of weight every week, which is why monthly targets are more encouraging.

• DON'T WEIGH YOURSELF MORE THAN ONCE A WEEK, IF AT ALL

The way you feel inside is the most important feature of losing weight. You should be able to tell whether you are losing weight by the general feel of your body and the clothes you wear. Weighing more than once a week will only show you the natural fluid fluctuations in the body and cause you to become reactive, not pro-active. Slight increases in weight may lead to a negative reaction, either of bingeing or of not eating sensibly. If you feel that weekly weight checks help to keep you motivated, then go ahead, but remember to use the same pair of scales and to weigh yourself at the same time of day.

• LEARN TO BE HAPPY WITH YOUR BODY SHAPE

An 'apple' with a rounded tummy and slim hips will never become a 'pear' with heavier hips and a flat stomach and vice versa. Learn to love the contours of your body as nature made them. Some women find it very frustrating that the weight always seems to go off the face and upper body before it goes from the hips and middle. The only way you will be able to significantly change the pattern of weight loss is to combine good eating habits with exercise. Discuss different exercises with a trained fitness professional, as the type of exercise will dictate to a great extent the way your body changes.

• EXERCISE

The prime reason that women go on diets is not to lose weight but to lose fat. Although it is perfectly possible to lose weight without exercising, it is doubtful that you will shed fat. Exercise can also develop muscles to

The only low-fat products I have in the kitchen are low-fat natural yoghurt and fromage frais. I use yoghurt to add a creamy taste to soups and baked vegetable dishes, and mix it with garlic and herbs to make salad or vegetable dressings. Fromage frais makes dips and pâtés. Either can be served with fruits and desserts in place of cream.

Don't add yoghurt to boiling liquids, as it may curdle. Let hot liquids cool very slightly, and stir the yoghurt into the dish just before serving.

support the fat and keep your body firmly contoured, but you may not notice a significant change in the amount you weigh, just the way your body feels and fits into clothes. A combination of exercise and good healthy eating is both energizing and empowering. I recommend that you do some form of aerobic exercise, lasting twenty to thirty minutes, at least three times a week. Good aerobic exercises are swimming, cycling, roller-blading, brisk walking, jogging and running. Whichever exercise you choose don't become obsessive about it, as this is as psychologically damaging as obsessive eating.

NUTRITIONAL TIPS

Losing weight should be a natural, gradual process, requiring only slight modification from the guidelines set out in Part One of this book. I suggest you read through the whole section, but to sum up:

• Eat plenty of fresh fruits and vegetables.

• Balance your meals. Most women need just one rich source of protein at their main meal and a small amount in another meal. A portion the size of a chicken breast is enough for the main meal. Your other meals should consist mainly of high-fibre carbohydrates, vegetables and fruits.

• Drink plenty of water.

• Make sure that your refrigerator and your cupboards contain good, healthy foods. This is an easy way to reduce the number of calories you eat; after all, you can't eat it if it's not there. Stock up with fresh fruit, vegetables, lean meats and poultry, fish, wholegrain breads and cereals, along with some yoghurt and good-quality cheeses. It also helps if you have a selection of spices and fresh and dried herbs to make your food more interesting.

• Make a list of what you need when shopping – and stick to it. Pat yourself on the back when you manage to get past the cash till without grabbing a chocolate bar. I have nothing against chocolate and I encourage my clients to have some, if they really consider it a treat food and enjoy every mouthful. But I'm not sure that a hastily grabbed bar is a real treat.

• Don't base your agenda on deprivation. Have three small meals a day, plus a couple of snacks. Don't try to skip meals or go for long periods without eating as this causes your body to become 'deprived' of essential nutrients. Hunger is not only a physical sensation, but also a psychological state: your brain tells you that you are hungry. If you deprive yourself you are far more likely to end up overeating and choosing something that isn't the best food in terms of nutritional value.

• Notice what you eat. Ideally lay the table first, then sit down and eat. Eating on the move or while you are doing something else, such as watching television, causes you to consume calories that are unnoticed and therefore wasted.

• REDUCE THE FAT CONTENT OF YOUR MEALS

No one can follow a completely fat-free diet; fat is one of the main carriers of flavour in food, and some fats are needed for various important functions in the body. However, most of us eat far too much fat, and the majority of women will lose weight if they keep their fat intake down.

• Choose lean dishes. Rather than eating pastries, fried or battered dishes or thick creamy sauces, choose lean proteins such as lean red meat, seafood with pasta, vegetable or bean casseroles, tomato sauces.

• If you don't have any choice over the menu, minimize the damage. There is no calorie difference between a large amount of a low-calorie dish and a small amount of a high-calorie dish. Just watch the amount you eat and remember that the high-calorie, fatty, sugary foods go whizzing through your stomach, without stimulating your stretch receptors (see page 8), so if you're not careful you could end up eating too much. If you are going to a function where the food will be rich, have some fresh fruit before you go, so you're able to control your appetite. It tends to be when you're desperately hungry that your conscious decision-making process is overridden by a drive to eat.

• Try to resist fatty foods such as pies, cakes, pâtés, cheese and rich sauces. They're not bad or forbidden foods, but if you do have them you should stick to a small helping and make up the bulk of the meal with vegetable or fruit accompaniments. For instance, rather than eating cheese on its own, accompany it with crisp sliced apples or grapes and a wholegrain biscuit. You may think this adds more calories, but the extra fibre keeps you full for longer and means you won't eat as much in your next meal.

• Food doesn't need to be smothered in butter, oil or creamy sauces. Experiment with herbs and spices as flavourings and blend ripe tomatoes with thyme, tarragon or basil for a delicious low-fat sauce. If you have a good-quality base ingredient such as a roast pheasant or a fillet of beef, leave it alone, don't drown it in a sauce just for the sake of it!

• Do not confuse cholesterol with total fat. Cholesterol is a type of fat found in eggs, shellfish and offal. However, these foods do not produce significant amounts of the type of cholesterol that can cause harm in our bodies. The damage is done by saturated fats such as butter, ghee, lard, cheese and excess fat on meat and poultry. See page 211 for more details.

• When you use fats, use as little as possible. I suggest you choose natural products such as olive, peanut or sunflower oil or butter, rather than a margarine or low-fat spread (unless you prefer the taste of a polyunsaturated sunflower margarine). The natural products have a delicious flavour which goes a long way, so you use less of them. The 'low-fat' spreads are only slightly lower in fat and their high water content means that you cannot cook with them. Hard margarines are to be avoided because many of them contain a type of fatty acid that may be dangerous to your health. A mistake often made is to think that margarines and oils have fewer calories than butter. They don't. Some of them

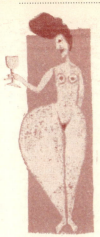

contain proportionally more calories, but many oils, such as olive, rapeseed, safflower and sunflower, are a better form of fat for many people because they do not produce cholesterol in the blood. I suggest you choose the fat you like and just use a small amount of it.

ALCOHOL AND WEIGHT LOSS

Alcohol in any form is a very calorific food, providing calories and very little else. It doesn't supply your body with any other major nutrient such as protein or fibre. However, some wines contain a certain amount of vitamins and minerals, as well as antioxidants – anthocyanins and tannins – which help to protect the arteries from cholesterol deposits (see page 213).

Ignore low-alcohol beers and wines, they're not worth putting in your mouth! Instead choose a really special wine that costs double the price you would normally spend, then you won't feel the need to overindulge! Savour every mouthful. It's best to have wine to accompany food, rather drinking before meals, as this may increase your appetite.

What is more, alcohol increases your appetite by lowering your blood sugar level. This may seem strange, as one would have thought that alcoholic drinks contain a lot of sugar and would therefore increase your blood sugar level. However, the alcohol prevents sugar that is normally stored in the liver, as glycogen, from breaking down. Therefore your sugar level lowers when you take alcohol into your body. The drop in blood sugar signals the hunger centre in your brain that you feel hungry.

It is best not to drink alcohol on an empty stomach. A small amount of your favourite wine can complement your food very well, but save it until you have a little food inside your stomach, to stop your sugar level dropping.

If you are happy to go without alcohol, then this would be an area where you could make a significant impact on reducing your calorie intake.

DIETS AND DRUGS

The slimming industry is big business, because so many people want to believe that there is a quick and easy way to lose weight. Drugs and 'slimming' drinks make almost magical claims, and there are all the diets that seem to promise that a particular combination of foods could make you lose weight. The draw-back with all these pills, powders and food fads is that they don't work in the long term. They are either so far removed from your natural eating habits that you feel you can only stick to them for a few weeks, or they make you lose weight in such an unnatural way that as soon as you eat anything normal the weight goes piling on. The only way to lose weight healthily is to understand why you are the weight that you are and how you can change your eating and lifestyle habits in a subtle, positive way.

There are several slimming drugs such as those based on amphetamines ('speed') and thyroxine (a synthetic or animal hormone) that are prescribed by highly questionable clinics and doctors to help you lose weight. These drugs either put you off your food or they increase your metabolic rate by increasing your heart rate. Unfortunately, when you take slimming drugs, the body begins to behave in a strange way. Many people suffer from a racing heart beat, a continual 'hyped-up' feeling, sickness and dizzy spells. All slimming drugs have adverse side effects and are potentially extremely harmful to your health. Of course the clinics are not going to tell you this; they just want quick results. But you should know that the majority of appetite suppressants are banned in Great Britain, therefore anyone prescribing them is in breach of the law.

Taking a drug doesn't really tackle the problem, it only provides a short-term solution. Try to change your long-term habits and approach to food rather than damage your health with a 'quick fix'.

WHAT IF YOU'VE TRIED EVERYTHING AND STILL CAN'T LOSE WEIGHT?

It is very often the case that the more times you have tried to lose weight by severely limiting your food intake, half-starving yourself or even resorting to using drugs, the harder it becomes to lose weight the next time you try. Just do your best. At the end of the day you can only do so much, and there has to come a point when you have to learn to love your body for what it is. Don't spend your life chasing after some unattainable dream, it's too short.

Having said this, I am yet to have a client who doesn't lose some weight. At the same time they begin to feel healthy and learn to love food and wine.

• IDEAS FOR AN ADVENTUROUS SLIMMING PROGRAMME

Garlic bean soup

Parsnip and apple soup

Chilled mint and cucumber soup

Carrot and orange soup

Pea, mint and lettuce soup

Baked garlic bruschetta

Tomato and tarragon vinaigrette

Pear and walnut salad with watercress

Christmas salad

Pasta bows with courgettes

Gado gado

Spicy fish kebabs

Prawn curry

Salmon and asparagus risotto

Duck breast with apricots

Garlic and herb chicken

Honey and mustard quail

Tropical dried fruit salad

Cinnamon apples and plums

Mixed berries in Grand Marnier

Pea, mint and lettuce soup

SERVES 3–4
- 15 g/½ oz butter
- 1 large onion, chopped
- 225 g/8 oz peas
- 500 ml/16 fl oz chicken stock
- ½ lettuce, chopped
- 2 tablespoons chopped fresh mint
- salt and pepper
- natural yoghurt (optional)
- small sprigs of mint or chopped chives, to garnish

Vegetable soups are a fabulous 'health food' for all occasions: packed with vitamins and minerals, high in fibre, low in fat and simplicity itself to make. They're great for weight watchers, comforting if you're feeling down, easy to eat if you don't fancy anything solid. You can swirl on some yoghurt, or enrich them with cream if you need to keep your strength up. The flavour combinations are infinitely versatile, but these are a few of my favourites.

Melt the butter in a saucepan and cook the onion gently until softened.

Add the peas and most of the stock, and bring to the boil.

Add the lettuce and mint and simmer for 5 minutes.

Purée in a liquidizer, then return the soup to the pan and season to taste. Add more stock if the soup is too thick. Serve hot or chilled.

Stir in some natural yoghurt for an extra creamy texture, or swirl it on top for a pretty effect. Garnish with mint or chives.

TIP *This can be frozen very successfully, but don't add the yoghurt until you come to reheat the soup.*

Parsnip and apple soup

SERVES 6
- 2 tablespoons olive oil
- 450 g/1 lb parsnips, peeled and sliced
- 2 Granny Smith apples, peeled and sliced
- 900 ml/1½ pints vegetable stock
- salt and pepper

Ideal comfort food for a winter day; you could add a pinch of curry powder for extra flavour.

Heat the oil in a saucepan and cook the parsnips and apples gently until softened.

Add the vegetable stock and bring to the boil. Cover the pan and simmer until parsnips are tender, about 25 minutes.

Purée briefly in a liquidizer; this soup should not be completely smooth. Season to taste and serve hot.

TIP *If you like, you could cut another apple into tiny dice and sprinkle them over the soup before serving. Alternatively, swirl a little apple purée on top, or sprinkle with chopped parsley.*

Carrot and orange soup

SERVES 4
- 15 g/½ oz butter
- 1 onion, chopped
- 6 carrots, peeled and chopped
- grated zest and juice of 1 orange
- 1 bay leaf
- 500 ml/16 fl oz vegetable stock
- salt and pepper
- chopped parsley or chives, to garnish

I first thought of this soup as perfect for when you have a cold: it is no trouble to make and slips down easily if you have a sore throat. Its lovely bright orange colour announces that it is high in beta-carotene, a powerful antioxidant that can help fight off heart disease, cancer and signs of ageing.

Melt the butter in a saucepan and cook the onion and carrots gently until softened.

Add the orange zest, bay leaf and stock and bring to the boil. Simmer for 30 minutes.

Remove the bay leaf and add the orange juice. Purée in a liquidizer. Taste and season if required. Reheat gently and serve hot, garnished with parsley or chives.

Garlic bean soup

SERVES 4–6
- 2 tablespoons virgin olive oil
- 1 onion, coarsely chopped
- 8–10 large garlic cloves, peeled
- 600 ml/1 pint vegetable or chicken stock
- 2 large cans (400g/14oz) haricot, cannellini or black-eyed beans
- salt and pepper
- natural yoghurt and chopped fresh herbs (chives, coriander, parsley), to garnish
- wholemeal croûtons (optional)

Garlic has many health-giving properties: it can help prevent cancer, heart disease and the common cold. This soup, served with a wholegrain roll, is a perfect meal in a bowl.

Heat the oil in a saucepan and cook the onion and garlic over a low heat until softened.

Add the stock and half the beans, bring to the boil and simmer for 20–30 minutes.

Purée in a liquidizer until smooth. Add the remaining beans to the soup and season to taste. Reheat and serve hot, with a swirl of yoghurt and a sprinkling of herbs.

VARIATION: LENTIL SOUP *Use 200 g/7 oz brown lentils, soaked in water overnight (discard any that rise to the surface), or red lentils. Place them in a saucepan with 4 tablespoons olive oil, 2 crushed garlic cloves, 2 tablespoons chopped fresh basil and a good pinch of salt. Add 2 litres/3½ pints water, bring to the boil and simmer for 1½ hours, until the lentils are almost disintegrating. Serve hot, garnished with fresh basil.*

You could also add some chopped ham, leeks, carrots or mushrooms.

Spinach borscht

SERVES 6
- 2 potatoes, diced
- 3 small onions, finely chopped
- 2 sprigs of dill
- ¼ teaspoon freshly grated nutmeg
- 450g/1lb fresh spinach, washed,stemmed and finely chopped
- 2 tablespoons fresh lemon juice
- salt and pepper
- 2 eggs
- 6 tablespoons soured cream or low-fat natural yoghurt
- chopped fresh dill, to garnish

This Jewish soup is slightly tart and very refreshing. It is traditionally made with sorrel, but I like it with fresh spinach. High in iron, B vitamins and magnesium, this is a good choice if you're anaemic, have heavy periods, or are generally tired.

Place the potatoes, onions, dill and nutmeg in a saucepan with 900ml/1½ pints water. Bring to the boil and simmer for 5 minutes.

Add the chopped spinach, lemon juice, salt and pepper. Simmer for 15 minutes or until the potatoes are tender.

Remove from the heat and take out the sprigs of dill.

In a large bowl beat the eggs with 6 tablespoons cold water until light and fluffy. Gradually add about 300 ml/½ pint of the hot soup to the egg mixture, stirring constantly to avoid curdling. Add the egg mixture back into the soup, stirring well. Chill for at least 4 hours.

Just before serving, taste and adjust the seasoning and whisk in the soured cream or yoghurt. Garnish with dill.

Leek and potato soup

SERVES 4
- 1 tablespoon olive oil
- 1 tablespoon butter
- 1 onion, chopped
- 8 leeks, chopped
- 3 potatoes, peeled and sliced
- 600 ml/1 pint chicken stock
- salt and pepper
- 150 g/5 oz low-fat fromage frais
- 1 tablespoon finely chopped chives, plus extra to garnish
- freshly grated nutmeg

The potatoes in this comforting soup are a good source of the sort of carbohydrate that releases energy slowly into the body, preventing mood and energy swings.

Heat the oil and butter in a large saucepan. Add the onion and leeks and cook gently for about 10 minutes, until softened.

Add the potatoes, stock, salt and pepper and bring to the boil. Simmer for 30 minutes.

Purée in a liquidizer until smooth, then return to the pan and add the fromage frais, chives and nutmeg. Adjust the seasoning; this soup needs quite a lot of salt and pepper to bring out the flavours. Reheat and serve hot, sprinkled with chives.

VARIATION: SORREL SOUP *For a subtle and unusual soup, use 2 tablespoons butter instead of half oil, half butter. Omit the onion and replace with 175 g/6 oz roughly torn sorrel leaves.*

Chicken liver and tagliatelle soup

SERVES 6
- 6 chicken livers, washed and trimmed
- 40 g/1½ oz unsalted butter
- 1 litre/1¾ pints strong chicken or meat stock, preferably homemade
- 225 g/8 oz tagliatelle (preferably fresh for the best taste)
- 25 g/1 oz fresh, parsley chopped
- salt and pepper
- 25 g/1 oz Parmesan cheese, or mature Cheddar, grated

This is one of my favourite soups for those occasions when I fancy something quick and tasty, to leave me feeling revitalized, especially on wintry days. The chicken livers are one of the richest sources of iron in the diet. You could serve it with a baby spinach and cherry tomato salad for an extra boost of iron.

Chop the chicken livers into very small pieces and fry them lightly in the butter for 5 minutes. Remove from the heat and keep warm.

Bring the stock to the boil and add the tagliatelle. Boil until just tender, about 1–2 minutes.

Add the chicken livers, chopped parsley and seasoning to taste. Serve at once, topped with the grated cheese.

French onion soup

SERVES 6
- 2 tablespoons olive oil
- 2 onions, finely sliced
- 900 ml/1½ pints vegetable stock
- 1 teaspoon yeast extract
- 1 teaspoon mixed herbs
- salt and pepper
- wholemeal croûtons
- Cheddar cheese, grated

This is a variation on the classic Paris market porters' pick-me-up. The yeast extract is a good source of the B vitamins, and onions have some of the same, almost magical properties of garlic: decongestant, anti-cancer, anti-viral and anti-bacterial, to name but a few.

Heat the oil in a saucepan and fry the onions until golden brown.

Add the stock, yeast extract and herbs, and bring to the boil. Simmer for 15 minutes.

Season to taste and serve hot, sprinkled with the croûtons and grated cheese.

Clam chowder

SERVES 8–10
- 50 g/2 oz butter
- 2 onions, chopped
- 4 sticks of celery, chopped
- 3 garlic cloves, chopped
- 300 ml/½ pint clams, chopped
- 50 g/2 oz plain white flour
- 900 ml/1½ pints vegetable stock
- 275 g/10 oz potatoes, diced
- 600 ml/1 pint single cream
- 600 ml/1 pint semi-skimmed milk
- 1 tablespoon chopped fresh coriander leaves
- 1 tablespoon chopped fresh parsley
- 2 teaspoons Worcestershire sauce
- salt and pepper

Clams are a good source of zinc, a very useful nutrient, especially if you are trying to improve your immune system, skin, hair or sex life! However, this is quite a rich dish, so save it for special occasions.

Melt the butter in a saucepan, add the onions, celery and garlic and cook gently until softened.

Add the clams and fry for 2 minutes. Sprinkle the flour into the pan and cook, stirring, for 1 minute. Gradually add the stock, stirring constantly to prevent lumps. When you have incorporated all the stock, bring to the boil and simmer for 30–40 minutes.

Add the diced potatoes, cream, milk and herbs. Simmer for a further 10 minutes or until the potato is tender.

Just before serving, add a dash of Worcestershire sauce, then taste and adjust the seasoning.

Chilled mint and cucumber soup

SERVES 4
- 1 cucumber, peeled and chopped
- 1 garlic clove, crushed
- 1 spring onion, chopped
- 300 ml/½ pint low-fat natural yoghurt
- 3 tablespoons crème fraîche
- 2 tablespoons finely chopped fresh mint
- 1 teaspoon lemon juice
- 1 teaspoon ground coriander
- salt and pepper
- diced cucumber and sprigs of mint, to garnish

If you are pregnant or ill, soups are excellent for days when you don't fancy anything more substantial. The combination of mint and cucumber makes this a deliciously settling soup for those occasions when you're feeling nauseous. It also has the advantage that it doesn't require any cooking, so there are no smells to make you feel more sick.

Purée all the ingredients together in a liquidizer, then transfer to a large bowl. Season well and chill the soup thoroughly in the refrigerator before serving.

Garnish with mint and diced cucumber.

TIP *This can be kept in a covered container in the refrigerator for 2 days.*

Minestrone soup

SERVES 6–8
- ¼ Savoy cabbage, chopped
- 150 g/5 oz fresh spinach, washed, stemmed and shredded
- 50 g/2 oz prosciutto, or unsmoked back bacon, chopped
- 50 g/2 oz fresh parsley, chopped
- 2 garlic cloves, chopped
- 2 carrots, sliced
- 1 onion, sliced
- 2 courgettes, sliced
- 1 potato, peeled and sliced
- a piece of belly pork (optional)
- 450 g/1 lb canned cannellini or borlotti beans
- 2 tablespoons tomato purée
- 2 litres/3½ pints beef or lamb stock
- salt and pepper
- 275 g/10 oz long-grain rice
- 4 tablespoons freshly grated Parmesan cheese

This nourishing soup is a meal in itself, high in protein and fibre. It's a delicious way to eat beans, so it's good for preventing constipation.

Put the cabbage and spinach in a saucepan with a little water and simmer until soft. Remove from the heat and drain well.

Put the prosciutto or bacon in a large saucepan over a low heat. Add the parsley and garlic and fry for about 5 minutes.

Add the cabbage and spinach, stir, then add all the other vegetables, belly pork (if using) and drained, rinsed beans. Stir in the tomato purée and stock, cover the pan and simmer for 2 hours.

Taste and adjust the seasoning. Stir in the rice and cook for a further 15 minutes or until the rice is tender. Remove from the heat and stir in the Parmesan. Serve hot.

Smoked mackerel pâté

SERVES 4
- 225 g/8 oz smoked mackerel fillets, skinned, flaked and any bones removed
- 125 g/4 oz low-fat fromage frais
- 1 bunch of watercress, leaves only, chopped, plus extra to garnish
- finely grated zest and juice of ½ lemon or lime
- freshly ground black pepper

This is a very easy and delicious starter for a supper party. Mackerel is one of the oily fish that are rich in omega-3 fatty acids, which fulfil all sorts of vital functions within the body. They are particularly good for reducing blood cholesterol, and their anti-inflammatory properties may relieve arthritis. The watercress adds tons of vitamin C and some anti–cancer substances.

Mash the mackerel in a bowl and beat in the fromage frais.

Stir in the watercress and lime or lemon zest, and add juice to taste. Season with pepper; you should not need salt.

Spoon the mixture into a serving dish, cover and refrigerate for at least 2 hours.

Serve chilled, with hot toast, garnished with watercress.

TIPS *I prefer the texture of this pâté when made by hand, but you could simply throw all the ingredients into the food processor.*
The pâté can be kept in the refrigerator for a couple of days.

Smoked salmon ramekins

SERVES 4
- 2 eggs, separated
- 2 teaspoons lemon juice
- few drops of anchovy essence
- salt and pepper
- 1 tablespoon powdered gelatine
- 150 ml/5 fl oz fish stock
- 225 g/8 oz smoked salmon, finely chopped (ideally in a food processor)
- dill or watercress to garnish
- 8 tablespoons liquid aspic (optional)

Lovers of good food will be delighted to know that salmon is one of the healthiest of fish. Like mackerel, herrings and sardines, it contains oils that have been shown to reduce the risk of heart disease, arthritis and certain cancers.

Place the egg yolks in a bowl with the lemon juice, anchovy essence, salt and pepper. Place the bowl over a saucepan of hot water and beat until slightly thickened. Leave to cool, beating from time to time.

Dissolve the gelatine in the fish stock and beat into the egg mixture. Stir in the chopped salmon.

Whisk the egg whites until stiff and lightly fold into the salmon mixture until they are evenly mixed.

Divide the mixture between four ramekin dishes and chill for 30 minutes.

Garnish with dill or watercress and spoon over the aspic, if using. Chill until set.

Fish terrine

SERVES 4
- 450 g/1 lb haddock fillets
- 900 ml/1½ pints fish stock
- 25 g/1 oz butter
- 25 g/1 oz plain white flour
- 3 tablespoons milk
- 2 eggs, separated
- 85 ml/3 fl oz double cream
- 2 tablespoons chopped fresh parsley
- 1–2 teaspoons anchovy essence
- 1–2 teaspoons lemon juice
- salt and pepper
- 3–4 tablespoons fresh white bread-crumbs, toasted

This delicate terrine can be served as a first course or light lunch. Since it can be made a day or two ahead it is a good thing to have in the refrigerator if you are pregnant or suffer from cancer or migraine, with occasional 'bad head days'.

Preheat the oven to 160°C/325°F/Gas 3. Poach the fish in the stock until tender. Remove the fish and reserve the liquid. Mash the fish until quite smooth.

Melt the butter in a saucepan, stir in the flour and cook, stirring, for 1 minute. Put the milk in a measuring jug and add some of the fish liquid to make 150 ml/5 fl oz. Stir this into the flour and butter. Keep stirring while you add the fish.

Beat the yolks with the cream; add to the fish mixture with the parsley. Season to taste with anchovy essence, lemon juice, salt and pepper.

Whip the egg whites until thick. Fold into the fish mixture.

Sprinkle the breadcrumbs into an oiled 450 g/1 lb loaf tin. Add the fish mixture. Cover with oiled foil and bake in a bain-marie for 1–1¼ hours or until set and risen.

Serve warm or cold.

Baked garlic bruschetta

TO SERVE 2:
- 1 large whole bulb of garlic for (preferably not 'wet' new garlic)
- olive oil
- butter (optional)
- chopped thyme or rosemary (preferably fresh)
- salt and pepper
- French bread or ciabatta

Garlic is a wonderful natural medicine, with anti-viral, anti-bacterial, anti-cancer and anti-blood-clotting properties. Baking tempers the pungency of the garlic and brings out the sweeter, softer flavours.

Remove the outermost, papery leaves of the garlic. Slice off the tops of the bulbs so that each clove is open at the top. Pierce each clove with a sharp knife so the steam can be released.

Set the garlic bulbs in an earthenware garlic roaster or a small baking dish. Drizzle a little olive oil over each bulb and dot with butter if liked. Sprinkle with the herbs, salt and pepper. Cover the dish and put into a cold oven set at 150°C/300°F/Gas 2 for about 30 minutes.

Remove the lid and bake for a further 30 minutes or so, basting occasionally with olive oil, until the husks are golden brown.

Spread the soft baked cloves on to slices of hot French bread or Italian ciabatta.

TIP *The garlic bulbs can be microwaved at full power for 2 minutes or a little longer for a softer consistency. However, they will not have the mellow, roasted, nutty flavours of the traditional oven-baked garlic.*

Goats' cheese and aubergine crostini

SERVES 2
- 1 small aubergine, cut into thin rounds
- olive oil
- a little sun-dried tomato sauce or tomato purée (or canned chopped tomatoes, drained)
- 1 garlic clove, halved
- 1 small wholemeal baguette, sliced diagonally
- 100 g/3½ oz firm goats' cheese, sliced
- basil leaves, olives or shavings of Parmesan cheese, to garnish

The cheese provides calcium and protein, the bread provides fibre; served with a salad this makes a well-balanced lunch.

Brush each slice of aubergine with olive oil, then spread over a small amount of tomato sauce or purée. Place under a hot grill for 3–5 minutes or until softened and browned. Turn, brush the other side with oil and tomato and grill until browned.

Rub the garlic clove over each slice of baguette, brush with oil and toast lightly on both sides.

Place a slice of aubergine on each piece of baguette. Top with goats' cheese and return to the grill until the cheese is melted. Serve immediately, garnished with basil, olives or Parmesan shavings.

TIP *Increase the quantities and serve these crostini with two or three of the other starters on this page and the next for easy, healthy party food.*

Caramelized artichoke and tomato toasts

SERVES 4
- 1 large can (400 g/14 oz) artichoke hearts
- 1–2 garlic cloves, finely chopped
- 1 tablespoon olive oil
- 1 tablespoon finely chopped fresh basil
- salt and pepper
- 4 tomatoes, halved
- 3 teaspoons tomato purée
- 4 wholegrain rolls, halved

An easy and impressive dish to serve as an after-theatre supper or for Sunday brunch. It is low in fat, and its lovely Mediterranean flavours will perk up a jaded appetite.

Preheat the grill. Drain the artichoke hearts thoroughly and cut each one in half.

Mix the garlic with the oil and brush on to a nonstick baking sheet. Sprinkle the artichokes with half the basil and a little salt and pepper, and place on the baking sheet.

Spread the halved tomatoes with tomato purée and the remaining basil and place on the baking sheet.

Cook under the hot grill for a few minutes until they are beginning to brown.

Place one or two halved artichokes and a halved tomato on each roll, then return to the grill to brown.

Leave to cool for a few minutes before serving.

VARIATION *Place a slice of goats' cheese or soft blue cheese (e.g. blue Brie or Roquefort), on top of the tomato-filled roll before returning it to the grill.*

Chicken liver pâté

SERVES 3–4
- 100 g/3½ oz butter
- 1 small onion, finely chopped
- 1 garlic clove, crushed
- 225 g/8 oz chicken livers, washed and trimmed
- 1 tablespoon sherry
- 1 tablespoon rosemary
- salt and pepper
- clarified butter, to seal (optional)

Chicken livers are an excellent source of iron. I would recommend this recipe for all women, unless you are pregnant (liver should be avoided for the full nine months) or watching your weight, since it's quite high in fat.

Melt 15 g/½ oz of the butter in a saucepan and cook the onion and garlic gently until softened. Increase the heat, add the livers and fry quickly in the pan for about 2 minutes or until sealed and browned.

Leave to cool slightly, then tip into a food processor, add the remaining butter and process until smooth. Add the sherry and rosemary and season to taste.

Push through a sieve to remove any gristle and spoon into ramekin dishes or one large dish. Cover with clarified butter to seal and refrigerate for at least 2 hours.

Serve chilled, with melba toast.

TIPS *To make clarified butter, melt 175 g/6 oz unsalted butter over a low heat. Skim off the solids that have risen to the surface, then pour the butter into a clean container, leaving behind the solids at the bottom of the pan.*

This pâté can be kept in the refrigerator for 3–4 days, or frozen.

Guacamole

SERVES 2
- 1 ripe avocado pear, mashed
- 1 teaspoon fresh lemon or lime juice
- 1 large garlic clove, crushed
- 4 drops of hot chilli sauce, e.g. Tabasco
- ¼ teaspoon each of salt and pepper

This is a perfect little appetizer to 'kickstart' the taste buds when you don't really feel like eating. Avocados are high in monounsaturated fat and can help your body fight cancer, cardiovascular disease and ageing.

Mix all the ingredients together and serve as a dip with tortilla chips or crisps, or with strips of crisp red pepper.

Hummus

SERVES 2–3
- 200 g/7 oz dry chick peas
- 1 teaspoon bicarbonate of soda
- 2 teaspoons salt
- 100 g/3½ oz tahini (sesame paste)
- 125 ml/4 fl oz lemon juice
- 2 garlic cloves, crushed
- extra virgin olive oil, chopped fresh parsley and paprika, to garnish

If you have the time, homemade hummus is far superior to ready-made. It is high in fibre, and the tahini is a good source of calcium, for healthy bones and teeth. Serve it with crisp raw vegetables and warm wholemeal pitta bread.

Wash the chick peas well, cover with water and soak overnight.

Rinse the chick peas well, place in a saucepan and add fresh water to cover the chick peas by 5 cm/2 inches. Add the bicarbonate of soda and 1 teaspoon of the salt. Bring to the boil, then simmer gently for about 45 minutes. If a foam forms, skim it off. At the end of this time the chick peas should be very tender. If they are still firm, leave to simmer for a little longer.

When cooked, drain in a sieve and leave to cool for about 1 hour.

Place the cold chick peas in a food processor with the tahini, lemon juice, crushed garlic and 1 teaspoon salt. Blend until thick and smooth. If the mixture is too thick, add a little water or more lemon juice. Taste and add more salt, lemon juice or garlic if you like.

Spoon the hummus into a serving dish. To serve, sprinkle with olive oil, parsley and paprika.

Brie and porcini tart

SERVES 4
- 100 g/3½ oz dried porcini mushrooms (ceps), broken into pieces
- 25 g/1 oz butter
- 225 g/8 oz short-crust pastry
- 175 g/6 oz ripe Brie
- 175 ml/6 fl oz single cream
- 3 eggs
- 1 egg yolk
- 1 teaspoon English mustard
- salt and pepper

This dish is lovely hot or cold and is particularly versatile, being suitable for a picnic, or as a starter or lunch dish. It's a terrific way to meet some of your calcium requirements.

Preheat the oven to 190°C/375°F/Gas 5.

Soak the porcini in a little boiling water for 20 minutes. Drain well, then sauté lightly in butter.

Line a flan ring with the pastry and bake blind (see tip) for 15 minutes. Remove the beans and paper and bake for a further 5 minutes or until the pastry case is lightly golden brown.

Blend all the remaining ingredients in a food processor and pour into the pastry case. Add the mushrooms and bake in the oven for 15 minutes or until golden brown and just firm. Serve hot or cold.

TIP *To bake a pastry case blind, place a piece of greaseproof paper on top of the pastry and cover it with dried beans or rice.*

Apple, dolcelatte and walnut strudel

SERVES 4
- **40 g/1½ oz butter**
- **1 leek, thinly sliced**
- **2 garlic cloves, crushed**
- **2 apples, diced**
- **50 g/2 oz mushrooms, sliced**
- **50 g/2 oz walnuts**
- **salt and pepper**
- **8 sheets of filo pastry**
- **25 g/1 oz ground almonds**
- **85 g/3 oz dolcelatte cheese, crumbled**

This very unusual first course or light supper dish is surprisingly simple to make: great when you want to impress someone with a romantic meal.

Preheat the oven to 180°C/350°F/Gas 4.

Melt 15 g/½ oz of the butter in a saucepan and cook the leek and garlic gently until softened.

Add the apples and mushrooms and cook for about 2 minutes.

Add the walnuts, season to taste and mix well.

Melt the remaining butter. Lay a sheet of filo pastry on a floured surface and brush lightly with melted butter, then sprinkle with a little of the ground almonds.

Repeat with all the sheets of pastry and then pile the vegetable mixture in the centre. Sprinkle with the cheese and roll up the pastry.

Brush the top with a little melted butter and sprinkle with the remaining ground almonds. Bake for 15 minutes or until golden.

Serve warm, with a crisp leafy salad.

TIP *You can use other blue cheeses, such as Stilton or Roquefort.*

Grapefruit, smoked salmon and avocado salad

SERVES 4
- 2 ruby grapefruit, segmented
- 2 avocados, peeled and thinly sliced
- 100 g/3½ oz lightly smoked salmon, cut into 2.5 cm/1 inch wide strips

VINAIGRETTE
- 6 tablespoons virgin olive oil
- 3 tablespoons white wine vinegar
- 1 teaspoon Dijon mustard
- salt and pepper

With its combination of oily fish and the antioxidant substances in the grapefruit and avocado, this is a delicious way to lower blood cholesterol.

Arrange the grapefruit segments, avocados and salmon in overlapping semi-circles on four plates. Whisk the vinaigrette ingredients together and drizzle over the salads.

Radicchio and grape salad

SERVES 4
- 1 head of radicchio
- 1 small head of curly endive
- ½ a lettuce or 1 Little Gem or Density lettuce
- 1 large can (400 g/ 14 oz) artichoke hearts, sliced
- 175 g/6 oz French beans, lightly cooked and cut into 2.5 cm/ 1 inch lengths
- 50 g/2 oz shelled broad beans
- 100 g/3½ oz green grapes, halved
- 1 punnet of mustard and cress, snipped and rinsed
- 125 ml/4 fl oz vinaigrette (see above)

Everyone should aim to have five helpings of vegetables and fruit a day. This salad, full of varied colours and textures, provides a generous helping!

Rinse and dry the radicchio, endive and lettuce. Trim the radicchio and put it in a salad bowl. Tear the endive and lettuce into pieces and add to the radicchio with the sliced artichoke hearts, French beans, broad beans, grapes and mustard and cress.

To serve, toss gently and serve the vinaigrette in a separate bowl or jug.

Grilled vegetable salad

SERVES 6

- 150 ml/5fl oz herb vinaigrette (see left; add ½ tablespoon each of finely chopped fresh chives and parsley and 1 small garlic clove, finely chopped)
- 2 corn cobs, husked
- 3 courgettes, cut lengthways into 5 mm/¼ inch slices
- 2 red peppers, cut lengthways into 5 mm/¼ inch slices
- 12 asparagus spears, trimmed
- 8 spring onions, trimmed
- 2 heads of chicory
- 2 heads of radicchio
- 2 Little Gem lettuce
- 450 g/1 lb large mushrooms
- 4 tablespoons finely chopped fresh herbs (basil, parsley, dill, chives)

Cooking the vegetables quickly over high heat means they remain full of vitamins and minerals.

Place all the ingredients for the vinaigrette in a screw-topped jar and shake well. Set aside.

Heat the barbecue or grill to very hot. Grill the corn, turning it until it is lightly browned all round. Leave to cool, then scrape off the kernels into a salad bowl. Place the courgettes, peppers, asparagus, spring onions, chicory, radicchio and lettuce on the grill, about 8 cm/3 inches from the heat. Cook for about 4 minutes or until slightly charred.

Remove the vegetables from the grill and chop into 2.5 cm/ 1 inch pieces. Place in the salad bowl.

Grill the mushrooms until just cooked, brushing them lightly with the vinaigrette. Add the mushrooms to the salad bowl, together with the herbs and a little dressing. Toss and serve, warm or cold.

Pear and walnut salad with watercress

SERVES 4
- 50 g/2 oz walnuts, chopped
- 2 heads of Cos lettuce
- large bunch of rocket
- 2 bunches of watercress
- 3 ripe Comice pears, cored and sliced
- freshly ground black pepper

WALNUT VINAIGRETTE
- 2 tablespoons sherry vinegar
- 2 small shallots, finely chopped
- salt
- 3 tablespoons light olive oil
- 2 tablespoons walnut oil

Here's a great-tasting way to get a generous helping of vitamins, minerals and fibre.

Preheat the oven to 190°C/375°F/Gas 5.

Prepare the vinaigrette by mixing together the sherry vinegar, shallots and a little salt. Whisk in the oils to emulsify. Set aside.

Toast the walnuts in the oven for 10 minutes or until they begin to brown. Set aside to cool.

Rinse and dry the lettuce, rocket and watercress.

Toss the salad leaves, pears and walnuts with the vinaigrette. Sprinkle with black pepper and serve at once.

VARIATION *Make this into a light lunch by crumbling some blue cheese over the top and serving warm wholemeal or walnut bread as an accompaniment.*

Chicken with melon, grapes and asparagus

SERVES 4
- 4 chicken breasts
- 50 ml/2 fl oz white wine
- 2 garlic cloves, crushed
- 1 Cantaloupe melon, cut into chunks
- 1 small bunch of seedless grapes, halved
- 1 bunch of asparagus, cooked and cut into 5 cm/2 inch pieces
- 2 sticks of celery, finely chopped
- 50 g/2 oz Gruyère cheese, coarsely grated
- mixed salad leaves (curly endive, crisp lettuce, watercress), to serve

LEMON AND WINE DRESSING
- juice of 1 lemon
- 3 tablespoons olive oil
- 1 garlic clove, crushed
- salt and pepper
- 1 tablespoon dry white wine

This salad is refreshing, yet settling, so I often recommend it to women suffering from cancer, indigestion or fatigue.

Whisking the dressing ingredients together until smooth. Set aside.

Place the chicken breasts in a saucepan. Add the wine, garlic and enough water to just cover the chicken. Bring to the boil, then reduce the heat, cover and simmer for 5 minutes. Turn the breasts over and simmer for another 5 minutes or until cooked. Lift the chicken out of the stock and leave to cool.

Once the chicken is completely cool, chop into small pieces.

Place the chicken, melon, grapes, asparagus, celery and cheese in a large bowl and pour over the dressing. Toss together well and season to taste.

Serve on a bed of mixed salad leaves, accompanied by warm or cold new potatoes.

Christmas salad

SERVES 4
- 225 g/8 oz lean bacon, chopped into small strips
- 2 garlic cloves, crushed
- 450 g/1 lb spinach
- 12 cherry tomatoes (red or yellow), grilled
- 12 quails' eggs, boiled
- freshly grated nutmeg
- 4 basil leaves, chopped
- lemon dressing (see Warm goats' cheese salad, page 336) flavoured with coarse-grain mustard

With vitamins and minerals from the spinach and tomatoes, protein from the bacon and egg, and garlic to keep your arteries clear, this is a lovely starter or after-theatre supper.

Heat a nonstick pan, add the bacon and garlic and fry until golden and crisp. Drain on a paper towel.

Wash the spinach thoroughly and place in a large saucepan over medium-high heat, stirring frequently until it begins to wilt.

Place the wilted spinach in a bowl with all the remaining ingredients and toss together. Serve at once.

VARIATION: WARM SALAD OF SPINACH AND FRENCH BEANS WITH PANCETTA *First, lightly boil some French beans, drain and refresh in cold water. Use pancetta instead of bacon and omit the garlic. Remove the pancetta from the pan and add 3 tablespoons walnut oil, 2 tablespoons raspberry vinegar and 1 tablespoon honey. Tear the washed spinach into bite-sized pieces and add to the pan, with the beans. Stir until just wilted, then serve on warmed plates. Scatter the pancetta on top, with 2 tablespoons toasted pine nuts.*

Tabbouleh

SERVES 6-8
- 100 g/3½ oz burghul (bulgar or cracked wheat)
- 3 bunches of flat-leaf parsley
- 1 bunch of fresh mint
- 1 bunch of spring onions
- 3 firm ripe tomatoes, diced
- juice of 3 lemons
- 2 teaspoons salt
- ½ teaspoon black pepper
- 4 tablespoons extra virgin olive oil
- ½ teaspoon seven spices (can be found in Lebanese food shops)
- 1 Cos lettuce

Parsley is rich in vitamins A and C, iron, calcium and potassium. In this recipe you get the chance to use it in abundance.

Rinse the burghul in cold water, then place in a bowl, cover with water and leave to soak for 30 minutes.

Squeeze the burghul with your hands to extract excess water and spread on a tea towel while you prepare the other ingredients.

Wash the parsley and mint and dry in a salad spinner. Discard the thick stalks from the parsley and all the mint stalks, chop the leaves coarsely and place in a salad bowl.

Trim the spring onions, leaving about 5 cm/2 inches of the green parts, and chop finely. Add to the salad bowl together with the tomatoes. Add the burghul to the salad bowl and mix well.

Mix the lemon juice with the salt and pepper.

Just before serving, add the seasoned lemon juice and the olive oil. Toss well and season with seven spices, adding more lemon juice or salt if you like. Serve with Cos lettuce leaves.

Artichoke and avocado salad

SERVES 2
- 225 g/8 oz broccoli, cut into small florets
- about 30 g (a small pack) lambs' lettuce
- about 30 g (a small pack) rocket
- 3 sticks of celery, cut in thin diagonal slices
- 1 large can (400 g/ 14 oz) artichoke hearts, drained and halved
- chopped fresh herbs (dill, parsley), to serve

AVOCADO DRESSING
- juice and grated zest of 1 lime
- 1 avocado, peeled
- 3 tablespoons low-fat natural yoghurt
- 1 tablespoon virgin olive oil
- salt and pepper

Avocados are full of the special fats that can fight off damaging free radicals, thus they can help your skin, your arteries and other cells within the body.

Blanch the broccoli florets in boiling water, drain and refresh in cold water. Drain well.

Place the broccoli, lambs' lettuce, rocket, celery and artichokes in a bowl and toss gently.

Blend all the dressing ingredients together in a liquidizer.

To serve, drizzle the dressing over the salad and sprinkle with chopped herbs.

Tomato and tarragon vinaigrette

- 225 g/8 oz canned chopped tomatoes or ripe fresh tomatoes, skins and seeds removed
- 2 garlic cloves, chopped
- 2 tablespoons red wine vinegar
- ½ teaspoon coarse-grain mustard
- salt and pepper
- 1 tablespoon virgin olive oil
- 1½ level tablespoons chopped fresh tarragon

This flavourful, versatile dressing goes beautifully with crisp lettuces such as Cos, or with peppery watercress or rocket salads. I also like to serve it with hot or cold poached salmon or rainbow trout. For an elegant finish, garnish with fresh whole tarragon leaves.

If you use fresh tomatoes they must be ripe and full flavoured, as this dressing needs a substantial tomato base. Chop the tomatoes roughly.

If you use canned tomatoes, drain off a little of the juice if they look watery.

Put the tomatoes into a liquidizer or food processor with the garlic, vinegar, mustard, and a little salt and pepper. Blend for a few seconds, so the tomatoes are reduced to a pulp, but still have some texture. With the machine running, gradually blend in the oil. Add the chopped tarragon and blend again, very briefly. Taste and adjust the seasoning.

TIP *This can be refrigerated in a sealed jar for a few days.*

Warm goats' cheese salad

SERVES 4
- 4 Little Gem lettuce, separated
- handful of baby spinach leaves
- ½ cucumber, sliced
- 100 g/3½ oz cherry tomatoes, quartered
- 85 g/3 oz mangetout, blanched
- 4 asparagus stalks, blanched and cut in half
- fresh coriander, finely chopped
- fresh parsley, finely chopped
- fresh basil, finely chopped
- 50 g/2 oz pine nuts, toasted
- 4 individual goats' cheeses

LEMON DRESSING
- 4 tablespoons olive oil
- 1½ tablespoons lemon juice
- 1 garlic clove, crushed
- salt and pepper

You'll feel full of energy after eating this salad, either as a first course or a small meal.

Whisk together the dressing ingredients. Preheat the grill.

Rinse and dry the salad leaves and arrange on four plates. Arrange the cucumber, tomatoes, mangetout, asparagus, herbs and nuts on top.

Place the cheeses on a baking sheet and grill until slightly browned, but not falling apart. Place on top of the salad, drizzle with dressing and serve at once.

Warm duck breast salad with apricots

SERVES 4
- 1 duck breast,
  roasted and sliced,
  kept warm in foil
- 15 g/½ oz butter
- 2 red onions, sliced
- 6 spring onions,
  thinly sliced
- 2 red peppers, diced
- 2 yellow peppers,
  diced
- large bunch of baby
  spinach
- 400 g/14 oz canned
  apricots, drained,
  quartered, juice
  reserved for
  the dressing

APRICOT DRESSING
- 2 garlic cloves,
  chopped
- 1 teaspoon chopped
  fresh ginger
- 4 teaspoons lemon
  juice
- 2 teaspoons soy
  sauce

Bright colours and oriental flavours make this salad perfect to satisfy any appetite. Amazingly, as long as the duck is lean and well-roasted, this is a good choice for women on a weight loss programme.

Heat the butter in a frying pan, add the onions, spring onions and peppers and cook until softened.

Add the spinach and cook until just wilted.Place the vegetables in a salad bowl.

To make the dressing, add the garlic to the pan and sauté gently. Add the ginger, lemon juice, reserved apricot juice and soy sauce and heat through.

Arrange the duck and apricots on the vegetables and pour over some of the dressing. Serve at once.

Cheese fluff

SERVES 2 (SMALL
PORTIONS)
• 2 egg whites
• 50 g/2 oz mature or
  smoked Cheddar
  cheese, finely grated
• pinch of English
  mustard powder
• salt and pepper
• 2 slices of whole-
  meal bread (walnut
  or olive breads are
  delicious

A comforting cheesy dish to pick you up when you're feeling down. It's a favourite in my family, and my brother likes to round it off with a dollop of brown sauce!

Beat the egg whites until stiff and stir in the cheese, mustard and seasoning.

Toast the bread on one side only, spread the egg mixture on to the untoasted side and grill until lightly golden. Serve at once.

TIP *Choose a well-made genuine Cheddar from Somerset: Keen's or Montgomery's are very good.*

Eggs Benedict

SERVES 2 (GENER-
OUS PORTIONS)
• 4 slices of cooked
  ham or 4 rashers
  of back bacon
• 4 thick slices of
  white bread
• 4 eggs
• 50 g/2 oz unsalted
  butter

HOLLANDAISE
SAUCE
• 3 tablespoons white
  wine vinegar
• piece of mace
• 1 small bay leaf
• 2 egg yolks
• 100g/3½ oz butter,
  cut into cubes
• pinch of English
  mustard powder
• salt and cayenne
  pepper

A luxurious supper dish for when you want to indulge yourself and your partner. Eggs provide vitamin E, zinc and protein.
The easiest way to make hollandaise sauce is in a liquidizer or food processor. Because the eggs are not cooked, it is important that the butter is very hot.

Trim the ham to fit the bread or fry the bacon rashers in a little butter until crisp.

To make the sauce, put the vinegar, mace and bay leaf in a small saucepan. Bring to the boil, then simmer over a low heat until reduced to 1 tablespoon. Remove the spices.

Pour the reduced vinegar into a liquidizer, add the egg yolks and blend well. Heat the butter in a small saucepan until it is bubbling. With the liquidizer running at high speed, pour the butter on to the eggs in a steady stream and blend until smooth. Season and keep warm.

Poach the eggs and toast the bread. Butter the toast, cover each slice with ham or bacon and top with a poached egg. Pour over the warm sauce and serve at once.

Tomato, pesto and olive omelette

SERVES 2
- 1 garlic clove, crushed
- ½ onion, finely chopped
- 1 tablespoon pesto
- 2 tomatoes, halved
- 50 g/2 oz goats' cheese
- 50 g/2 oz olives, pitted and chopped
- 4 eggs
- 4 tablespoons milk
- ½ teaspoon English mustard
- 1 teaspoon butter
- fresh basil, to garnish

If you're feeling weak and tired, through illness or depression, this is a perfect pick-you-up. Serve with a spinach or watercress salad and olive ciabatta rolls for a light meal or pre-or after-theatre supper.

Preheat the grill. Mix the garlic and onion with the pesto and spread this on to the surface of the halved tomatoes. Grill the tomatoes until they are brown at the edges. Leave to cool slightly.

Chop the goats' cheese into small pieces and mix with the pitted olives.

Beat the eggs together with the milk and mustard.

Heat a frying pan and add the butter. When it foams, pour in the egg mixture and cook on one side, until lightly browned. Place the tomatoes and cheese/olive mixture on the omelette and fold over to heat the filling through gently.

Garnish with basil and serve hot.

TIPS *Plum tomatoes have a good flavour, so choose them when in season. For a slightly different flavour, use a blue cheese such as Roquefort.*

Spinach and goats' cheese soufflé

SERVES 4

- 300 ml/½ pint semi-skimmed milk
- 25 g/1 oz butter
- 25 g/1 oz plain white flour
- 4 eggs, separated
- 100 g/3½ oz goats' cheese
- 1 garlic clove, finely chopped
- 100 g/3½ oz spinach, washed, cooked and finely chopped
- ½ teaspoon freshly grated nutmeg
- 1 teaspoon Dijon mustard
- salt and pepper

This scrumptious dish is rich in calcium and is effortless to eat.

Preheat the oven to 200°C/400°F/Gas 6.

Butter a soufflé dish and line with nonstick baking paper, which should extend 5 cm/2 inches above the rim.

Put the milk, butter and flour in a saucepan over a low heat and whisk, using a balloon whisk, until thick and smooth. Beat in the egg yolks, crumbled cheese, garlic, spinach, nutmeg, mustard, and salt and pepper to taste.

The mixture can be prepared up to this stage several hours in advance. Cover with clingfilm until nearly ready to serve.

Whisk the egg whites until stiff and fold into the mixture, first adding 1 tablespoon of whites to lighten the mixture.

Fill the prepared soufflé dish and bake for 20–30 minutes or until risen. Serve at once.

Spinach and watercress roulade

SERVES 4
- 250 g/9 oz frozen spinach
- small bunch of watercress
- 50 g/2 oz butter
- 2 tablespoons plain white flour
- 100 ml/3½ fl oz semi-skimmed milk
- 4 eggs, separated
- 40 g/1½ oz Parmesan cheese, grated
- ½ teaspoon freshly grated nutmeg
- salt and pepper

MUSHROOM FILLING
- 150 g/5 oz wild mushrooms, thinly sliced
- 25 g/1 oz butter
- 2 garlic cloves, crushed
- 200 g/7 oz cream cheese

This impressive-looking roulade is packed with vitamins, protein, calcium and zinc.

Preheat the oven to 180°C/350°F/Gas 4.

Grease and line a Swiss roll tin with nonstick baking paper.

Thaw the spinach in a saucepan over a low heat, until all the water has evaporated. Tear the watercress leaves into small pieces, discarding the stalks.

Melt the butter in a saucepan, add the flour and cook, stirring, for 1 minute. Add the milk and bring to the boil, stirring until it thickens. Beat in the egg yolks, cheese, nutmeg, salt and pepper, spinach and watercress. Remove from the heat.

Whisk the egg whites until stiff and fold into the spinach mixture, then pour into the lined tin.

Bake for about 20 minutes, until set and golden. Turn on to a wire rack and cover with a tea towel.

Sauté the mushrooms with the butter and garlic. Mix with the cream cheese and spread over the roulade. Roll up and serve at once.

Potatoes with basil

SERVES 4

- 1 kg/2¼ lb new potatoes
- large handful of fresh basil leaves
- 150 ml/5 fl oz low-fat natural yoghurt
- 1 tablespoon lemon juice
- 1 tablespoon clear honey
- salt and pepper

Most of the vitamins in potatoes are near the skins, an added benefit of this high-fibre carbohydrate salad.

Scrub the potatoes in their skins. Plunge into boiling water and simmer for 10–15 minutes or until just tender. Leave to cool.

Finely chop the basil and mix with the yoghurt, lemon juice and honey. Season to taste.

While the potatoes are still slightly warm, stir them into the basil sauce. Chill in the refrigerator. Mix again before serving.

Gruyère potatoes

SERVES 4

- about 800 g/1¾ lb evenly shaped potatoes, about 6 cm/2½ inches long, peeled
- a little butter
- 300 ml/½ pint low-fat natural yoghurt
- 1 teaspoon Dijon mustard
- 2 teaspoons chopped fresh chives
- 2 teaspoons finely chopped fresh parsley
- ¼ teaspoons paprika
- salt and pepper
- 85 g/3 oz Gruyère cheese, grated

This is so creamy you'd never guess it was made with yoghurt.

Preheat the oven to 180°C/350°F/Gas 4.

Trim the potatoes so they are all the same size, then place in a pan with a little salt and cold water to cover. Bring to the boil and simmer for 5 minutes. Drain well.

Butter a casserole or soufflé dish about 18 cm/7 inches in diameter and 8 cm/3 inches deep.

Arrange the potatoes in the dish so they are standing upright and packed in firmly so they cannot move.

Mix together the yoghurt, mustard, herbs, paprika, salt and pepper and pour over the potatoes. Sprinkle the cheese over the top.

Place in the oven and bake for 1–1¼ hours or until the potatoes are tender and the cheese is golden brown. Serve warm, as an accompaniment to roast beef, grilled steak or grilled salmon.

Broccoli with roasted tomatoes

SERVES 2
- 450 g/1 lb fresh plum tomatoes
- 4 tablespoons virgin olive oil
- 1 garlic clove, finely chopped
- 12 black olives, pitted finely chopped
- 1 tablespoon chopped fresh parsley
- 1 teaspoon chopped fresh marjoram
- balsamic vinegar
- salt and pepper
- 250 g/9 oz broccoli, cut into small florets

Broccoli is something of a wonder-vegetable, packed with anti-cancer compounds, and vitamins and minerals to promote healthy blood, bones and skin.

Preheat the grill. Halve the tomatoes and brush lightly with olive oil. Place under the hot grill for a few minutes until nicely browned. Chop them roughly and mix with the virgin olive oil, garlic, virgin olive oil, olives and herbs. Add balsamic vinegar and salt and pepper to taste.

Cook the broccoli in lightly salted boiling water for about 30 seconds. Drain well and combine with the tomato mixture. Adjust the seasoning to taste. You may like to add a little more vinegar. Alternatively, add a good squeeze of lemon juice and some finely slivered lemon zest instead of more vinegar.

Tomatoes stuffed with olives, garlic and parsley

SERVES 2
- 4 large ripe tomatoes
- salt and pepper
- 2 slices of whole-meal bread
- 1-2 garlic cloves, halved
- olive oil
- 50 g/2 oz fresh parsley, chopped
- 8 black olives, pitted and finely chopped
- shavings of Parmesan cheese (optional)

This method of baking tomatoes incorporates fibre, calcium and antioxidants in a delicious Mediterranean supper dish.

Cut the tomatoes in half, score the cut surface with a sharp knife, press in some salt and, when it has dissolved, turn the tomatoes upside down on a plate and leave them for 1–2 hours.

Cut the crusts off the bread and rub the bread on both sides with the garlic. Sprinkle with olive oil and leave to soften.

Mix the parsley with the olives and bread; season well.

Squeeze the juice and pulp from the tomatoes and press in the bread and parsley mixture.

Put the tomatoes into a gratin dish, sprinkle with more olive oil and cook under the grill, slowly at first, then closer to the heat to brown the surface. Serve at once, with shavings of Parmesan cheese on top, if desired.

Spiced red cabbage with apple

SERVES 4
- 1 red cabbage, finely shredded
- 2 Cox's or other well-flavoured dessert apples, cored and finely sliced
- 125ml/4fl oz red wine
- 100 ml/3½ fl oz unsweetened apple juice
- 2 garlic cloves, crushed
- 1 teaspoon honey
- ½ teaspoon ground ginger
- salt and pepper

This cabbage dish, rich in fibre and antioxidants, is a good accompaniment to roast meats and oily fish such as grilled mackerel or sardines.

Preheat the oven to 150°C/300°F/Gas 2.

Place the cabbage and apples in a large casserole dish. Mix the other ingredients together and pour over the cabbage. Put a knob of butter on top, cover and place in the oven for 2 hours.

Check every so often that the liquid has not evaporated and top up if necessary.

Aubergines au gratin

SERVES 2 AS A LIGHT MEAL, 4 AS AN ACCOMPANIMENT
- 2 aubergines, sliced obliquely into 1 cm/ ½ inch thick pieces
- 100 ml/3½ fl oz fresh tomato coulis or tinned thick tomato juice mixed with a little tomato purée
- 3 garlic cloves, finely chopped
- 50 g/2 oz wholemeal breadcrumbs
- 4 tablespoons chopped fresh parsley or basil
- salt and pepper
- 2 tablespoons extra virgin olive oil
- a small buffalo mozzarella cheese, sliced

This way of cooking vegetables turns a relatively low-calorie, high-fibre food into a nourishing dish, good for anyone who needs to keep up their energy levels.

Preheat the oven to 190°C/375°F/Gas 5.

Plunge the aubergines into boiling salted water and cook for 3 minutes. Drain very thoroughly, then arrange in a large, flat, lightly oiled baking dish.

Spread each aubergine slice thickly with tomato coulis and sprinkle with the garlic, breadcrumbs and chopped parsley or basil. Season and drizzle with olive oil. Bake for 40 minutes.

Cover the aubergines with the slices of mozzarella and return to the oven until the cheese has melted. Serve hot or cold.

VARIATIONS *Add some chopped ham, bacon or sausage to this dish to make a change. Instead of aubergines you could use halved courgettes or peppers, or sliced marrow.*

Grilled peppers with garlic cheese croûtons

SERVES 6

- 6 red and yellow peppers, halved
- 75 g/3 oz garlic cream cheese (e.g. Boursin - full fat or light, or make your own by mixing cream cheese with crushed garlic)
- 18 slices of ciabatta or Italian sun-dried tomato or olive bread, lightly toasted

BASIL AND GARLIC DRESSING

- 2 teaspoons lemon juice
- 1½ tablespoons red wine vinegar
- 1 garlic clove, finely chopped
- 1 tablespoon finely chopped fresh basil
- 3 tablespoons virgin olive oil
- salt and pepper

The bright colours of the peppers announce that they are high in beta-carotene, to build up your immune system. Serve as a light meal.

Grill the peppers until the skins blister and begin to blacken. Leave in a covered bowl until cool enough to handle, then peel and cut into 1 cm/½ inch slices. Set aside.

Make the dressing by mixing the lemon juice, vinegar, garlic and basil. Add the oil and beat until emulsified. Season to taste.

Put the peppers in a bowl and pour the dressing over. Leave to marinate for 2–3 hours.

Drain the peppers and place them on serving plates. Spread the cheese on the bread and arrange on the plates with the peppers.

Vegetarian chilli

SERVES 6
- 2 tablespoons olive oil
- 1 onion, chopped
- 3 garlic cloves, finely chopped
- ½ jalapeno chilli pepper, trimmed and finely chopped
- 3 carrots, diced
- 1 sticks of celery, diced
- ½ red or green pepper, chopped
- 2 large cans (400 g/ 14 oz) kidney beans, drained
- 1–2 teaspoons chilli powder
- 2 tablespoons cumin (ground or seeds)
- ½ teaspoon salt
- 2 large cans (400 g/ 14 oz) tomatoes, lightly drained and chopped
- 2 courgettes, thickly sliced
- 100 g/3½ oz Cheddar cheese, grated

A high-fibre dish that will surely ease constipation. The jalapeno chilli makes it a little hot, but you could use a milder chilli. Be careful when chopping chillies, as even a tiny amount of the juices can really sting your skin.

Heat the oil in a large saucepan and cook the onion, and fresh chilli and garlic gently until softened. Add the carrots, celery and peppers and cook until all are softened.

Add the beans, chilli powder, cumin, salt, tomatoes and 4 tablespoons water. Cover and simmer for about 20 minutes.

Stir in the courgettes and simmer for a further 5 minutes, until the courgettes are just tender.

Serve hot, topped with grated cheese, accompanied by corn chips or warm crusty wholegrain bread.

Yam biriyani

SERVES 6
- 2 tablespoons sunflower oil
- 200 g/7 oz basmati or brown rice
- pinch of saffron strands
- 2 teaspoons turmeric
- salt and cayenne pepper
- 4 hard-boiled eggs, chopped
- 2 onions, finely chopped
- piece of fresh ginger, chopped
- 1 teaspoon each of ground cumin, coriander and cinnamon
- 2 sweet potatoes, peeled and cut into 1 cm/½ inch dice
- 1 carrot, diced
- 50 g/2 oz French beans, chopped
- 50 g/2 oz peas
- 2 tomatoes, diced
- 50 g/2 oz raisins
- 25 g/1 oz flaked almonds, toasted

Americans call them yams, we call them sweet potatoes.

Preheat the oven to 180°C/350°F/Gas 4.

Heat 1 tablespoon of the oil in a frying pan and fry the rice until coated with oil. Add the saffron, turmeric, salt and 200 ml/7 fl oz hot water. Bring to the boil, cover and simmer for 25 minutes.

When the rice is cooked, add the chopped hard-boiled eggs and set aside.

Heat the remaining oil in a saucepan and add the onions and spices. Cook gently until the onion is softened.

Add a little water, the sweet potatoes, carrot and beans and sauté for a few minutes. Add the peas, tomatoes and raisins and a little salt and cayenne pepper. Season.

Place half the rice in an ovenproof dish, top with the vegetables and the remaining rice. Cover and bake for 30 minutes. Serve hot, sprinkled with toasted almonds.

Gado gado

SERVES 4
- 2 shallots, chopped
- 3 garlic cloves, chopped
- 1 teaspoon virgin olive oil
- 2 teaspoons ground coriander
- 1 teaspoon ground cumin or 4 teaspoons garam masala
- 1 teaspoon turmeric
- 150 ml/¼ pint vegetable stock
- 600 g/1¼ lb canned chopped tomatoes
- 2 tablespoons tomato purée
- 4 courgettes, chopped
- 125 g/4 oz wild mushrooms, sliced
- 2 carrots, diced
- 4 celery sticks, diced
- 8 cauliflower florets
- dash of red wine
- 4 tablespoons crunchy peanut butter

I have taken the flavours of the Malaysian salad as inspiration for this spicy, peanutty vegetable casserole. Serve it with whole-grain rice, pasta or noodles. It is high in fibre and relatively low in calories.

Sauté the shallots and garlic in the olive oil, add the spices and sweat for 5 minutes. Add the stock, tomatoes and tomato purèe and simmer for 15 minutes.

Add all the vegetables and a dash of red wine and simmer for a further 10 minutes.

Stir in the peanut butter and cook for a further 10 minutes or until the vegetables are just cooked, but still firm to the bite.

TIP *This can be refrigerated or frozen very successfully; in fact the flavours improve on reheating.*

Pasta bows with courgettes

SERVES 4
- 4 courgettes, sliced
- salt and pepper
- 3 tablespoons olive oil
- 1 garlic clove, crushed
- ¼ teaspoon cayenne pepper
- 450 g/1 lb pasta bows (farfalle)
- freshly grated Parmesan cheese, to serve

Pasta is a very comforting and settling food to eat, and is quick to cook, so it's good for indigestion sufferers, or when you're pregnant or a little headachy or nauseous and just want something simple.

Place the courgettes in a colander and sprinkle with salt to draw out the excess water. Leave for 30 minutes, then rinse with cold water.

Heat the oil in a large frying pan and sauté the garlic. Add the cayenne pepper and courgettes and sauté for a further 5 minutes.

Meanwhile, boil the pasta until it is al dente, in other words it still has a little firmness. Drain well.

Tip the pasta into the frying pan, mix well, season and sprinkle with Parmesan. Serve hot or cold.

Pasta with wild mushrooms

SERVES 2–4
- 25 g/1 oz dried wild mushrooms
- 225 g/8 oz fresh mushrooms (preferably wild)
- 200 g/7 oz dried pasta shapes
- 2 tablespoons olive oil
- ½ small onion, chopped
- 2 garlic cloves, finely chopped
- 2 sprigs of thyme
- 1 bay leaf
- 300 ml/½ pint single cream
- 2 teaspoons chopped fresh parsley
- 2 teaspoons chopped fresh marjoram
- salt and pepper

The combination of dried and fresh mushrooms gives this dish a good depth of flavour.

Cover the dried mushrooms with 85 ml/3 fl oz boiling water and leave to soak until they have softened, about 20 minutes. While the mushrooms are still in the liquid, make sure that they are completely clean. Remove the mushrooms and pat dry, reserving the soaking liquid. Strain the liquid through a coffee filter and set aside. Slice the mushrooms.

Clean the fresh mushrooms thoroughly, removing any tough parts of the stems. Slice.

Put the pasta on to boil, but make sure that it doesn't overcook.

In another pan, heat the olive oil and cook the onion and garlic gently until the onion is light golden brown. Add the dried and fresh mushrooms, thyme and bay leaf.

Add the cream and bring slowly to the boil. Add the strained mushroom liquid, herbs and seasoning.

Drain the cooked pasta and tip into a large bowl. Add the sauce and stir well. Serve at once, with black pepper.

Baked pasta with ratatouille sauce

SERVES 4

- 3 tablespoons olive oil
- 1 large onion, chopped
- 1 large aubergine, diced
- 3 courgettes, sliced
- 2 large red peppers, chopped
- 1 large can (400 g/ 14 oz) chopped tomatoes
- 500 ml/16 fl oz tomato juice
- 2 garlic cloves, finely chopped
- 1 teaspoon oregano
- 1 teaspoon chopped fresh basil
- salt and pepper
- 450g/1lb pasta shells
- 8 tablespoons fresh wholemeal breadcrumbs
- 125g/4 oz cheese, grated (mature Lancashire is good)

A lovely combination of pasta and Mediterranean vegetables, which is easy, satisfying and nutritious.

Preheat the oven to 180°C/350°F/Gas 4.

Heat the oil in a large saucepan and cook the onion and aubergine gently until softened.

Add the courgettes and peppers and fry for a few minutes, stirring occasionally. Add the tomatoes, tomato juice, garlic, herbs and seasoning and simmer for 20 minutes.

Meanwhile, cook the pasta shells. Drain well and mix with the ratatouille. Tip the mixture into a large ovenproof dish.

Mix the breadcrumbs with the grated cheese and sprinkle over the pasta mixture.

Bake in the oven for 15–20 minutes, or heat through in the microwave.

Pasta vongole

SERVES 2
- 1 kg/2¼ lb fresh small clams in their shells
- 3 tablespoons olive oil
- 1–2 garlic cloves, chopped
- salt and pepper
- 200 g/7 oz spaghetti
- 2 tablespoons chopped fresh parsley

Spaghetti with clams is rather messy to eat, but for supper for two it can be fun. The clams are a good source of zinc, which is good for your skin – and your libido!

Put the cleaned clams in a saucepan with 1 tablespoon of the olive oil. Cover the pan and shake over moderate heat to open the clams; this will take 6–8 minutes. Discard any that do not open after this time. Drain, reserving the liquid.

Heat the remaining oil, add the garlic and fry. Add the clams and mix quickly. Add the reserved clam liquid, bring to the boil and remove from the heat; keep warm.

Boil the spaghetti until it is al dente (just cooked but still with a little firmness). Drain and mix with the clams. Serve at once, sprinkled with parsley and black pepper.

Smoked cheese and olive pasta

SERVES 2–4
- 50 g/2 oz fresh wholemeal breadcrumbs
- 2 teaspoons virgin olive oil
- 1 onion, finely chopped
- 1 garlic clove, finely chopped
- 1 apple, peeled, cored and chopped
- 2 teaspoons Dijon mustard
- 225 g/8 oz dried pasta shapes
- 225 g/8 oz smoked cheese (e.g. Applewood Cheddar), grated
- 75 g/3 oz olives, pitted and chopped
- large bunch of parsley, finely chopped
- salt and pepper

This is both settling and high in energy, so even if you can only manage a small portion, it can benefit you a lot.

Spread the breadcrumbs on a lightly oiled baking sheet. Place under the grill and toast gently until the breadcrumbs are golden brown and crisp. Set aside.

Heat the oil in a frying pan and cook the onion, garlic and apple gently until soft and golden brown. Add the mustard and keep warm.

Put the pasta on to boil, but make sure that it doesn't overcook.

Meanwhile, put the grated cheese, olives and parsley in a large bowl.

Drain the cooked pasta well and tip into the bowl with the cheese. Add the breadcrumbs and the onion mixture. Toss well and season to taste. If the cheese does not melt you could place it over a very low heat for a couple of minutes, stirring constantly to prevent it from sticking. Serve hot.

Smoked haddock spinach pasta

SERVES 4
- 1 kg/2¼ lb fresh spinach, washed and stemmed
- salt and pepper
- 175 g/6 oz dried pasta shapes (shells are good because they allow some sauce to nestle inside!)
- 25 g/1 oz butter
- 275 g/10 oz smoked haddock (preferably un-dyed)
- ¼ teaspoon grated nutmeg
- a dash of fresh lemon juice
- 85 ml/3 fl oz double cream
- 75g/3 oz Pecorino cheese

The smoked fish and pecorino makes this dish quite strongly flavoured, so even when you've lost a lot of your sense of taste with a cold you should be able to taste it.

Put the wet spinach in a large saucepan and cook over a low heat, shaking the pan, until the spinach has reduced in volume and made its own liquid. Add ½ teaspoon salt and cover the pan. Cook gently for 5–8 minutes, then drain the spinach thoroughly in a fine sieve, squeezing out as much liquid as possible.

Meanwhile, boil the pasta until it is al dente, in other words it still has a little firmness. Drain well.

Chop the spinach roughly. Melt the butter in a saucepan, add the chopped spinach, smoked haddock and nutmeg and heat through until the fish becomes pale and flaky, about 2 minutes. Squeeze in a little lemon juice, then stir in the cream. Add the pasta, mix thoroughly and season to taste.

Place in a hot serving dish and grate the cheese over the top.

Oysters with cream and Parmesan

PER PERSON:
- 4 oysters
- 4 tablespoons single cream
- 4 tablespoons freshly grated Parmesan cheese
- freshly ground black pepper

Oysters have always been regarded as an aphrodisiac, and there is some truth in the rumour, since they are high in zinc, which is needed for our sex hormones. It also boosts the body's immune system and is good for the skin. Serve as a starter or, if you allow 6 oysters each, you could make it a light supper.

Preheat the grill. Open the oysters, remove the beards and loosen the oysters from the shells. Place the oysters on a grill rack lined with crumpled foil.

Pour 1 tablespoon cream over each oyster, sprinkle with cheese and season lightly with pepper. Place under the hot grill and cook for 3–4 minutes or until the cheese is golden brown and bubbling. Serve at once.

Spicy fish kebabs

SERVES 4
- 2 red peppers, cut into 4 cm/1½ inch squares
- 2 courgettes, sliced
- 150 g/5 oz button or wild mushrooms
- 20 scallops
- 12 king prawns
- 2 thick fish fillets (monkfish, halibut, hake), cut into 5 cm/ 2 inch squares

MARINADE
- 3 tablespoons olive oil
- 2 teaspoons curry powder
- 2 teaspoons honey
- 1 tablespoon lemon juice

Fish and shellfish are low in fat and high in useful minerals, so they're great for weight watchers. These kebabs can be grilled on an outdoor barbecue or on a special ridged chargrilling pan. Or you could grill them under a conventional grill.

Thread the vegetables and fish and vegetables on to wooden skewers. Place in a shallow dish and brush with the marinade. Cover and leave in the refrigerator overnight, ready to barbecue or grill the next day.

Smoked mackerel and spinach fishcakes

SERVES 4

- 2 smoked mackerel, about 150g/5oz each
- 2 teaspoons olive oil
- 125 g/4 oz cooked spinach
- 50 g/2 oz butter
- 4 potatoes, peeled, boiled and mashed
- 2 eggs, beaten
- 2 tablespoons finely chopped fresh dill
- ½ teaspoon freshly grated nutmeg
- salt and pepper
- 150 ml/5 fl oz natural yoghurt

Heat the grill and place the smoked mackerel underneath, drizzled with olive oil. Cook for about 3 minutes on each side. Carefully flake the fish off the skin.

Place the spinach in a saucepan with a tiny knob of butter and dry out over medium heat.

Place the mackerel and spinach in a bowl with the butter, mashed potatoes, egg, dill, nutmeg, salt and pepper. Add yoghurt to mix to a fairly firm consistency; if it is too sloppy the fishcakes will not hold their shape.

Take a large egg-size amount of mixture in your hands and form into a flat cake; you should make 4 large fishcakes.

Place under the grill and cook for 5–10 minutes, turning once. Serve hot.

Prawn curry

SERVES 4

- 1 tablespoon vegetable oil
- 1 onion, finely chopped
- 2 garlic cloves, crushed
- 1 tablespoon medium-strength curry powder
- 2 large cans (400 g/ 14 oz) chopped plum tomatoes
- 3 tablespoons finely chopped fresh coriander, plus extra to garnish
- 2 tablespoons fresh lemon juice
- 500 g/1 lb 2 oz cooked and peeled Dublin bay prawns

A low-fat dish with tons of flavour.

Heat the oil in a large frying pan and fry the onion and garlic until soft. Add the curry powder and cook for 2 minutes.

Add the tomatoes, coriander and lemon juice, cover and bring to the boil. Reduce the heat and simmer for 10 minutes or until the tomatoes are very tender.

Add the prawns and heat through. Serve hot, with boiled rice. Garnish with coriander.

Salmon and asparagus risotto

SERVES 2–4

- 2 tablespoons olive oil
- 2 small shallots, finely chopped
- 1 garlic clove, crushed
- thin strip of lemon rind
- 8 cm/3 inch piece of fresh lemon grass
- 1 cm/½ inch cube of fresh ginger
- salt and pepper
- 250 ml/8 fl oz chicken or vegetable stock
- 200 g/7 oz arborio rice
- dash of dry white wine
- 350 g/13 oz fresh salmon fillet, cut into chunks
- 12 asparagus tips
- 2 tablespoons natural yoghurt
- freshly grated Parmesan cheese

Heat half the oil in a saucepan and cook the shallots gently for 3 minutes.

Add the garlic, lemon rind, lemon grass, ginger and salt and pepper.

Add the stock and 600 ml/1 pint water, bring to the boil and simmer for 10 minutes. Leave to stand for 30 minutes, then strain.

Heat the remaining oil in a large frying pan and fry the rice until translucent. Add the lemon grass stock, bring to the boil and simmer for 15 minutes.

Add the wine, salmon and asparagus and simmer for 5 minutes or until the liquid has been absorbed by the rice.

Just before serving, season to taste, stir in the yoghurt and sprinkle with grated Parmesan.

Salmon and lemon lasagne

SERVES 4
- 25 g/1 oz butter
- 50 g/2 oz plain white flour
- 600 ml/1 pint semi-skimmed milk
- grated zest of 2 lemons
- salt and pepper
- ½ teaspoon freshly grated nutmeg
- 1 tablespoon chopped fresh dill
- 450 g/1 lb spinach pasta sheets, blanched and drained
- 175 g/6 oz poached salmon, flaked
- freshly grated Parmesan cheese

Preheat the oven to 180°C/350F/Gas 4.

Melt the butter in a saucepan, remove from the heat and stir in the flour and milk. Return to the heat and bring to the boil. Add the lemon zest, salt, pepper and nutmeg and simmer for 5 minutes. Remove from the heat and stir in the dill.

Grease an ovenproof dish and cover the bottom with pieces of pasta.

Spread some of the sauce over the pasta and then sprinkle some salmon over this.

Continue to make layers in this way until you have three layers of pasta. Finish with a layer of sauce sprinkled generously with Parmesan cheese. Bake in the oven for 40 minutes. Serve with a crisp green salad or fresh green vegetable such as broccoli.

Salmon and celery kedgeree

SERVES 4
- 2 tablespoons olive oil
- 1 yellow pepper, diced
- 6 sticks of celery, finely chopped
- 1 shallot, finely chopped
- 1 teaspoon ground cumin
- 1 teaspoon ground coriander
- 350 g/13 oz basmati rice
- salt and pepper
- 600 ml/1 pint fish stock
- 275 g/10 oz salmon fillet
- 300 ml/½ pint semi-skimmed milk
- 2 eggs, hard-boiled and cut into quarters
- 2 tablespoons finely chopped fresh parsley

Heat the oil in a large frying pan, add the pepper, celery and shallot and cook gently until soft.

Add the spices and stir with the vegetables to release the aromas. Add the rice, salt and pepper and stir around the pan.

Add the stock, bring to the boil and simmer gently for 15 minutes or until the liquid has been absorbed.

Place the salmon in a saucepan and cover with the milk. Poach the salmon gently. When cooked, transfer to a plate and flake, removing the bones.

Add the flaked salmon and quartered eggs to the cooked rice, mix together gently and serve hot.

VARIATION *Instead of fresh salmon, you could use smoked salmon or smoked mackerel. For added colour, use ½ a yellow pepper and ½ a green pepper.*

Smoked fish casserole

SERVES 4

- 225 g/8 oz each of smoked haddock and cod fillets, cut into chunks
- 4 tablespoons plain white flour
- salt and pepper
- 7 tablespoons olive oil
- 1 onion, finely chopped
- 6 garlic cloves, crushed
- 3 potatoes, cut into cubes
- 1 can(185 g/6½ oz) red pimentos, cut into strips
- 4 ripe tomatoes, skinned and roughly chopped
- 2 tablespoons white wine vinegar
- 750 ml/1¼ pints dry white wine
- 750 ml/1¼ pints fish stock or water
- 3 bay leaves
- 2 hard-boiled eggs, sliced, to garnish

Toss the fish in seasoned flour. Heat 4 tablespoons of the oil in a frying pan and fry the fish for 10 minutes, until pale. Set aside.

Add the remaining oil to the pan and fry the onion and garlic until soft. Increase the heat and add the potato cubes and two-thirds of the pimento strips; fry for 5 minutes. Tip into a flame-proof casserole.

Add the tomatoes to the frying pan, then add the vinegar, wine, stock, bay leaves and salt and pepper to taste. Bring to the boil, then pour over the potatoes. Cover and simmer for 30 minutes or until tender.

Add the fish and simmer for a further 20 minutes or until the fish is tender and the potatoes soft. Season to taste and garnish with the reserved pimento strips and egg. Serve in shallow soup plates, with wholegrain rolls and a crisp green salad, dressed with fresh parsley.

Monkfish and mussel paella

SERVES 4-6
- 1 kg/2¼ lb fresh mussels
- 150 ml/5 fl oz dry white wine or water
- pinch of saffron strands
- 900 ml/1½ pints fish stock, hot
- 6 tablespoons olive oil
- 1 kg/2¼ lb monkfish fillets, cut into chunks
- 1 onion, chopped
- 2 garlic cloves, crushed
- 1 can(185 g/6½ oz) red pimentos, cut into strips
- 2 large ripe tomatoes, roughly chopped
- 350 g/13 oz Valencia or risotto rice
- salt and pepper
- 100 g/3½ oz cooked peas
- lemon wedges and chopped fresh parsley, to garnish

In Spain there are many versions of this rice dish. This one is based on fish.

Scrub the mussels and rinse in cold water, discarding any with broken or open shells. Place in a large saucepan with the wine or water and cook over high heat for 3–4 minutes, shaking the pan occasionally, until the mussels open. Tip into a colander over a bowl, to collect the cooking liquid. Discard any mussels that remain closed.

Put the saffron in a small bowl and pour over 2–3 tablespoons of the hot stock. Leave to infuse for 20 minutes.

Heat the oil in a paella pan or large frying pan and fry the monkfish for 5 minutes. Remove with a slotted spoon and set aside.

Add the onion, garlic and pimento strips to the pan and fry for 10 minutes over a high heat. Add the tomatoes and fry for 5 minutes or until quite thick.

Add the rice and stir until it is coated with the onion mixture. Return the monkfish to the pan, then pour in the fish stock, the strained mussel cooking liquid, the saffron and seasoning. Cook briskly for a few minutes, then lower the heat and cook for 15–20 minutes without stirring, until the rice and fish are tender.

Remove most of the mussels from their shells, keeping a few in shells. Add the shelled mussels and peas to the rice. Stir and add more stock if necessary.

Turn off the heat, cover with a tea towel and leave to stand for 3–4 minutes. Serve at once, garnished with the reserved mussels in shells, lemon wedges and parsley.

Honey and mustard quail

SERVES 4
- 4 Bramley apples
- 8 quail
- 3 teaspoons honey
- 5 teaspoons Dijon mustard
- salt and pepper

I like to serve quail either at a dinner party or for a summer lunch, as an alternative to red meat.

Preheat the grill.

Peel and core the apples and slice into rings. Place the apple rings in a heatproof dish and place the quail on top.

Mix the honey and mustard together and brush over the quail. Sprinkle with salt and pepper and place under the hot grill to cook the quail thoroughly, turning them from time to time.

Serve hot, with new potatoes and a green leafy vegetable such as steamed spinach, or a tossed green salad.

TIP *Test whether the bird is cooked by piercing it with a sharp knife; the juices should run clear. The flesh should be a uniform brown colour and not pink.*

Chicken stroganoff with tarragon

SERVES 4
- 50 g/2 oz butter
- 4 large boneless, skinless chicken breasts, sliced into 1 cm/½ inch strips
- 8 sprigs of tarragon, with leaves stripped
- a dash of brandy or sherry
- 125 ml/4 fl oz double cream
- 125 ml/4 fl oz low-fat natural yoghurt
- salt and pepper
- lemon juice

Chicken's mild flavour tends to be better tolerated than red meat when you're pregnant or feeling ill. You can make this dish with all cream but I prefer to use half yoghurt to give it a slightly lighter, sharper taste.

Melt the butter in a shallow frying pan and add the chicken and tarragon. Cook over high heat, stirring frequently, until the chicken is slightly coloured on all sides, about 3 minutes.

Pour in the brandy or sherry, cream, and yoghurt. Let it simmer for a few minutes to thicken and finish cooking the chicken. Season to taste and add a good squeeze of lemon juice. Taste again, to make sure you have the right balance of flavours.

Garlic and herb chicken

SERVES 6

- 1 tablespoon sunflower oil
- 6 large boneless, skinless chicken breasts
- salt and pepper
- 3 whole bulbs of garlic
- ¾ tablespoon each fresh thyme and rosemary (or ½ teaspoon dried)
- about 150 ml/5 fl oz dry white wine
- 50 g/2 oz fresh parsley, chopped

Garlic boosts the immune system and prevents heart disease. This light dish is perfect for an easy lunch or supper.

Preheat the oven to 180°C/350°F/Gas 4.

Heat the oil in a frying pan over medium heat and fry the chicken gently until golden brown. Season to taste.

Separate the cloves of garlic and remove the papery outer skin, but do not peel.

Lay the chicken pieces in a casserole. Place the garlic on top and among the pieces of chicken, and sprinkle with thyme and rosemary. Add wine to cover the chicken. Cover the casserole and bake for 1 hour, until the liquid is reduced and the garlic soft.

Serve hot, sprinkled with parsley. This dish can be served with rice, either brown or white basmati, or comforting creamed potato or tagliatelle pasta.

Coconut chicken

SERVES 4

- 1 tablespoon
  sunflower oil
- 1 large onion,
  finely chopped
- 3 garlic cloves,
  finely chopped
- 4 cm/1½ inch piece
  of fresh ginger,
  finely chopped
- 6 cardamom pods
- 10 cloves
- 1 cinnamon stick
- 2 tablespoons
  ground almonds
- 4 boneless, skinless
  chicken breasts,
  cut into small pieces
- 50 g/2 oz wild
  mushrooms, sliced
- 200 ml/7 fl oz
  coconut milk
- ¼ teaspoon turmeric
- salt and pepper
- 2 tablespoons low-
  fat natural yoghurt
- 2 tablespoons finely
  chopped fresh
  coriander
- toasted coconut
  flakes, to garnish

A special dinner party dish which charms even red meat eaters.

Heat the oil in a large saucepan and gently cook the onion, garlic and ginger until softened. Add the cardamom, cloves and cinnamon and cook for a few minutes before adding the almonds.

Lower the heat a little and add the chicken, stirring frequently until the meat turns white. Add the mushrooms and then the coconut milk, turmeric, salt and pepper and bring to the boil. Reduce the heat and simmer for 30 minutes.

Add the yoghurt and adjust the seasoning. Serve hot, sprinkled with coriander and roasted coconut flakes.

Somerset steak and cider pie

SERVES 4

- 1 kg/2¼ lb lean stewing steak
- 1 tablespoon vegetable oil
- 1 large onion, sliced
- 450 ml/15 fl oz beef stock
- 300 ml/½ pint dry cider
- 2 teaspoons chopped fresh thyme
- 1 teaspoon ground allspice
- salt and pepper
- 450 g/1 lb carrots, thickly sliced
- 450 g/1 lb turnips or parsnips, thickly sliced
- 200 g/7 oz filo pastry
- 225 g/8 oz Bramley apple, chopped
- melted butter for brushing

Preheat the oven to 150°C/300°F/Gas 2.

Trim the meat and cut into cubes. Heat the oil in a flameproof casserole. Add the meat and fry until brown. Drain on paper towels.

Lower the heat under the casserole and add the onion. Fry for 5 minutes.

Return the meat to the casserole and add the stock, cider, thyme, allspice and salt and pepper to taste. Bring to the boil and cover. Transfer to the oven and cook for 1 hour.

Blanch the carrots, turnips or parsnips in boiling water for 3 minutes. Add the vegetables and apples to the casserole and stir. Return to the oven for a further 1 hour or until the meat is tender. Turn into a pie dish and leave until cold.

Heat the oven to 220°C/425°F/Gas 7. Brush the sheets of filo pastry with melted butter and lay on the pie. Bake for 30 minutes or until golden.

Serve hot with dark green leafy vegetables and new potatoes boiled in their skins.

Winter vegetable and oxtail pie

SERVES 4
- ½ tablespoon
  vegetable oil
- 1 kg/2¼ lb oxtail
  steak, trimmed and
  cut into small
  bite-sized pieces
- 1 large onion,
  finely chopped
- 2 garlic cloves,
  finely chopped
- 2 sticks of celery,
  finely chopped
- 1 large courgette,
  thinly sliced
- 450 ml/15 fl oz
  beef stock
- 300 ml/½ pint
  red wine
- 2 teaspoons chopped
  fresh thyme
- 1 teaspoon
  ground allspice
- 1 teaspoon
  English mustard
- salt and pepper
- 450 g/1 lb carrots,
  thickly sliced
- 225 g/8 oz parsnips,
  thickly sliced
- 300 g/11 oz
  puff pastry
- beaten egg for
  glazing

This pie is perfect for days when you need something substantial. Oxtail is rich in iron, protein and zinc.

Preheat the oven to 150°C/300°F/Gas 2.

Heat the oil in a flameproof casserole. Add the oxtail and fry until brown. Drain on paper towels.

Add the onion, garlic and celery and fry for 5 minutes. Add the courgette and fry for another 1–2 minutes.

Return the meat to the casserole and add the stock, wine, thyme, allspice, mustard, salt and pepper. Bring to the boil and cover. Transfer to the oven and cook for 1 hour.

Blanch the carrots and parsnips in boiling water for 3 minutes. Add to the casserole and cook for a further 1 hour or until the meat is tender. Turn into a pie dish and leave until cold.

Heat the oven to 220°C/425°F/Gas 7. Roll out a pastry lid for the pie and decorate. Brush lightly with beaten egg and bake for 30 minutes, until golden brown. Serve hot.

Minted meatballs with yoghurt sauce

SERVES 4

- 2 aubergines
- 225 g/8 oz minced lamb
- 225 g/8 oz minced lean beef
- 1 onion, chopped
- 2 garlic cloves, chopped
- 100 g/3½ oz fresh white breadcrumbs
- 4 heaped table-spoons chopped fresh mint
- 1 teaspoon ground allspice
- salt and pepper
- olive oil for shallow frying
- 450 ml/15 fl oz beef stock, hot
- 2 tablespoons tomato purée
- 150 ml/5 fl oz natural yoghurt
- 1 tablespoon cornflour

Preheat the oven to 200°C/400°F/Gas 6.

Skewer the aubergines and grill for 10–15 minutes. Peel off the skins with a knife. Chop the flesh roughly, then place in a food processor with the lamb, beef, onion and garlic. Blend to a fine paste. Add the breadcrumbs, half the mint, the allspice and salt and pepper to taste. Mix, then chill in the refrigerator for at least 2 hours.

Form the mixture into small balls and fry in very hot oil until brown.

Transfer to an ovenproof dish. Mix the hot beef stock with the tomato purée and pour over the meatballs. Cover and cook for 1 hour.

Drain the liquid from the meat-balls into a jug. Whisk the yoghurt and cornflour together and gradually whisk in the liquid. Bring to the boil and simmer until thickened. Pour some sauce on to each plate and arrange the meatballs on top. Sprinkle with mint and serve hot, with the remaining sauce in a jug.

Sausage and bean casserole

SERVES 8

- 2 tablespoons
  olive oil
- 2 onions, finely
  chopped
- 2 garlic cloves
- 1 kg/2¼ lb good-
  quality lean pork
  sausages, cut into
  small pieces
- 225 g/8 oz lean
  smoked bacon, cut
  into small pieces
- 2 teaspoons medium-
  strength mustard
- 2 tablespoons
  plain flour
- 600 ml/1 pint
  beef stock
- 2 cans (400 g/14 oz)
  baked beans
- 1 can (400 g/14 oz)
  chopped tomatoes
- a dash of
  Worcestershire sauce

This is quick comfort food to cheer you up on a cold winter's evening.

Heat the oil in a large casserole.

Add the onions and garlic and cook gently until the onions are light golden brown. Add the sausages and bacon and cook until golden brown.

Stir in the mustard and sprinkle over the flour. Slowly add the stock and the remaining ingredients and bring to the boil. Simmer for 30–40 minutes. Adjust the seasoning to taste. Serve with jacket potatoes, warmed bread, pasta or rice.

Sausage, tomato and potato pie

SERVES 4
- 450 g/1 lb potatoes, peeled and boiled
- 6 tablespoons single cream
- 100 g/3½ oz strong mature cheese (Cheddar, Gouda, Emmenthal)
- 2 teaspoons Dijon mustard
- salt and pepper
- 450 g/1 lb good-quality lean sausages
- 2 onions, thinly sliced
- 2 garlic cloves, finely chopped
- 1 tablespoon olive oil
- 1 large can (400 g/14 oz) chopped tomatoes
- 2 tablespoons tomato purée
- 1 tablespoon chopped fresh basil
- grated Parmesan or sliced Mozzarella cheese

This is very easy to make. Enriched with cream and cheese to keep up your energy levels.

Preheat the oven to 190°C/375°F/Gas 5.

Mash the potatoes with the cream, mature cheese, mustard and seasoning to taste.

Grill the sausages until golden brown. Slice and set aside.

Gently fry the onions and garlic in the olive oil until golden brown and soft. Add the tomatoes, tomato purée and fresh basil. Bring to the boil and simmer for 8 minutes.

In a large ovenproof dish, arrange layers of the sausage, tomato and potato mixtures, finishing with potato. Top with Parmesan or mozzarella and bake in the oven for 20–25 minutes or until the pie is golden brown on top and heated through.

Tropical dried fruit salad

SERVES 4
- 50 g/2 oz dried banana
- 50 g/2 oz dried mango
- 50 g/2 oz dried pineapple
- 50 g/2 oz dried prunes
- 100 g/3½ oz dried apricots
- 300 ml/½ pint pineapple juice
- 1 cinnamon stick
- 2 tablespoons Tia Maria

A luxurious and intriguingly flavoured dessert that's low in calories and high in fibre.

Put all the fruit into a large saucepan and cover with the pine-apple juice. Add the cinnamon stick and bring almost to the boil. Simmer for 15 minutes or until the fruit is soft. Leave to cool for at least 1 hour.

Add the Tia Maria and reheat gently.

Transfer to a sealed container and leave to macerate for several hours to enrich the flavours. Serve with a spoonful of low-fat fromage frais or low-fat natural yoghurt.

Oranges in caramel

SERVES 4-8
8 seedless oranges
Grand Marnier (optional)
175 g/6 oz granulated sugar

Oranges are high in vitamin C. Burying them in a haze of caramel is a lovely way to serve them. It certainly beats taking a pill!

Carefully pare the rind from the oranges. Cut the rind into needle-fine shreds and blanch in boiling water for 30 seconds. Drain and set aside.

Peel the oranges, making sure all the pith is removed. Keeping the shape of the fruit, cut the oranges into slices, check that there are no pips, and secure with cocktail sticks. Place in a serving bowl and scatter over the shreds of rind. If you like, sprinkle the oranges with Grand Marnier.

Put the sugar in a small saucepan and add 125 ml/4 fl oz hot water. Place over medium heat and stir until the sugar has dissolved. Increase the heat and boil, without stirring, until a light golden caramel forms.

Pour most of the caramel over the oranges; pour a little on to a lightly oiled baking tray, for decoration. (If you are experienced in sugar spinning I suggest you spin the sugar over the oranges: it looks beautiful.)

Chill the oranges for 1 hour. Just before serving, decorate by crushing the remaining caramel over the oranges.

Fruit compote

SERVES 4
- 225 g/8 oz dried or fresh fruit (apricots, peaches, pears, prunes, figs)
- 300 ml/½ pint water
- 1 clove
- 1 cinnamon stick
- grated zest of 1 lemon and 1 orange

This compote can be stored in the refrigerator for days; dip into it whenever you need a fruit boost.

It's high in fibre and organoleptic value: the colours, shapes and 'mouth feel' of the different fruits are very satisfying to eat. Serve the compote on its own or with cereals, yoghurt, ice cream or crème fraîche, or in winter with hot, fresh custard.

If using dried fruit, soak overnight in the water, with the clove, cinnamon, lemon and orange zest.

The next day, put all the ingredients into a saucepan and bring to the boil. Simmer for 30 minutes or until the fruit is tender, and then remove the cinnamon stick and clove. Chill before serving.

VARIATION: MIXED BERRIES IN GRAND MARNIER
This easy dessert offers a perfect source of vitamin C.
Use seasonal fruits (blueberries, strawberries, raspberries, blackberries, or soft fruits such as peaches, apricots and mango). Place the fruits in a bowl and sprinkle with Grand Marnier or Cointreau. Leave to macerate for several hours.

Serve chilled, decorated with mint leaves and dusted with icing sugar.

Mixed fruits with a butterscotch sauce

SERVES 6-8
- Allow approximately 125-150 g/4-5 oz of fruit per person. Choose a colourful selection such as strawberries, peaches, kiwi fruits or bananas

BUTTERSCOTCH SAUCE
- 75 g/3 oz butter
- 175 g/6 oz soft light brown sugar
- 2 tablespoons golden syrup
- ½ teaspoon vanilla essence

In this refreshing variation on fruit salad the fibre content of the fruits helps the body to absorb the sugary sauce more slowly, hence it shouldn't cause a headache or migraine. It is a perfect dish for a supper party, served in elegant glass bowls.

Make the butterscotch sauce by placing all the ingredients in a saucepan and bringing them slowly to the boil. Take care not to let the sauce burn, as the sugar can easily 'catch'. Simmer gently for 3 minutes and then remove from the heat.

Slice the fruits into bite-sized pieces and divide between the serving bowls.

Just before serving, trickle a small amount of butterscotch sauce over the fruits.

TIP *Surplus sauce can be kept in the refrigerator in an airtight jar and then reheated gently over a low heat.*

Fresh figs filled with almond cream

SERVES 4
- 100 g/3½ oz ricotta cheese
- 75 g/3 oz reduced fat cream cheese
- 2 tablespoons skimmed milk
- 25 g/1 oz almonds, finely chopped (optional)
- 18 ripe figs
- 2 teaspoons finely chopped fresh mint
- honey

A delicious way to boost your calcium intake. The almonds supply a number of vitamins and minerals, especially vitamin E.

Mix the ricotta, cream cheese and milk together. Push the mixture through a fine sieve into a bowl. Add the nuts at this stage if you wish. Form the mixture into a ball and wrap in a dampened tea towel. Chill in the refrigerator.

Slice the stems off the figs and make two cuts in each from top to bottom, stopping just before the base of the fig. Press each fig at the base, which will make it open up. Spoon some cheese mixture into each fig. Serve sprinkled with mint and drizzled with a little honey.

Blackberry and raspberry fool

SERVES 4
- 225 g/8 oz blackberries
- 225 g/8 oz raspberries
- 50 g/2 oz caster sugar
- 50 g/2 oz double cream
- 50 g/2 oz low-fat fromage frais
- fresh mint leaves
- icing sugar

Reserve 4 blackberries and 4 raspberries to decorate.

Gently blend the remaining fruits together with a spoon, so they are soft and pulpy. Push them through a sieve to remove the pips.

Stir the sugar into the fruit purée and fold in the double cream and fromage frais. Place in individual sundae or wine glasses. Chill for at least 1 hour.

Just before serving, decorate each fool with a blackberry and raspberry, and a mint leaf to set off the rich colours. Gently shake a little icing sugar over the top to give a frosted effect.

Vanilla poached peaches

SERVES 4
- 8 ripe peaches (preferably white peaches)
- 500 ml/16 fl oz water
- 500 ml/16 fl oz white wine
- 200 g/7 oz caster sugar
- 1 vanilla pod
- 1 orange, thinly sliced
- ½ lemon, thinly sliced

Remove the stalks from the peaches and place them in a stainless steel saucepan. Add the water, wine, sugar and vanilla pod. (There should just be enough liquid to cover the fruit.) Add the orange and lemon slices.

Slowly bring the liquid to the boil, reduce the heat, cover and simmer gently for 20–30 minutes. You must not allow the peaches to boil, as the fierce heat will damage the flesh and cause the syrup to brown. Remove from the heat and leave the peaches to cool in their syrup.

When the peaches are completely cool, remove them using a slotted spoon. Gently remove the skins and place the peaches in a glass bowl. Add the orange and lemon slices and strain the syrup over them. Cover and chill for at least 8 hours before serving.

VARIATION: POACHED PEARS WITH GINGER *Peel 4 firm Comice or Naji pears, leaving the stalks on. Place in a saucepan with 300 ml/½ pint white wine, 75 ml/3 fl oz water, 50 g/2 oz sugar, rind of ½ lemon, a vanilla pod and a 2 cm/¾ inch piece of fresh ginger, chopped. Simmer until the pears are tender. Serve hot or cold, with a raspberry or apricot coulis.*

Lemon syllabub with a strawberry surprise

**SERVES 2 (GENER-
OUS PORTIONS)**
- 1 lemon
- a little brandy
- 75 g/3 oz caster
  sugar
- 150 ml/5 fl oz
  sweet white wine
- 300 ml/½ pint
  double cream
- 75 g/3 oz strawber-
  ries, thinly sliced,
  plus extra to deco-
  rate (optional)

This dessert, rich in vitamin C and calcium, provides a colourful
and easy to swallow dessert, a perfect end to a dinner party.

Peel the zest from the lemon in thin strips and set aside. Squeeze
the lemon juice. Add a little brandy to the juice, to make 50 ml/
2 fl oz.

Add the zest and leave to infuse, covered, for several hours.

Strain the liquid and add the sugar, stirring until it has
dissolved. Add the wine.

Whip the cream until stiff and add the liquid very slowly,
whisking continuously.

Place the strawberries in the bottom of the serving glasses and
pour the mixture on top. Chill for several hours.

Decorate with a thin twist of lemon zest, or sliced strawberries
and some washed strawberry leaves if you have them.

Blackberries and ricotta pancakes

**MAKES 8 X 15CM/
6 INCH PANCAKES**
- 100 g/3½ oz white
  plain flour
- pinch of salt
- 2 eggs, beaten
- 250-300 ml/
  8-10 fl oz milk
- 2 dessertspoons
  sunflower oil
- 25 g/1 oz flaked
  almonds
- a little butter

BLACKBERRY FILLING
- 275 g/10 oz ricotta
  cheese
- 2 dessertspoons
  clear honey
- 1 dessertspoon
  crème de cassis
- 300 g/13 oz fresh or
  frozen blackberries

Put the flour and salt in a large bowl. Make a well in the centre,
add the eggs and gradually whisk in the milk. Stir in the oil and
almonds and leave to rest in the refrigerator for at least 20
minutes.

Blend the ricotta, honey and cassis in a food processor. Stir in
the blackberries.

Heat a knob of butter in a small frying pan and when hot add
a half ladleful of pancake mixture. Swirl until the pancake is
even. Cook gently until the underside is golden brown. Toss and
cook the other side. Stack the pancakes under a warm towel.

Spread the ricotta mixture over half of each pancake and fold
the other half over.

VARIATION *Mix 100 g/3½ oz buckwheat flour, 100 g/3½ oz
rice flour, 25 g/1 oz caster sugar, ½ teaspoon bicarbonate of
soda, ¼ teaspoon tartaric acid and ¼ teaspoon salt. Beat in
25 g/1 oz margarine and 2 eggs. Gradually add 275 ml/9 fl oz
milk or water to make a smooth mixture. Leave to rest and cook
as above.*

Apricot filo tart

SERVES 8
- 150 g/5 oz butter
- 175 g/6 oz filo pastry
- 100 g/3½ oz caster sugar
- 2 eggs, beaten
- 50 g/2 oz plain flour
- 150 g/5 oz ground almonds
- 1 tablespoon Cointreau
- 425 g/15 oz fresh or canned skinned apricot halves
- 1 tablespoon apricot jam
- chopped pistachio nuts to decorate

The combination of apricots and almonds fuels your body with beta-carotene, vitamin E, calcium and potassium.

Preheat the oven to 220°C/425°F/Gas 7.

Melt 15 g/½ oz of the butter and brush over the sheets of filo pastry. Grease a 28 cm/11 inch diameter loose-bottomed flan tin and line with the filo sheets, making sure they overlap.

Cream the remaining butter with the sugar until pale and light. Beat in the eggs little by little, beating well to avoid curdling. Fold in the flour, almonds and Cointreau and spread the mixture over the pastry.

Arrange the apricot halves, round side up, on top of the nut mixture.

Place in the oven for 10 minutes, then reduce the temperature to 190°C/375°F/Gas 5 and bake for a further 25 minutes or until the pastry is golden.

Heat the jam in a small saucepan with a drop of water and brush this over the apricots to glaze. Sprinkle with chopped pistachio nuts and serve warm or cold.

Cinnamon apples and plums

SERVES 4
- 4 Bramley apples, peeled, cored and sliced
- 6 Victoria plums, stones and skin removed
- 2 teaspoons sugar
- dash of white wine and water
- 1 cinnamon stick

A fruity winter dish for dessert or a high fibre snack.

Place all the ingredients in a small saucepan and simmer gently for 15–20 minutes or until the fruit is soft.

Remove the cinnamon stick. Stir the fruits gently to break up any large lumps of fruit.

Serve warm or chilled, with cream, yoghurt or custard. It is also nice to roast some sunflower seeds, tossed in a little brown sugar, under the grill until they are golden brown. Sprinkle on top of the stewed fruit.

Chilled gingered rhubarb

SERVES 4
- 450 g/1 lb rhubarb, cleaned and cut into 2.5 cm/1 inch pieces
- 500 ml/16 fl oz water
- 200 g/7 oz caster sugar
- 2 cinnamon sticks
- 1 piece of fresh ginger, chopped
- grated zest and juice of 3 oranges

Chilled fruit can be very refreshing yet satisfying at the same time, especially with the addition of spices.

Place the rhubarb in a saucepan with the water and sugar, add the cinnamon sticks and ginger and bring to the boil. Reduce the heat and simmer very gently for about 20 minutes, or until the rhubarb is tender.

Strain the rhubarb and set aside. Boil the cooking liquid to reduce until very syrupy. Add the orange zest and juice. Pour over the rhubarb and chill well before serving.

Serve with thick Greek yoghurt and a shortbread biscuit.

Apple and fig crumble

SERVES 6
- 100 g/3½ oz plain wholemeal flour
- 50 g/2 oz caster sugar
- 50 g/2 oz unsalted butter
- 4 Bramley apples, peeled, cored and sliced
- 6 dried or fresh figs, diced
- 2 tablespoons soft brown sugar
- 1 teaspoon ground cinnamon or allspice

Preheat the oven to 220°C/425°F/Gas 7.

Place the flour and caster sugar in a large bowl and lightly rub in the butter until the mixture forms coarse crumbs.

Put the prepared fruit into an ovenproof dish. Sprinkle with the brown sugar and spices, then sprinkle the crumble mixture on top. Bake in the oven until golden brown. Serve warm.

VARIATIONS *Try other combinations of fruits, such as plum and blackberry in the autumn, rhubarb and strawberry in early summer; either of these two combinations would be enhanced by the addition of the grated zest and juice of an orange.*

For a crunchier oaty topping, mix 50 g/2 oz porridge oats, 15 g/½ oz wholemeal flour, 25 g/1 oz ground hazelnuts, 50 g/2 oz light muscovado sugar, ½ teaspoon ground cinnamon and ¼ teaspoon ground ginger and rub in 50 g/2 oz butter.

Prune and bitter chocolate tart

SERVES 4-6
- 175 g/6 oz prunes, pitted
- 100 g/3½ oz good-quality plain chocolate
- 20 cm/8 inch diameter baked sweet shortcrust pastry case
- 2 eggs
- 50 g/2 oz soft brown sugar
- 50 g/2 oz butter, melted
- grated zest and juice of 1 lemon

A luxurious way to increase your fibre intake.

Preheat the oven to 190°C/375°F/Gas 5.

Chop the prunes and the chocolate and place in the pastry case.

Beat together the eggs, sugar, butter, lemon zest and juice, and pour the mixture into the pastry case. Bake in the preheated oven for 25 minutes, or until the custard is just firm. Serve warm with cream, vanilla ice cream, fromage frais or fresh vanilla custard.

Bread and butter pudding

SERVES 4
- 8 soft wholemeal or white rolls
- 100 g/3½ oz unsalted butter
- 50 g/2 oz demerara sugar
- 50 g/2 oz sultanas
- 50 g/2 oz raisins
- 2 eggs
- 2 egg yolks
- 3 tablespoons caster sugar
- 300 ml/½ pint milk
- 300 ml/½ pint cream
- vanilla essence
- apricot glaze (optional)

Classic comfort food to cheer you up when you're feeling low. It's very nutritious if you need to build up your strength – the eggs provide protein and iron, the milk and cream add calcium.

Preheat the oven to 180°C/350°F/Gas 4.

Butter a pie dish. Cut the rolls in half and spread with the butter. Put a layer of bread in the bottom of the dish. Scatter with the demerara sugar and dried fruits. Repeat, finishing with a top layer of bread, buttered side uppermost.

Mix together the eggs, yolks, caster sugar, milk, cream and vanilla. Pour this mixture over the layered bread to fill the dish. Set in a bain-marie and bake for 30–40 minutes or until the custard is set and the top is browned. Brush with the apricot glaze, if using.

Coconut ice cream

SERVES 4
- 200 ml/7 fl oz condensed milk
- 200 ml/7 fl oz natural yoghurt
- 200 ml/7 fl oz coconut milk
- freshly grated nutmeg
- 1 teaspoon vanilla essence

This ice cream takes a little more effort as you need to mix it twice. It is worth the effort though. It is lovely on its own or with fresh or poached fruits. I can particularly recommend it with mango.

Mix all the ingredients together and pour into a plastic container. Freeze for 3 hours.

Blend the mixture in a food processor or with a hand blender, to break up any ice particles and create a smooth consistency.

Return to the freezer for at least a further 3 hours before serving.

Brown bread ice cream

SERVES 4
- 1 vanilla pod
- 600 ml/1 pint whipping cream
- 4 egg yolks
- 100 g/3½ oz caster sugar
- 175 ml/6 fl oz double cream
- 4 tablespoons brown breadcrumbs
- 50 ml/2 fl oz brandy

This ice cream is really easy to make as it doesn't require an ice cream churn or machine.

Infuse the vanilla pod with the whipping cream over a gentle heat for 15 minutes. Beat the egg yolks and sugar together and pour on the warm cream. Stir well, then return the mixture to the pan to thicken. Leave to cool.

Whip the double cream and fold into the custard base.

Brown the breadcrumbs in a moderate oven. Leave them to cool and then stir into the ice cream. Add the brandy and freeze for a minimum of 4 hours.

A butterscotch or caramel sauce would go very well with this dish.

VARIATION: PRALINE ICE CREAM *To make the praline, put 75 g/3 oz unblanched almonds and 75 g/3 oz sugar in a heavy-based saucepan over a low heat to toast the almonds and caramelize the sugar. Turn on to an oiled baking sheet and leave to cool. Crush into a coarse powder and fold into the ice cream mixture. Freeze.*

Flapjacks

MAKES 6–8
- 150 g/5 oz butter
- 75 g/3 oz brown sugar
- 75 g/3 oz golden syrup or black treacle
- 225 g/8 oz porridge oats
- pinch of salt

Deliciously sticky, yet eminently sensible, flapjacks are perfect snack food. They're portable, they keep well, and the oats are a good source of fibre, which slows the release of sugar into the body.

Preheat the oven to 190°C/375°F/Gas 5.

Melt the butter, sugar and syrup or treacle in a saucepan, but be careful not to let it boil. Stir in the porridge oats and the salt and mix thoroughly.

Press the mixture into a 20 cm/8 inch round shallow tin and bake for 25 minutes or until golden brown.

Remove from the oven and mark into slices. Leave to cool before attempting to remove from the tin and leave until cold before cutting. Store in an airtight container.

VARIATIONS *Add 75 g/3 oz chopped dried apricots, prunes, figs, raisins, coconut, nuts, or chopped lemon and orange peel.*

Fig and ginger parkin

MAKES A 1 KG/ 2¼ LB LOAF CAKE
- 225 g/8 oz whole-meal self-raising flour
- ½ teaspoon bicarbonate of soda
- 2 teaspoons ground ginger
- 100 g/3½ oz butter
- 100 g/3½ oz brown sugar
- 4 tablespoons black treacle
- 2 tablespoons milk
- 1 egg
- 50 g/2 oz dried figs, chopped

This very sustaining cake has a double boost of iron, from the black treacle and the figs. The figs also act as a gentle laxative.

Preheat the oven to 180°C/350°F/Gas 4. Grease and line a 1 kg/2¼ lb loaf tin.

Sift the flour, bicarbonate of soda and ginger into a bowl.

Melt the butter, sugar and treacle in a saucepan until dissolved.

Leave to cool slightly, then stir in the milk, egg and figs. Add the liquid to the flour mixture and beat well.

Pour the mixture into the prepared tin. Bake for 45 minutes or until a skewer inserted into the centre comes out clean.

TIP *This is best if you store it in an air-tight container for at least 24 hours before you devour it. It keeps well for several days.*

Barabrith

MAKES A 1 KG/
2¼ LB LOAF CAKE
• 300 g/11 oz mixed
  dried fruit
• 75 g/3 oz brown
  sugar
• grated zest of 1 lemon
• 400 ml/14 fl oz hot
  tea
• 350 g/13 oz whole-
  meal plain flour
• 2 teaspoons baking
  powder
• 2 teaspoons mixed
  spice
• 1 egg

Place the fruit, sugar, lemon zest and tea in a bowl and soak overnight.

Preheat the oven to 190°C/375°F/Gas 5. Grease and line a 1 kg/2¼ lb loaf tin.

Strain the fruit and reserve the liquid. Put the remaining ingredients into a bowl and add the fruit and enough of the liquid to make a soft consistency. Pour into the prepared tin. Bake for 45 minutes or until risen and firm. Cool and serve with butter, if desired.

Boston brownies

MAKES 16
• 50 g/2 oz butter
• 50 g/2 oz plain
  chocolate
• 175 g/6 oz caster
  sugar
• 75 g/3 oz white
  self-raising flour
• pinch of salt
• 2 eggs, beaten
• ½ teaspoon
  vanilla essence
• 50 g/2 oz shelled
  walnuts, chopped
• 25 g/1 oz chopped
  dates or dried figs

Keep these cookies in the cupboard for afternoon snacks or serve them with ice cream for a seductive supper.

Preheat the oven to 180°C/350°F/Gas 4. Grease and flour a 20 cm/8 inch square shallow tin.

Melt the butter and chocolate in a bowl over a pan of hot water and stir in the sugar.

Sift the flour and salt into a bowl and stir in the chocolate mixture, beaten eggs, vanilla essence, walnuts and dates or figs. Beat the mixture until smooth, then spoon into the prepared tin. Bake for about 35 minutes.

Leave in the tin to cool slightly before cutting into squares.

Date and walnut cake

SERVES 8–12

- 225 g/8 oz chopped dates
- 150 ml/5 fl oz boiling water
- 1 teaspoon bicarbonate of soda
- 75 g/3 oz butter
- 225 g/8 oz sugar
- 1 egg, beaten
- 1 teaspoon vanilla essence
- 275 g/10 oz wholemeal self-raising flour
- ½ teaspoon salt
- 50 g/2 oz chopped walnuts, plus extra for topping

TOPPING

- 2 tablespoons butter
- 5 tablespoons soft brown sugar
- 2 tablespoons single cream

A rich and heavenly combination, full of fibre and with a little folic acid from the dates.

Put the dates in a bowl and soak in the boiling water and bicarbonate of soda for 2 hours.

Preheat the oven to 190°C/375°F/Gas 5. Grease and line a 23 x 13 cm/9 x 5 inch cake tin.

Cream the butter and sugar together until light and fluffy. Gradually beat in the egg and vanilla essence. Stir in the flour, salt and walnuts. Add the date mixture and mix thoroughly. Spoon into the prepared tin and bake for 35 minutes.

Make the topping by melting the butter and sugar together in a saucepan and adding the cream. Simmer for 3 minutes. Pour over the warm cake and sprinkle with walnut pieces.

Fig and orange cake

**MAKES A 20 CM/
8 INCH CAKE**
- 225 g/8 oz dried figs
- juice and grated zest
  of 1 orange
- 225 g/8 oz butter
- 225 g/8 oz brown
  sugar
- 3 eggs, beaten
- 350 g/13 oz whole-
  meal self–raising
  flour

If you get tired in the afternoon, have a slice of this cake with a warm drink or a glass of fresh fruit juice or iced tea.

Soak the figs in the orange juice overnight.

Preheat the oven to 190°C/375°F/Gas 5. Grease a 20 cm/8 inch round deep cake tin.

Cream the butter and sugar together and gradually beat in the eggs. Add the fig mixture and fold in the flour and orange zest. Pour the mixture into the cake tin and bake for 30–45 minutes or until a skewer inserted into the centre comes out clean.

Banana cake

**MAKES A 1 KG/
2¼ LB LOAF CAKE**
- 225 g/8 oz white
  self–raising flour
- ¼ teaspoon bicar-
  bonate of soda
- 50 g/2 oz caster
  sugar
- 50 g/2 oz butter
- 2 eggs
- 3 ripe bananas
- 4 tablespoons milk

TOPPING
- 50 g/2 oz curd
  cheese
- grated zest of ½
  lemon and a dash
  of juice
- 25 g/1 oz caster
  sugar

Preheat the oven to 180°C/350°F/Gas 4. Place all the cake ingredients in a food processor and process for a few minutes.

Pour into a greased 1 kg/2¼ lb loaf tin and bake for 1¼ hours or until a skewer inserted into the centre comes out clean.

Make the topping shortly before you intend to eat the cake. Mix the topping ingredients together until thoroughly blended, but don't over-mix, as the acidity of the lemon can cause the mixture to curdle a little.

If you want a longer lasting topping, you could make a simple glacé icing with icing sugar, lemon juice and just enough water to make a spreadable coating.

TIP *I like a banana cake to be moist, so as soon as I take it out of the oven I put it into an airtight tin to cool completely. The steam from the cake keeps it moist. If you prefer a drier cake you can leave it to cool on a wire rack. Banana cake keeps very well for 2–3 days, if stored in an airtight tin.*

Fruit cake

MAKES A 20 CM/
8 INCH CAKE
- 175 g/6 oz butter,
  softened
- 175 g/6 oz caster
  sugar
- 75 g/3 oz sultanas
- 75 g/3 oz seedless
  raisins
- 25 g/1 oz glacé
  cherries, chopped
- 50 g/2 oz dried figs,
  chopped
- 350 g/13 oz whole-
  meal self-raising
  flour
- pinch of salt
- 1 teaspoon mixed
  spice
- 3 tablespoons milk
- 3 eggs

Preheat the oven to 180°C/350°F/Gas 4. Grease a 20 cm/8 inch round cake tin and line with buttered greaseproof paper.

Mix the butter and all the dry ingredients in a bowl, then add the milk and eggs and beat with a wooden spoon for 2–3 minutes, until well mixed. Turn into the prepared tin and level the top.

Bake in the centre of the oven for about 1½ hours. The cake is cooked when a warm skewer inserted into the centre comes out clean. Leave the cake in the tin for 15 minutes before turning out on to a wire rack to cool.

Lemon cake

MAKES AN 18 CM/
7 INCH CAKE
- 100 g/3½ oz butter
- 175 g/6 oz caster
  sugar
- 2 eggs, beaten
- 4 tablespoons semi-
  skimmed milk
- 1 teaspoon baking
  powder
- grated zest and juice
  of 1 lemon
- 175 g/6 oz white
  self-raising flour
- 3 tablespoons caster
  sugar for the topping

A deliciously lemony cake to tempt jaded appetites. The sugary topping makes it just a little different from a normal lemon sponge.

Preheat the oven to 190°C/375°F/Gas 5. Grease and line an 18 cm/7 inch round cake tin.

Cream the butter and sugar together until pale and fluffy. Add the eggs a little at a time, beating well after each addition to prevent curdling. Add the milk, baking powder and lemon zest. Sift the flour into the creamed mixture and mix lightly. Spoon into the tin and bake for 15 minutes.

Mix the caster sugar for the topping with the lemon juice in a small bowl. Remove the cake from the oven and pour the sugar mixture over the cake. Return the cake to the oven and bake for a further 5 minutes or until golden brown.

Carrot cake

MAKES AN 18 CM/
7 INCH CAKE
- 175 g/6 oz carrots,
  washed and any
  tough peel removed,
  grated
- 2 eggs
- 100 g/3½ oz sugar
- 85 ml/3 fl oz
  olive oil
- 100 g/3½ oz
  wholemeal
  self-raising flour
- 1 teaspoon ground
  cinnamon
- ½ teaspoon ground
  nutmeg
- 50 g/2 oz raisins
- 50 g/2 oz sultanas

LEMON AND
ORANGE ICING
- 40 g/1½ oz butter
- 75 g/3 oz brown
  sugar
- grated zest of
  ½ orange and
  ½ lemon
- 25 g/1 oz chopped
  walnuts

Boost your beta-carotene levels with this moist, high-fibre cake.

Preheat the oven to 190°C/375°F/Gas 5. Line an 18 cm/7 inch round cake tin with nonstick baking paper.

Whisk the eggs and sugar together until light and fluffy. Gradually whisk the oil into the egg mixture. Once all the oil is incorporated add the remaining ingredients.

Pour into the tin and bake for 20 minutes or until the cake is golden brown and firm to the touch; a warm skewer inserted into the centre should come out clean. Leave on a wire rack to cool.

Make the icing by beating the butter and sugar together, then beating in the orange and lemon zest. Spread over the cooled cake and decorate with walnuts.

Oatcakes

MAKES 8
- 75 g/3 oz plain flour
- ½ teaspoon bicar-
  bonate of soda
- 75 g/3 oz brown
  sugar
- 75 g/3 oz porridge
  oats
- 75 g/3 oz butter
- 1 tablespoon golden
  syrup

These crisp little biscuits are high in a type of fibre that is particularly good for keeping the arteries clear. I recommend them as an easily portable snack to stave off hunger pangs in a healthy way.

Preheat the oven to 160°C/325°F/Gas 3.

Sift the flour and bicarbonate of soda into a bowl and add the sugar and oats.

Melt the butter and syrup in a saucepan over a low heat and pour into the dry mixture. Form the mixture into a ball, then roll out to 2 cm/¾ inch thick and cut into rounds. Place on a lightly oiled baking sheet and bake for 15 minutes or until golden brown.

VARIATIONS *You could roast some sesame, pumpkin, or sunflower seeds and incorporate these into the mixture or sprinkle on top of the biscuits. They keep well in an airtight tin.*

Staffordshire oatcakes

MAKES 6–8
- 50 g/2 oz oat flour
- 175 g/6 oz
  porridge oats
- pinch of salt
- ¼ teaspoon bicar-
  bonate of soda
- 50 g/2 oz butter
- 3 tablespoons
  molasses

These oatcakes are more like pancakes. They are high in fibre, with molasses for an iron boost. Try them warm, drizzled with golden syrup.

Preheat the oven to 190°C/375°F/Gas 5.

Mix the oatflour, oats, salt and bicarbonate of soda together.

Melt the butter and molasses in a saucepan over a low heat. Add to the dry ingredients and mix together. Drop spoonfuls of the mixture, spaced well apart, on to a baking sheet and bake for 10 minutes.

Soft sesame bread

**MAKES A 450 G/
1 LB LOAF**

- 1 large banana
- 125 g/4 oz tofu
- 1 egg
- 150 ml/5 fl oz milk
- 150 g/5 oz rice flour
- 50 g/2 oz cornflour
- 25 g/1 oz soya flour
- 1 teaspoon bicar-
  bonate of soda
- 1 teaspoon cream
  of tartar
- ½ teaspoon tartaric
  acid
- pinch of salt
- 1 tablespoon olive oil
- 1 teaspoon caster
  sugar
- 50 g/2 oz sesame
  seeds, for topping

These four breads are all wheat-, gluten-and yeast-free.

Preheat the oven to 190°C/375°F/Gas 5.

Liquidize the banana, tofu, egg and milk and transfer to a bowl.

Mix the dry ingredients together. Fold into the purée together with the olive oil.

Line a 25 cm/10 inch square shallow tin with nonstick baking paper and pour in the mixture. Sprinkle with sesame seeds and bake for 35–40 minutes.

Check the centre is cooked by inserting a skewer; it should come out clean.

TIP *Gluten-free breads are best served warm from the oven. Otherwise serve toasted.*

Potato bread

**MAKES A 450 G/
1 LB LOAF**

- 75 g/3 oz peeled potato
- 1 egg
- 150 ml/5 fl oz milk
- 50 g/2 oz cornflour or cornmeal
- 100 g/3½ oz rice flour
- 1 teaspoon bicarbonate of soda
- 1 teaspoon cream of tartar
- 1 teaspoon tartaric acid
- pinch of salt
- 1 tablespoon olive oil
- 1 teaspoon caster sugar

This is lovely served with soups or made into warm sandwiches.

Preheat the oven to 220°C/425°F/Gas 7.

Boil the potato until soft, drain and liquidize. Add the egg and milk to the potato and blend again. Transfer to a bowl.

Mix the dry ingredients together. Fold into the purée together with the olive oil.

Line a 25 cm/10 inch square shallow tin with nonstick baking paper and fill with the mixture.

Bake for 35 minutes, or until a skewer inserted into the centre of the bread comes out clean.

VARIATIONS *For a flavoured savoury bread you could add 2 crushed garlic cloves or some chopped fresh herbs, such as parsley, tarragon, chives or dill.*

Rice bread

**MAKES A 450 G/
1 LB LOAF**
- 1 large apple,
chopped
- 1 egg
- 150 ml/5 fl oz water
or milk
- 100 g/3½ oz rice
flour
- 100 g/3½ oz
potato flour
- 25 g/1 oz soya
flour (optional)
- 1 teaspoon bicar-
bonate of soda
- ½ teaspoon
cream of tartar
- ¼ teaspoon
tartaric acid
- pinch of salt
- 1 tablespoon olive oil
- 1 teaspoon caster
sugar

Besides having no wheat, gluten or yeast, this bread, and the
buck-wheat bread (right), can be made without milk.

Preheat the oven to 220°C/425°F/Gas 7.
   Liquidize the apple, egg and water or milk and transfer
to a bowl.
   Mix the dry ingredients together. Fold into the purée together
with the olive oil.
   Line a 25 cm/10 inch square shallow tin with nonstick baking
paper and fill with the mixture.
   Bake for 35 minutes, or until a skewer inserted into the centre
of the bread comes out clean.

VARIATIONS *To give any of these breads a crunchy crust,
sprinkle the top with pumpkin, sunflower, sesame or poppy seeds
before you bake the bread.*

Buckwheat bread

**MAKES A 450 G/
1 LB LOAF**

- 100 g/3½ oz grated carrot
- 1 egg
- 150 ml/5 fl oz water or milk
- 100 g/3½ oz buck-wheat flour
- 100 g/3½ oz rice flour
- 1 teaspoon bicar-bonate of soda
- ½ teaspoon cream of tartar
- ¼ teaspoon tartaric acid
- pinch of salt
- 1 tablespoon olive oil
- 1 teaspoon caster sugar
- 25 g sugar

Preheat the oven to 220°C/425°F/Gas 7.

Liquidize the carrot, egg and milk and transfer to a bowl.

Mix the dry ingredients together. Fold into the purée together with the olive oil.

Line a 25 cm/10 inch square shallow tin with nonstick baking paper and pour in the batter.

Bake for 35 minutes, or until a skewer inserted into the centre of the bread comes out clean.

TIP *All these breads can be cooked in a frying pan, covered with the lid. You need to turn the bread frequently.*

Subject index

Recipe index

Special thanks to all my friends and associates, especially,
Tim Adkin, Jim Ainsworth, Andrew Barr, Hasan Basar,
John and Tom Cussen, Caroline Elston, John Fingleton,
Anthony and Katingo Giannoulis, Terry Gibson, Helen Gourley,
Susan Haynes, Jill, Naji and Adli Halabi, Michael Harding,
Jamie Harrison, Lucy Holmes, Dr Susan Horsewood-Lee,
Jess Koppel, Fiona Lindsay, Eleanor Lines, Laura Marriott,
Judith McGuire, Daniel Pudles, Maggie Ramsay, Mary Renouf,
Sir Tim Rice, Chris Rose, Lyn Rutherford, Linda Shanks,
Dr Andrew Scurr, Dr Martin Scurr, Dr Richard Staughton,
Margaret Vinton, Gilly Waugh.

*And to the memory of Auntie May, Uncle Tom, Dadda, Mary
Harrison and Graham Fletcher. I wish they were still with us.*

....

The Coeliac Society
PO Box 220
High Wycombe
Bucks HP11 2HY

The Vegetarian Society
Parkdale
Dunham Road
Altrincham
Cheshire WA14 4QG

The Soil Association
86 Colston Street
Bristol BS1 5BB

Specialist Cheese Makers
Association
Milk Marque Ltd
The Brampton
Newcastle Under Lyme
Staffordshire ST5 0QS